SOAKING UP THE RAYS

MANCHESTER
1824
Manchester University Press

Soaking up the rays

Light therapy and visual culture in Britain, c. 1890–1940

TANIA ANNE WOLOSHYN

Manchester University Press

Published byManc hester University Press
Altrincham Street, Manchester M1 7JA
www.manchesteruniversitypress.co.uk

British Library Cataloguing-in-Publication Data
A catalogue record for this book is available from the British Library

ISBN 978 1 7849 9512 6 hardback
ISBN 978 1 5261 1598 0 open access

DOI: http://dx.doi.org/10.9760/MUPOA/9781526115980

First published 2017

Typeset by Out of House Publishing

To the special Henrys of my life:

Sir Henry Wellcome, Professor Henry Jones Jr, and Master Henry Cleaves

Contents

Illustrations

Plates

Figures

Acknowledgements

THERE are so many people who have helped, supported, and inspired me, and I am delighted to be able to express my gratitude here.

I want to begin by thanking my family and friends – why should they always come last in these things? – especially my parents, Lynn and Nick Woloshyn; my in-laws, Colin and Janet Cleaves; my husband/best friend/personal copy-editor, Simon Cleaves; and our son, Henry. They truly understand how long a journey this has been and have been incredibly supportive, patient, and loving.

This book is the product of four years of research and collaborations, supported by a Wellcome Trust research fellowship in the Medical Humanities (grant #WT098912MA) and based in the Centre for the History of Medicine (CHM) at the University of Warwick. Everyone at the Wellcome and the CHM has been caring, generous with their time, and critical when it counts. I have been struck by the tremendous warmth, openness, and support of the Wellcome team, not least Dan O'Connor, Crestina Forcina, Chris Hassan, and Cecy Marden. At the CHM I am particularly grateful to my mentor, Hilary Marland, as well as to Tracy Horton and Sheilagh Holmes for all they have done. My research has been kindly assisted by excellent staff at many archives, libraries, and museums, notably the British Library, John Rylands Library, Florence Nightingale Museum, Greater Manchester County Archives, Hampshire Records Office, Leamington Spa Art Gallery and Museum, London Metropolitan Archives, Medical Museion, Modern Records Centre, Royal London Hospital Archives, Science Museum, Scottish Borders Council Archives, Thackray Medical Museum, and Wellcome Library. The generosity and aid of many private collectors, heirs, and rights-holders have enabled reproduction of the images, with particular thanks to Duncan Forbes, Martine Gagnebin, Nicolai Howalt, William Thuiller, Imogen Gray, Jeremy Smith, Philippa Smith, Wolfgang Suschitzky, and Heather Anthony, as well as the staff at the National Galleries of Scotland, London Metropolitan Archives, and the Wellcome Library. Excerpts from Chapter 5 originally appeared in my essay, 'Regenerative Tanning: Pigmentation,

Neo-Lamarckian Eugenics and the Visual Culture of the *Cure de Soleil*', in *Picturing Evolution and Extinction: Regeneration and Degeneration in Modern Visual Culture*, edited by Fae Brauer and Serena Keshavjee (2016) and is published with the permission of Cambridge Scholars Publishing.

Many colleagues of mine have provided invaluable feedback over the years on my research, and this book would be a rambling mess without them: Roberta Bivins, Fae Brauer, Anthea Callen, Simon Carter, Annie Jamieson, Ludmilla Jordanova, Richard Hobday, Nicolai Howalt, Mary Hunter, Greg Lynall, Alice Mah, Hilary Marland, Natasha McEnroe, Melissa Miles, Martin Moore, Katherine Rawling, Natasha Ruiz-Gómez, John Stanislav Sadar, and Tanya Sheehan. I would particularly like to single out Keren Hammerschlag for graciously reading – and re-reading – the chapters of the book, encouraging its clarity and confidence. Thank you also to the staff at Manchester University Press and Out of House Publishing, the Little Red Pen's Liz Hudson, and the anonymous peer reviewers, who have clipped, shaped, and conditioned this unkempt manuscript into a shiny, finished book. Lastly, several influential teachers and peers in my long education deserve special mention: Caroline Alexander, Barbara Allison, Mitchell Frank, Helen Foster, Janice Helland, Vojtech Jirat-Wasiutynski, Carol Payne, and Carl Widstrand. Thank you to everyone for making me the scholar, author, and person I am today.

1

Consuming light

> It is only within quite recent times that the question of utilizing the sun's rays for the purpose of the prevention or cure of disease, or other objects of health, has been seriously considered and practically applied. Like most of the greatest things in life, the very simplicity and obviousness of the method – at any rate the principle of it – seems to have concealed the secret. It is the obvious thing that invariably escapes our notice. In our moments of idealism we talk of 'hitching our wagon to a star'. May we not, in a more prosaic and material spirit, harness our bodies to the Sun?[1]
>
> (Edward J. Deck, 1926)

> The treatment of some diseases by exposure of the skin to the action of light, natural or artificial, has in a marvellously short space of time leaped from the obscure position of a somewhat contemptuously neglected specific to the status of one of the most valued and even invaluable weapons in the medical armoury.[2]
>
> (Royal Institute of British Architects [RIBA], 1933)

In May 1928, *The Times* published a forty-page supplement entitled, 'Sunlight and Health', replete with photographs, illustrations, and advertisements. Readers' eyes were greeted with smiling faces, bronzed skin, and lithe nude and semi-nude figures in open fields and on busy beaches, or indoors under gleaming lamps and shafts of light (Figs. 1.1–1.4). These images represent bodies consuming therapeutic light – soaking up its rays – and the natural surroundings and technological paraphernalia enabling such exposures. Together they offer a salient point of entry into the history and visual culture of light therapy in Britain during the early twentieth century, the subject of this book. This supplement, which collapsed medical and popular conceptions of light therapy, evinces the central role light played in notions of health, disease, pleasure, and risk at the time, and which persist today.

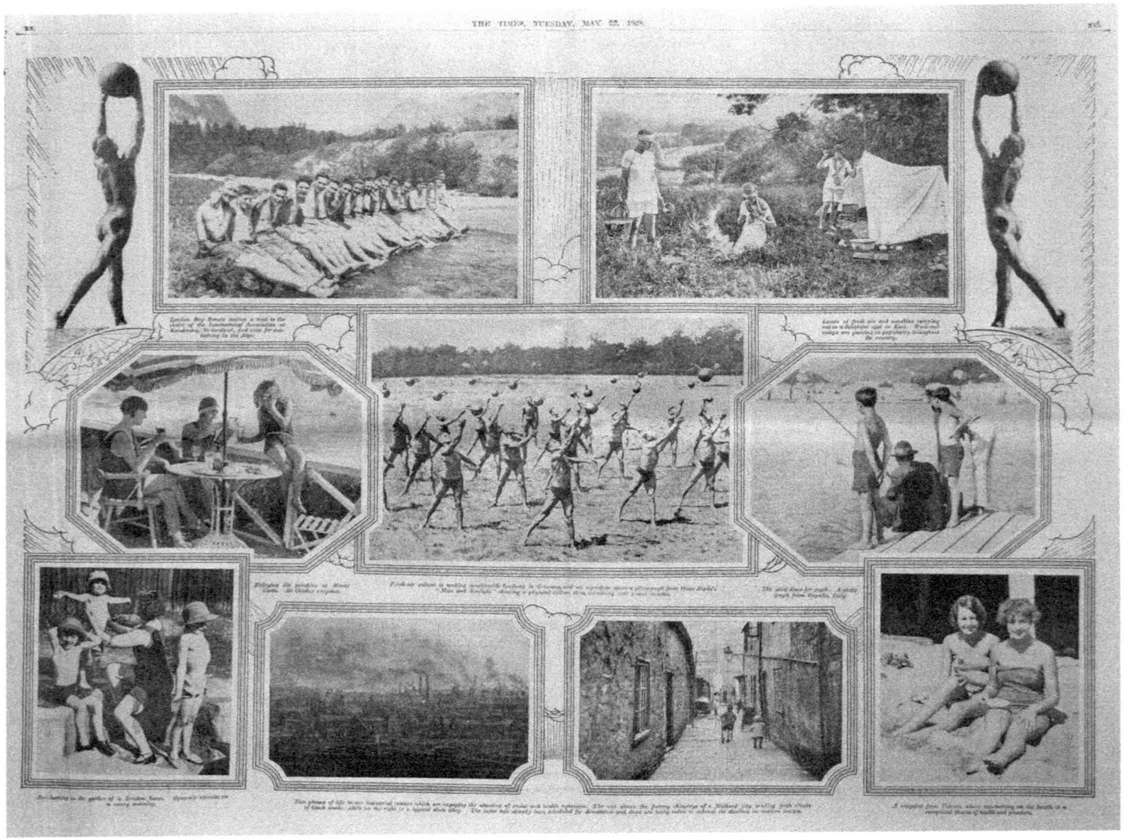

Figure 1.1 'Seeking health in the rays of the sun.'
In the *Times* supplement, 22 May 1928, pp. xx–xxi.

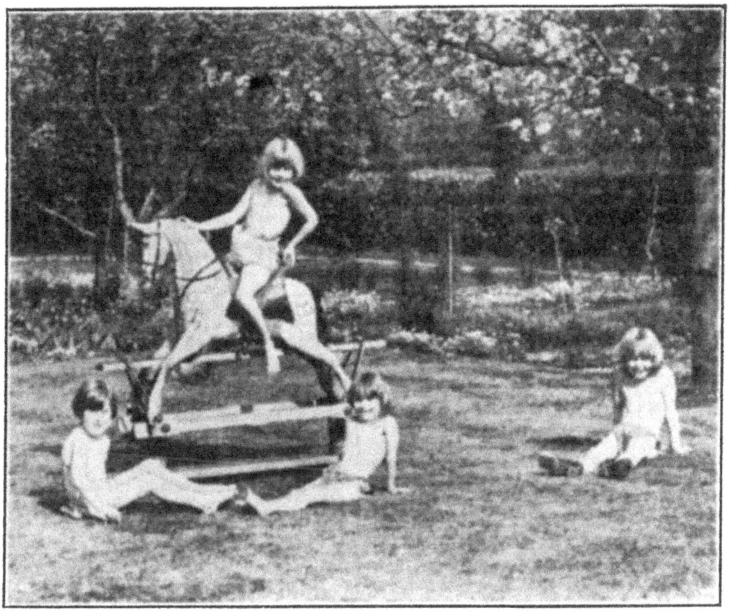

Figure 1.2 'Little patients in the gardens of the country branch of the Royal National Orthopaedic Hospital at Brockley Hill, Stanmore, Middlesex.' In 'Light Treatment in Hospitals', *Times* supplement, 22 May 1928, p. xxxi.

'Light therapy' encompassed a variety of methods and approaches. Bodies consumed therapeutic light in one of two ways: outdoors in the natural sunshine, known as heliotherapy; or indoors with artificial, electrical substitutes, known variously as phototherapy, artificial sunlight therapy, ray therapy, or actinotherapy. The latter method commonly used carbon arc, tungsten arc, or mercury vapour lamps, which produced different outputs of infrared, visible, and ultraviolet rays. Most prized among these was the ultraviolet. Referred to as 'chemical' or 'actinic' rays – notably for their use in photography – the ultraviolet rays were understood to disinfect and heal lesions and wounds by virtue of being bactericidal; to regenerate blood by increasing phosphorus, calcium, and haemoglobin levels; and to stimulate the production of vitamin D, the 'sunshine vitamin'.

To this end, both natural and artificial light were used to combat various illnesses, from the serious to the superficial. Although the effectiveness of light therapy was questioned, its use was widespread, as noted by RIBA in 1933 (see epigraph). Light therapy treated a multitude of ailments such as forms of tuberculosis, skin diseases, and deficiency disorders like rickets. It was also used to stimulate hair growth, correct the mental functioning of 'backward' children, restore 'normal' menstrual flow,

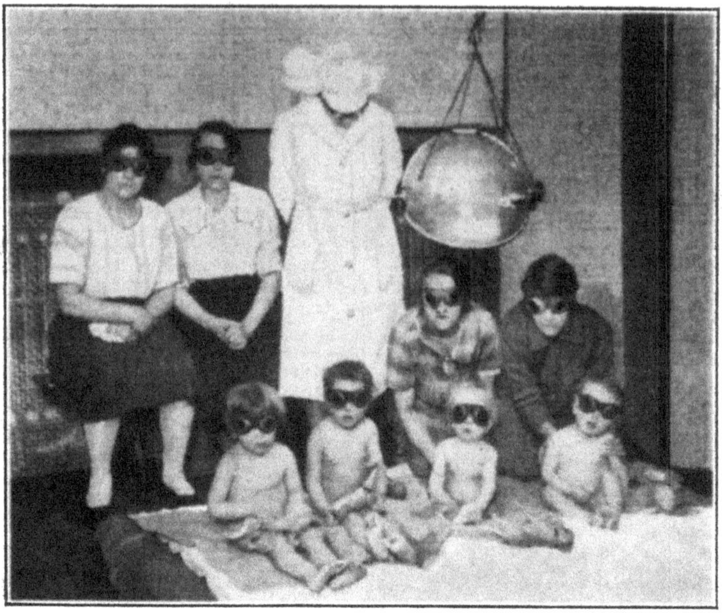

Figure 1.3 'A corner of the ultra-violet ray clinic at Bethnal Green, showing children undergoing treatment. The patients come from large families, living in one room.'
In Leonard Hill, 'Ultra-violet Radiation of Its Measurement', *Times* supplement, 22 May 1928, p. xv.

and increase lactation in nursing mothers. Therapeutic light was aimed onto football players, actors on Drury Lane, miners, athletes, and soldiers too, but most of all onto children. Light therapy took place in hospitals, sanatoria, spas, and in private and public clinics, at schools and factories, on the beach, and in the home.[3] It could be expensive (home-use lamps were pricey) or free when physicians or medical officers of health sent poor children and adults to council-run or charitable clinics.

By 1928, when *The Times* distributed 'Sunlight and Health', light therapy had reached its zenith in popularity, both among the public and the medical profession. Although almost 200 clinics existed in England at this time, the supplement authors described light therapy as in its infancy, awash with 'fragmentary and insufficient' knowledge.[4] The reasoning behind the supplement's publication was the 'wide dissemination of the information' that 'must hasten the coming of established and authenticated knowledge'.[5] In other words, *The Times*' editors intended the supplement to enable, not merely reflect, the widespread acceptance and legitimisation of therapeutic light – to cement the so-called innate connection between sunlight and health within the minds of its readership. This was no small feat. Light

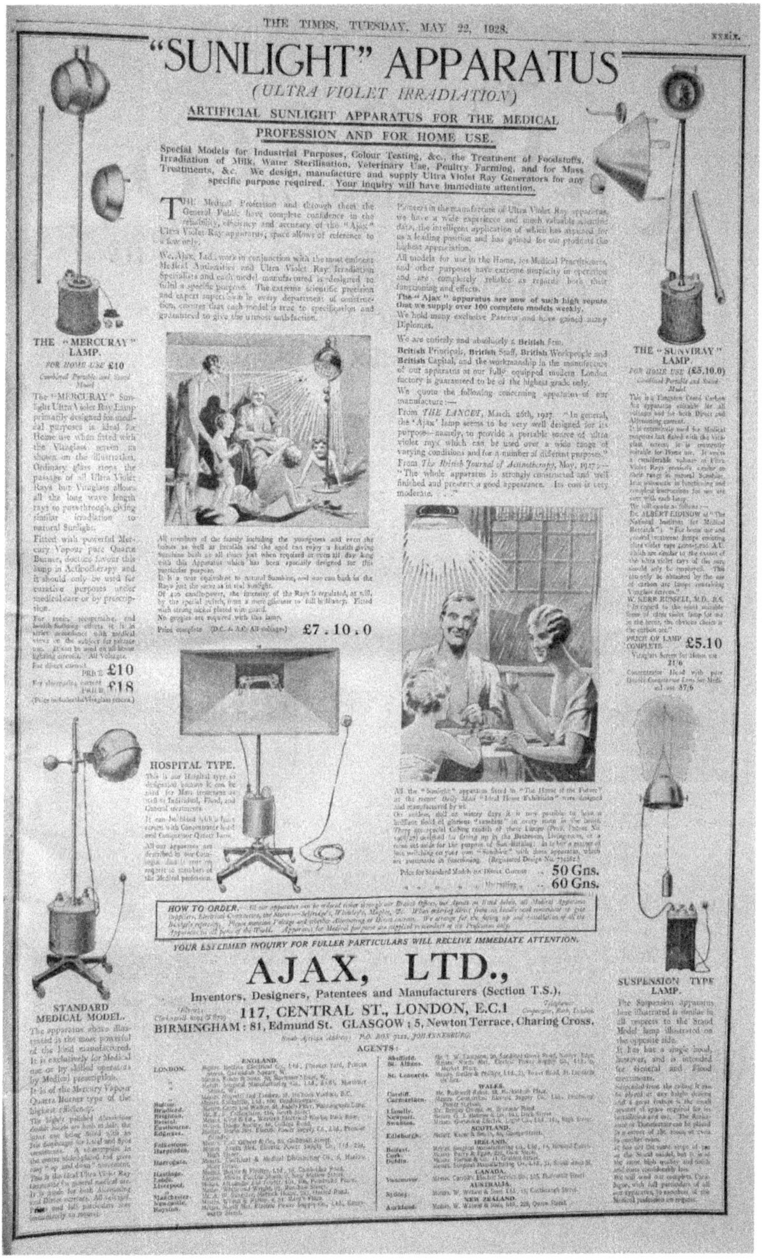

Figure 1.4 Advertisement for 'Sunlight' apparatus, Ajax Ltd (London). In the *Times* supplement, 22 May 1928, p. xxxix.

therapy was a self-styled 'modern' and progressive form of medical treatment that never possessed a stable or unchallenged reputation, however popular. As this book argues, the British population's relationship with sunlight, especially ultraviolet light, was complex and contentious, and remains so to this day, as evidenced by continued concerns about sun safety, skin cancer, rickets, and depression.

Throughout the 1928 supplement, ultraviolet light was described as a source of essential nutrition, able to combat rickets by stimulating the production of vitamin D: 'light is a food', declared the opening article.[6] Manufacturers advertised an array of home-use and clinical lamps, propounding to nourish Britain's 'sun-starved' citizens (e.g., Fig. 1.4). Other products offered unfettered access to sunlight through their own transparency: 'Vita' glass windows and 'Celanese' fabric were permeable to ultraviolet radiation, allowing for bodily exposure to sunlight even when indoors and clothed.[7] Those who could not access ultraviolet radiation directly, via sunshine or electrical devices, were advised to consume it through irradiated foodstuffs: an Allenburys' infant food advertisement claimed it was impregnated with vitamin D as a result of being exposed to a mercury vapour lamp.[8] As the supplement's writers made clear:

> Sunlight has become, for the whole world, a commodity rather than a mere stimulus. For sunlight can be absorbed into the body either through the skin or by way of the digestive tract. The conception of 'a place in the sun' is giving way to the conception of a 'ration of sunlight', something to be possessed and consumed.[9]

By correlating an increase in death rates to the winter months, the journal's medical correspondent concluded that 'light is, literally, life'.[10]

When read alongside the images interspersed throughout its pages, such a declaration indicates, at first glance, that the supplement acted as an endorsement for this nascent therapy, one with particularly striking 'legs': the numerous images of attractive and scantily clad women, men, and children 'harnessed to the sun', to quote Dr Edward Deck (1872–1952; see epigraph), produced an effective visual rhetoric wholly dependent on bodily representation, linking sunlight with health, beauty, and erotic promise (Fig. 1.1).

Messy messages

Yet closer examination of the illustrated texts and advertisements unsettles any stable or clear reading of the supplement as a whole; contradictions emerge and confound as competing voices and interests – medical, popular, commercial – topple onto each other. The first article in the supplement, 'A New Science', advised readers against the adoption of irradiated foodstuffs, despite its overall enthusiasm for light therapy: 'Cases have been reported in which, after the use of irradiated food, symptoms of a more or less distressing type have manifested themselves', the author notes. 'It is probable that in this, as in other directions, "what is one man's food is another man's poison".'[11] This article was placed in close proximity to both Allenburys' irradiated infant food advertisement and an article praising the British food industry for irradiating butter, bread, margarine, and milk to prevent rickets.[12] How were readers to know if Allenburys would act as a cure for their malnourished children and not a poison?

Advice from eminent authorities was no clearer when it came to the use of lamps. Professor Sidney Russ (1879–1963), the world's first hospital physicist, contributed an article on ultraviolet, X, and gamma rays to the supplement, warning readers that,

> Sources of ultra-violet radiation can now be obtained very easily, perhaps too easily, from those who represent that they have 'artificial sunlight' for sale. It is a bad term, for the radiation from none of these lamps resembles sunlight very closely, and they all contain some ultra-violet rays which normally never reach us [from the sun]. So it cannot be recognized too clearly that anyone using such lamps is using a source of rays with which man is yet quite unfamiliar, and how the body is going to react to repeated doses of these rays is not yet really known.[13]

Russ conducted pioneering research on radiation protection at Middlesex Hospital's Medical School while acting as the first chair of medical physics. The hospital was one of many noted in the supplement for employing light therapy for in-patients and out-patients. Others included the (Royal) London Hospital (the reputed first and most well known of hospitals to introduce light therapy in Britain, opening its light department in 1900), the Royal National Orthopaedic Hospital (Fig. 1.2), King's College Hospital (which reported an annual attendance to its sunlight department in 1927 of 81,000 patients), St Bartholomew's Hospital (reporting treating sixty different diseases with light therapy), Guy's Hospital, University College Hospital, St Mary's Hospital, and Charing Cross Hospital.

The last two featured reports addressing light therapy's precarious reputation. Dr Justina Wilson, in charge of the electro-therapeutic and light department at St Mary's, stated:

> light is not a specific remedy for every disease. It is comparatively costly and often inconvenient [...] Ultra-violet light is in its infancy in this country. It is the duty of the medical profession to see it is not brought into disrepute by unscientific persons. It is no mushroom growth; though new to us, this form of therapy is centuries old. It has stood the test of time. Physicians should neither, on the one hand, repudiate it *en bloc*, because some who give it have a

> bad technique and are ignorant of the qualities of the various sources of light; nor should they, on the other hand, be led to accept the extravagant claims made by many who apply it indiscriminately to all conditions.[14]

She was not the first to bring up the costliness of buying, running, and maintaining the electrical equipment. Already by 1903 Sydney Holland (1855–1931), chairman of the London Hospital, was quoted as saying, 'These machines eat money.'[15] Wilson was also not the first, nor the last, to express concern that physicians tended to take extreme views towards the therapy, some advocates describing its effects as bordering on the miraculous or fantastical.[16] The writer reporting on the Charing Cross Hospital further explained: 'The conclusion has been reached that the value of this treatment, properly carried out, is undoubted; but, like all other comparatively new treatments, light treatment has been over-praised and its promiscuous and improper use may lead to its being temporarily discredited in the public mind.'[17] The warning proved prophetic. Less than one year after *The Times* released its 1928 supplement, the very institution that had facilitated light therapy's growth, the Medical Research Council (MRC, founded in 1913), published a damning report undertaken by Dr Dora Colebrook (1884–1965). Attempting to prove whether the therapy's 'extravagant claims' were founded, Colebrook conducted two major controlled trials. The first trial involved adults receiving phototherapy for varicose ulcers. The second involved 300 schoolchildren, a third randomly selected to receive phototherapy to gauge whether ultraviolet light improved their general health and development.[18] In both cases she discovered that light therapy had little effect and, thus, little medical value. The MRC reports caused a particularly vocal outcry in medical and public presses such as the *British Medical Journal* (*BMJ*) and *The Times*, revolving around perceptions about correct technique, standardised practice, and visible results (see Chapter 2). Tensions between the therapy's scientific standardisation and its holistic attention to individual patients led practitioners to assert that, just like photography (the subject of Chapter 3), light therapy was both a science and an art.[19]

The offset statement above, from Charing Cross Hospital's reporter, is the last of the supplement, the remaining pages devoted to advertisements. The words of warning by Russ, Wilson, and this writer sit uneasily next to the advertisements for clinical and home-use lamps by manufacturers. As with irradiated foodstuffs, the supplement provided mixed messages when it came to accessing and consuming the ultraviolet radiation produced by lamps. Russ insinuated that the ultraviolet output of mercury vapour lamps was dangerously close to X rays and gamma rays, both known by the 1920s to be lethal. Indeed, as will be discussed in Chapter 4, ultraviolet radiation's carcinogenic potential was understood already by 1925, amidst the height of its popularity. Because of their similarities, ultraviolet radiation was frequently employed alongside X rays and radium in hospitals during the early twentieth century, an understudied aspect of light therapy's history.[20]

Hard selling

Turning to the advertisements, major manufacturers such as Hanovia (Slough) and Ajax (London) encouraged 'promiscuous' use of their wares with jovial figures in the height of fashion, with exposed flesh and glowing health (Fig. 1.4). Hanovia's 'Homesun' mercury vapour lamp, which opens Chapter 5, was advertised with illustrations of vigorous athletes, goggled nude and semi-nude children, irradiated milk, and even animals undergoing exposure. Its central vignette featured a nude boy, face tucked to chin and wearing requisite goggles, in front of the 'Homesun' in a private, darkened interior. The advertisement stated that, 'This treatment is now brought within the means of every householder, through the production of a portable Hanovia model … [N]ot to be confused with ineffective toys like small arc lamps. It is now delivered free to any address in Great Britain', with no mention of a medical certificate required.[21] The small arc lamps – those 'ineffective toys' – were advertised a few pages later by competing manufacturers.[22] The mercury vapour lamp, Hanovia's speciality, had the advantage of producing greater quantities and a higher range of ultraviolet radiation and so required very short exposure times in comparison to the carbon arc lamp, but the latter produced a spectrum close to that of sunlight and was thus considered safer and more 'natural'.

Ajax's advertisement included both carbon arc and mercury vapour lamps for sale, to the public and the medical profession simultaneously (Fig. 1.4). Old and young alike, healthy and ill, supposedly could safely expose their skin and eyes to Ajax's lamps. Two vignettes of illustrated adults and children were included, none of the figures wearing goggles to protect their delicate eyes from the ultraviolet light. Undisturbed by the glaring, pointed shafts of white light, they relax, play games, and enjoy meals while being exposed to the health-giving rays 'all day long'. Timed exposures were apparently unnecessary. Dressed fashionably and with the latest haircuts, they were depicted as part of a social class affluent enough to afford the initial cost of a full-size lamp (approximately £400 in today's money) as well as its ongoing electrical consumption and maintenance.[23] Similar models 'of the most powerful kind' were advertised along the borders for the medical profession or for 'skilled operators by medical prescription'. One hopes these were not the 'unscientific persons' who might bring light therapy into disrepute by 'promiscuous' or improper use, in spite of Ajax's encouragement that they do so.

It is not surprising that companies professed the superiorities of their own products against those of their competitors, as Hanovia did. Nor is it surprising that so many different advertisements appeared in the one supplement. After all, by the interwar years half the income of newspapers came from advertising.[24] What is surprising is that the articles, written by eminent physicians and scientists and *The Times*' editors, spoke directly against the advertisements surrounding them. How were readers to wade through such competing messages when it came to making informed, rational decisions about their health and that of their loved ones? Consuming light was, according to the supplement as a whole, at once a vital necessity and a risky practice.

Soaking Up the Rays explores these tensions within the history of light therapy in Britain with a particular focus on its visual culture, beginning with its earliest modern developments in the 1890s to its deeply embedded medical and public presence by the Second World War. British bodies were remarkably receptive to light's therapeutic potential: Britain's medical body quickly enlisted light's bactericidal properties to treat skin diseases such as lupus vulgaris (tuberculosis of the skin), and soon afterwards other external forms of tuberculosis attacking the bones, joints, glands, and spine;[25] Britain's social body, the public, proved a willing and active audience as popular newspapers such as *The Times* reported on the opening of light clinics and new hospital departments and provided a ready market to manufacturers for the sale of home-use lamps; and the body of the individual British patient, living in smoky urban centres and suffering from deficiency disorders such as rickets – the 'English disease' – was especially starving for light (Fig. 1.5).[26] As such, I mean the word 'receptive' here in two ways. The first refers to the open-mindedness and responsiveness of the medical community and the public, in relation to its nascent growth and acceptance through its visual, material, and textual dissemination. But I also use the word to think about the physical *taking on* or *taking in* of light, of bodies as photosensitive receptacles. The latter ultimately is bound to long-standing perceptions towards light, and especially ultraviolet light, as generative or regenerative, as active and activating, and as transformative in its powers.

Work/working/working through

How did practitioners, operators, and advocates conceptualise light to act upon the body, on its skin, organs, blood, and brain? How and why did they think light therapy worked? How was this imagined and imaged?

Even as late as the 1930s, a number of practitioners – physicians, nurses, masseuses, scientific researchers, alternative healers – confessed that the action of light on the body remained a perplexing mystery.[27] Focusing on the nitty-gritty details, such as exposure methods, the types of equipment, and the different rays, indicates that much speculation and research went into attempting to understand light's enigmatic but powerful effects on the body. Its riddles, put simply, did not remain unsolved for lack of effort. The MRC devoted a research body to the subject, the Committee on the Biological Actions of Light (CBAL, founded in 1922), which was

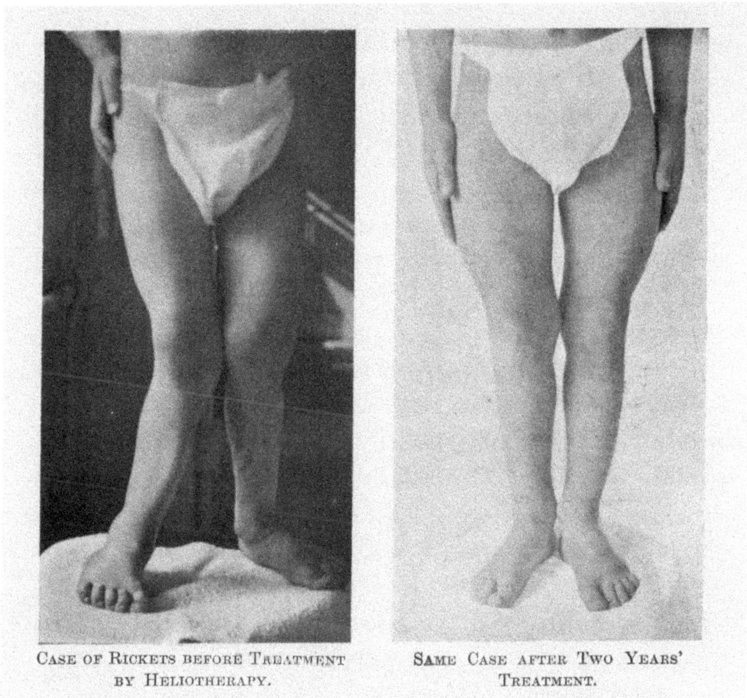

Figure 1.5 Before and after photographs of a child's legs with rickets, treated with heliotherapy for two years, detail. In Leonard Hill, *Sunshine and Open Air* (London: E. Arnold & Co., 1925), opposite p. 90. Wellcome Library, London CC BY-NC 4.0.

based at the National Institute for Medical Research (NIMR) under the direction of the highly respected physiologist Sir Leonard Hill (1866–1952) and his colleague Dr Albert Eidinow, and from which Colebrook's inflammatory reports later surfaced. At the NIMR, Hill and Eidinow undertook many experiments centring on light's actions on human and animal bodies, especially the skin (Chapter 2).

Light-therapy practitioners and researchers allocated enormous visual power to the skin to reveal the body's hidden interior processes under the influence of light's invisible wavelengths.[28] Solar erythema (sunburn) and pigmentation (suntan) were the most prominent of cutaneous reactions to actinic light, and their production on the patient's skin carried significant weight when it came to guiding light dosages, and even indicating the patient's prognosis. The patient who tanned well, for example, was perceived to be on the road to recovery. Both passive and active, the skin was transformed by the rays, being photosensitive, and yet could also transform them: practitioners perceived that, once pigmented, the skin absorbed and altered wavelengths into different energies during subsequent exposures. As a medical correspondent explained in the *Times* supplement: 'There is ample proof that the skin does not behave as an inert substance in regard to radiation to which it is exposed, but acts as a vital tissue which reflects its activity on the body as a whole.'[29] The German practitioner Hugo Bach even described the skin as 'an organ of light-assimilation', both receptive to light and transformative of its energies.[30] Pliant, penetrable, and receptive, the skin soaked up the rays to become an active, charged organ. It also became aesthetically desirable in the process. Through 'promiscuous' exposures to sunlight, white bodies acquired glowing tans and, worryingly for some, with them the sexual energy of so-called 'primitive' dark bodies (Chapter 5).

Once absorbed, light was understood to affect the body's appetite, blood, organs, nervous system, and psyche. Metabolism was raised, natural immunity was stimulated, and muscle tone was improved.[31] Sickly, malnourished patients gained weight and the bones of rickety children straightened (Fig. 1.5). Tuberculous lesions expelled necrotic bone and tissue then closed with excellent scarring (cicatrisation), as did wounds and burns. For arthritic patients, the joints eased with the help of infrared light, which was known to penetrate deeply into the body and relieve congestion by increasing blood circulation. Psychologically, the light exhilarated the mind and enlivened the spirits, bringing feelings of happiness and well-being.[32] Equally destructive and stimulating, light was a natural panacea in the eyes of its most ardent proponents.

Was it successful and effective as a treatment? I am frequently asked this question. My questions are: does it matter, in order for the therapy to deserve historical analysis and contextualisation? And by what forms of 'proof' can the historian ascertain its efficacy? As Martin Edwards explained,

> Any retrospective attempt to examine 'effective' therapies in isolation from those we now deem 'ineffective' misses the point [...] Whether a treatment 'works' is a socially and culturally bound conclusion, and can be fiendishly difficult ... to assess. New therapies were widespread during the first half of the twentieth century, each held its own promise and had its own advocates, and each required some form of verification.[33]

In light therapy's case, the most convincing forms of proof were the photographs of patients, charts, graphs, and X rays; that is, visual documentation. Take, for example, the before and after photographs of a child patient in a 1921 *BMJ* article by Sir Henry Gauvain (1878–1945), the medical superintendent of the Lord Mayor Treloar Cripples' Hospital in Hampshire (Fig. 1.6). At Treloar's, Gauvain employed natural and artificial sunlight as well as seawater (balneotherapy) to treat children suffering from external forms of tuberculosis, like this child pictured. The caption indicated that she suffered from pulmonary tuberculosis as well as tuberculosis of the cranium,

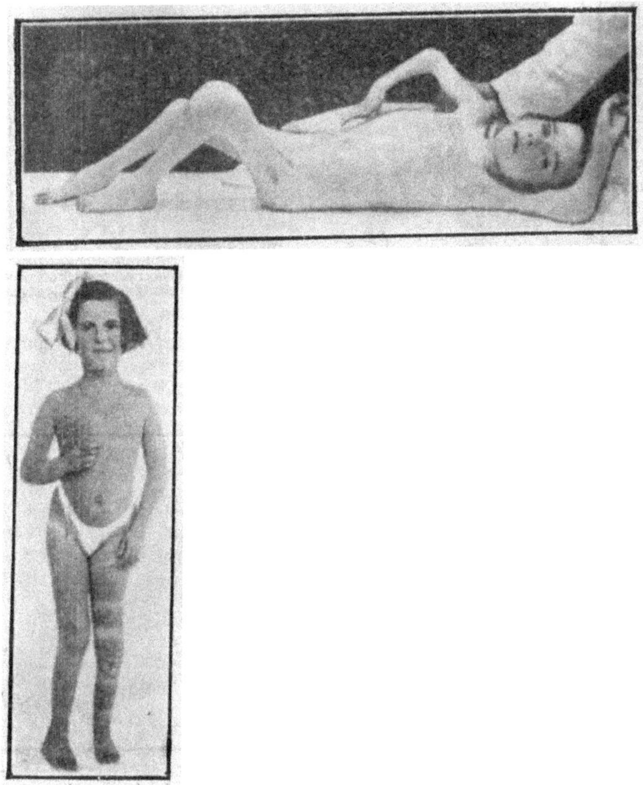

Figure 1.6 Before and after photographs of a patient suffering from multiple tuberculous lesions, treated by heliotherapy and balneotherapy. In Henry Gauvain, 'The General Principles of Treatment in Tuberculous Disease of the Bones and Joints in Children', *BMJ*, 26 November 1921, pp. 876–84, Figures 7 and 9. With permission from BMJ Publishing Group Ltd

elbows, wrists, knees, ankles, and mesentery, among other conditions. Unable to sit up independently, she was laid on a hospital bed supported by an adult carer, likely a nurse, in the before photograph. The after photograph presented her ambulant, plump, tanned, and happy. So dramatic was her transformation that she appears unrecognisable from her former diseased self.

Images like these quickly convinced medical colleagues and the public of light therapy's miraculous natural powers. But rather than look to this material for some kind of truth about whether light therapy really 'worked', let us treat them first and foremost as representations.[34] Strategic and standardised tactics were commonly employed to demarcate the treatment's effects: darkened interiors for the before image, often with obvious retouching to outline lesions and deformed joints; white exteriors for the after image, which highlighted the child's newly rounded contours and pigmented skin; facial expressions that mirrored physical states, notably the child's smile in the after image; and individualising, personal accoutrements, such as her neat hairstyle and pretty bow in the after image, which make the photograph act at once as a successful case record and a charming portrait.[35]

Recognising aesthetic strategies of representation does not imply such images were deliberate falsifications of the therapy's efficacies. It also does not mean that, by looking at these photographs, we cannot feel empathy for the patient's pain and relief in her recovery. It simply enables us the freedom to comprehend that these images had tremendous *work* to do, and that many contemporaneous viewers were convinced by their performance.[36] They are telling of practitioners' anxious investment in disseminating light therapy's *values* – its medical value or 'worth' and its social value or 'aim', as represented by its aesthetic values or 'luminosity' (relative lightness or darkness, particularly in relation to colour). In fact, as we will discover throughout this book, the images that are *not* convincing, that are resistant to interpretation, might be even more interesting than the ones that are.

Picturing light therapy

Soaking Up the Rays argues that the images and objects produced by practitioners and manufacturers did more than merely describe light therapy; they actively contributed to its very definition and, above all, visualised how light was conceptualised to act upon the body – and rarely in clear or simple ways. The history of light therapy's acceptance and appeal is thus complicated by its visual culture: damaged, overexposed, and heavily retouched photographs; saturated, hand-coloured pamphlets of suntanned bodies that appear more fluorescent orange than 'bronzed'; and montaged lamp advertisements that confound the boundaries between the invisible and visible.

These images are productive agents that communicate, and contributed to, practitioners' ambivalent and competing perceptions about light's benefits and risks. Using light therapeutically may have materialised at the forefront of modern medicine to widespread acclaim, but the therapy's emergence and legitimisation was not a straightforward process. Light therapy's 'discorded facts', as one author described them in 1925, deserve teasing out, as do the role of images amidst this discord.[37] The many images produced by the therapy's practitioners, manufacturers, and populists allow us to understand, in a far more nuanced way than texts alone, how much its legitimisation was dependent upon producing visual results and, to do that, by controlling light. The majority of light-therapy images are photographs, and photography is a *medium of light*. That the method of cure and its means of representation were dependent upon the same source makes light therapy a special case in the history of medicine.[38] With this in mind, I have written this book equally for medical historians and for scholars of visual culture.

In this book I focus especially on before and after photographs, documentary photographs of light clinics, and lamp advertisements, which provide alternative points of access into a contentious medical past. Selecting these particular images, as opposed to others, leads, however, to a simple but fundamental question: what exactly *is* an image of 'light therapy'?

Let us return to the heliotherapy images in the *Times* supplement (Figs. 1.1–1.2). Readers were presented with figures on holiday in the sunshine, both abroad and in Britain, or in the midst of physical culture exercises in the open air, involving adults and children, male and female. Boy scouts, beach-goers, well-to-do campers, families, hospital patients, Italian peasants, and German nudists were among the people pictured. Are they all equally practising the art of heliotherapy? And does that make all of these reproduced photographs images of light therapy? What did 'light therapy' mean during this period to its practitioners and enthusiasts, and what did it actually look like in practice?

The image from the Royal Orthopaedic Hospital's country branch in Middlesex depicts four child patients dressed only in loincloths, casually lying in the hospital gardens, one atop a large toy horse (Fig. 1.2). Aside from its stated location and the children's standard hospital apparel, there is little to suggest this depiction could be defined as 'medical photography'. Yet it is a typical representation of children undergoing heliotherapy during this period. The Treloar archives, for example, have hundreds of photographs like this one. When placed alongside the image of a mother and her three children, also outdoors in an English garden, in Figure 1.1 (lower left-hand corner), the similarities confound any clear separation between therapy and leisure, of heliotherapy as opposed to popular sunbathing. Yet the supplement's opening article forthrightly declared, 'Sunlight treatment is medical treatment in the strictest sense of that term and ought to be given only by physicians who have devoted special study to it.'[39] In Figure 1.2, the conspicuous absence of medical authorities (whether out of shot or acting as photographer) presents a rather different version of light therapy than the one encountered in the written word, a treatment strictly timed, monitored, and individualised to each patient.

The sheer variety of images in the supplement does little to clarify, and this is a crucial point. In its range and diversity the supplement challenges us to consider how light therapy and its rich visual culture were historically defined and articulated. Throughout its pages, discussion and visualisation of light's medical use was mixed – jumbled even – with its leisure use. Articles on Swiss sanatoria, rickets, and phototherapy departments in hospitals and clinics were interspersed with those on French and Spanish resorts, motorcar drives, and cruise ship voyages. Indeed, with its broad title, 'Sunlight and Health', the supplement playfully toyed with, and contributed towards, light's multivalent meanings.

At this point, I invite you to spend some time looking at the many images throughout this book.

What are your first impressions about the visual material? Through dissemination to various audiences I have learned that viewers find the images variously frightening, bizarre, charming, glamorous, silly, and pornographic. I acknowledge all of these descriptions, and feel it pertinent to mention that it is rare to come across a collection of images that can simultaneously delight and disturb, provoke guffaws of laughter and awaken sexual – even paedophilic – desire (see 'Exposing Children', below).

Images of radiant smiles, glowing tans, and revitalised bodies are juxtaposed with those of eerie 'séances', goggled nudes, and glaring lamps. The supplement's photograph of the Bethnal Green 'ultraviolet ray clinic' serves as an excellent example of depicting phototherapy (Fig. 1.3): patients arranged and posed, their goggled eyes face-forward and their flesh exposed; the nurse unassuming but characteristically present, the physician absent; and the lamp, given prominence in the composition as a piece of progressive and impressive technology but, significantly, not turned on. (Doing so would overexpose the negative, a curious problem in photographing light therapy discussed in Chapter 3.)

Undergoing a phototherapy session was described by some as a frightening experience, especially for children exposed in the nude to large carbon arc lamps, which erratically buzzed, smoked, and spluttered hot ash as the carbons burnt away. But while such scenes of séances – and practitioners did refer to exposures as *séances* ('sessions' or 'sittings') – may strike us as odd, novel, or downright weird today, many contemporaneous viewers, practitioners, and patients would have regarded them as normal, familiar, and even banal, however imposing the technological equipment.[40]

For those suppressing giggles or snorts at some of the more outrageous depictions (I am thinking particularly of the lamp advertisements, which feature heavily in Chapters 4 [Plate 1] and 5 [Plates 2–5]), I urge you to pay even closer attention to them. Carolyn Thomas de la Peña, analysing contemporaneous popular devices such as galvanic suspensory belts and prostate massagers marketed to men fearing sexual inadequacy, has perceptively cautioned against dismissing these seemingly ridiculous novelty items too lightly.[41] We might say the same for early forms of vibrators, as parodied in the film *Hysteria* (2011), or John Harvey Kellogg's treatments in the film *The Road to Wellville* (1994). Both films anachronistically trivialised and poked fun at popular medical devices intended to treat a range of mental and physical disorders that held considerable social currency at the time. Since one of light therapy's many applications was the treatment of sexual dysfunction, these other examples are not far off the mark. As for its images and objects, consider that their amusement value is a poignant indicator of the problematic nature of hindsight. Why else would they amuse? Simon Carter put it best in his 2007 book, *Rise and Shine*:

> At various points during my research for this book I became acutely aware that some of the material I was examining lends itself to mild ridicule or humour. When using archives I would sometimes come across an advertisement, photograph or description of a practice from the 1920s or 1930s that

> required the suppression of a guffaw to avoid the disapproving eye of a librarian. In the main body of this text I have tended towards sobriety. Historians of medicine have long warned about reinterpreting old maladies through a perspective provided by modern diagnostic categories, and in a similar way our re-interpretation of past practices using a modern humour idiom would not be in the spirit of a 'symmetrical' study – Latour may have urged us to 'follow the actors' but it's probably a bad idea to snigger while doing so.[42]

Perhaps we might describe them less as amusing than delightful or even *titillating*, since many of light therapy's images feature joyful nudes taking pleasure in being 'kissed' by the light (Figs. 5.13–5.16). Why in these images bodily exposure to light stimulates erotic pleasure, for the figures represented as well as for the viewer looking at them, is integral to historically contextualising the link between sunlight and sexuality, the focus of Chapter 5.

The 'art' of light therapy

There are long-standing art-historical precedents for imaging nudes in the sunlight, of mythical goddesses and biblical figures in pastoral or idyllic settings from the Renaissance onwards. Artists from Titian (1477–1576) to Pablo Picasso (1881–1973) treated the nude in the open air as standard aesthetic fare. By the early twentieth century, cultured British audiences and artists would have been familiar with the painted nudes and sunny landscapes of the Impressionists, the Neo-Impressionists, the Fauves, and the contemporaneous work of British artists such as Henry Scott Tuke (1858–1929) and Dame Laura Knight (1877–1970).[43] Biographers and art historians have repeatedly noted Tuke's primary interest: painting sunlight on nude male flesh out of doors, especially in Cornwall. He was referred to as a painter of sunshine, in his own time and today, and titled his works *Sunbathers* (1927, Collection of Sir Elton John), *Lovers of the Sun* (1923, private collection) and *To the Morning Sun [The Sunworshippers]* (1903, Hugh Lane Art Gallery, Dublin), which bear important similarities to the Symbolist art of German naturist, Fidus (Hugo Höppener, 1868–1948), especially the many versions of his *Lichtgebet (Prayer to the Light)*, c. 1894–1924.[44] Artist colonies based in Brig O'Turk and Cocksburnpath in Scotland, Newlyn in Cornwall, and Staithes in Yorkshire formed from the 1880s onwards, their members united in their passion for picturing the light, local colour, and open air of their environs.[45] Furthermore, as Linda Dalrymple Henderson, Pascal Rousseau, and Gavin Parkinson have shown, vanguard art of the early twentieth century was marked by a fascination with 'rays'.[46] Marcel Duchamp (1887–1968), František Kupka (1871–1957), and László Moholy-Nagy (1895–1946) were among many modern artists who explored visualising transparency, relativity theory, and the Fourth Dimension (Figs. 4.12–4.13).

But there were also artists who engaged directly with light therapy's visual dissemination. These included photographers Edith Tudor-Hart (1908–73, Chapter 3 Fig. 3.1), Bertram Park (1883–1972) and Yvonne Gregory (1889–1970, Fig. 5.14), illustrator Robert Gibbings (1889–1958, Fig. 5.10), and painter Beatrice Langdon (1898–1986, Plate 8). They feature in Chapters 3, 5, and 6, respectively. But if there was a formal or 'high' art of light therapy, it existed most dramatically in stone. Commemorating the work and life of light therapy's founder, the Danish physician and Nobel laureate Niels Finsen (1860–1904), is the sculpture *Mod lyset* (*Towards the Light*; 1904–9) by Rudolph Tegner (1873–1950; Fig. 1.7). It is not a representation of Finsen per se but one impregnated with Symbolist meaning about his therapeutic practices and achievements with light. Four figures – a man, two women, and a

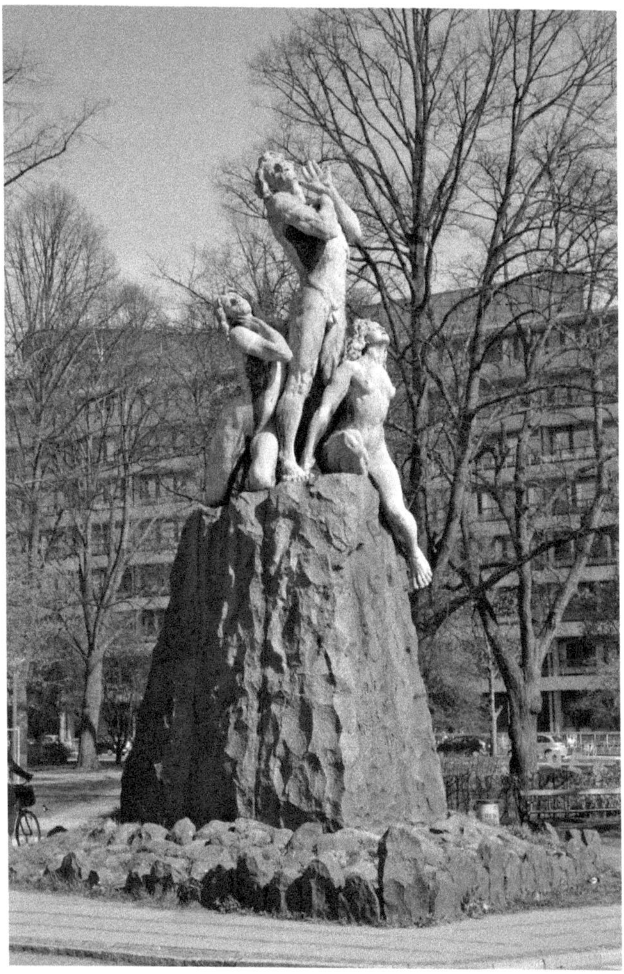

Figure 1.7 Rudolph Tegner, *Mod lyset (Towards the Light)*, 1904–9
Granite and bronze.
Corner of Blegdamsvej and Tagensvej, Copenhagen.
Author's photograph.

young boy (hidden behind) – enmesh in a tangled composition. The figures dramatically tilt their faces upwards with eyes closed to the sun, their poses reverent and even desperate for its benevolence to shine down on them. In their act of sun worship, the figures show clear affinities with those in Fidus's *Lichtgebet*, the Swedish Axel Emil Ebbe's *Solrosen* (*Sun-Rose*) sculptures (*c.* 1892 onwards), the German statues *Der Mensch* (*Man*) and *Gläserner Mensch* (*Transparent Man*) from the Dresden Hygiene Exhibitions of 1911 and 1930, and Roger Broders' poster *Le Soleil toute l'année sur la Côte d'Azur* (1931).[47] In their gesturing, Tegner's sculpted bodies go 'towards the light', an expressive metaphor for how Finsen's patients referred to attending their phototherapy appointments.[48]

The majority of the images that make up light therapy's visual culture, however, were produced by anonymous photographers, usually in the employment of a physician, institution, or press.[49] In some cases it was the physician or nurse who acted as photographer, taking casual snapshots of facilities, patients, and therapies. For me, the most interesting photographs are the ones that would normally be described as being of 'poor' quality, especially overexposed negatives and obviously retouched prints. They are the photographs hiding in archival boxes or reproduced in medical textbooks that are easily dismissed as damaged goods, marked by lens flare and 'black suns' (Figs. 3.10, 3.12–3.16). But it is the *damage* done to these material remnants that is of relevance here: they present to us photosensitive surfaces, akin to skin, burnt by the therapeutic light they sought to picture (Chapter 3). As physical objects made and marked by light, they make materially present the benefits and risks that light exposures could bring.

If, as Jennifer Tucker noted, 'Visual images are the stuff of science and an important way that science has defined itself … for hundreds of years', its definition through visual representation has not necessarily been stable, uniform, or fixed.[50] Revisiting the many images in the *Times* supplement and the question of what an image of light therapy exactly is, my answer is that in its definition there was nothing exact about it. Despite evident strategies of representation, for example particular lighting conditions, locations, patient poses, retouching, etc., the open and multivalent meanings of picturing bodies in the light lent this therapy tremendous scope for, and interest in, its visual dissemination. This is a rich and diverse collection, on par with the widespread, related popular and medical visual cultures of X rays, radioactivity, and electricity (see Chapter 4). Light therapy was imaged in specialist medical textbooks and journals, populist handbooks, illustrated newspapers, closed hospital records, tourist postcards, and avant-garde oeuvres. The same image could be found in these various sources, indicating that popular and medical audiences for the images were not always demarcated or fixed. That Ajax's advertisement (Fig. 1.4), Gauvain's patient portraits (Fig. 1.6), and Tegner's Finsen monument (Fig. 1.7) all fall within light therapy's visual culture indicates that its many proponents conceptualised what it was in many different ways – and that light's healing powers were at once medicalised, commodified, spiritualised, sexualised, and aestheticised.

The main images in this book (re)present light therapy's many faces, varying in medium and spanning four decades (Figs. 1.1, 2.1, and 3.1, and Plates 1, 3, and 8). The images' formal qualities and contexts provide new insights about the ambivalent meanings of sunburn, solarisation, radiation, and suntan among the medical community and their dissemination to the British public, *c.* 1890–1940.

Being methodical

Light therapy's invention, legitimisation, successes, and failures had as much to do with light's abilities to visualise as to heal. In fact, I argue in Chapter 3 that light therapy could not have existed without photography, both as an art (as a medium for visual representation) and a science (contributing significantly to the development of chemistry and light physics). The therapy's visual culture, which is predominately photographic, exemplifies the pivotal role played by photography as a means of modern image-making *and* knowledge-making, particularly for modern medicine.[51] Suggesting such things, and conducting the research to prove them, would be impossible without the influence and work of many excellent scholars. After all, publications, Ludmilla Jordanova poignantly wrote, are 'parts of elaborate conversations with other historians, living and dead'.[52]

The British history of light therapy has received little attention from medical historians, its visual culture none. The most thorough scholarly examination is sociologist Simon Carter's 2007 book, *Rise and Shine*. Exploring the emergence of a modern photophilia during the early twentieth century, Carter argued that a range of practices, technologies, and 'socio-technical artefacts' (sunlamps, sun creams, etc.) mediated the British body's relationship with sunlight, and continues to do so today. He stated that,

> the various associations between the sun and the body were then, as they still are, in a constant state of flux, and … [w]hile these associations often may have unravelled, at the same time this unravelling leaves its own traces that can continue to define our present relationship to the sun.[53]

Like Carter, I enjoy picking at these loose ties and finding these traces. Unlike Carter, I focus heavily on the visual material as well as the primary medical literature, giving far more weight to the medical profession's role in driving and normalising perceptions of sunlight as essential to health among the British public.[54] As Roger Cooter and John Pickstone asked, 'has any other profession [during the twentieth century] acquired such far-reaching influence in the governance of human life?'[55]

Scholars studying light therapy's history pay surprisingly little attention to its specific – and contested – methods, practices, and theories, preferring instead to examine its popular public appeal.[56] I propose that one cannot fully appreciate the latter without in-depth knowledge of the former. Above all, the historic role of images and objects has not undergone serious and methodical study. To carry out that study I have looked to influential scholars of art history and visual culture, especially those with interests in the history of medicine and the medical humanities.[57] Championing visual approaches to enrich our understanding of medicine, as Jordanova has called for, *Soaking Up the Rays* urges scholars with an interest in medical history to pay closer attention to its visual culture. This book approaches medicine's ephemera not as simple vessels reflecting established medical beliefs but as complex mediating agents that complicate, nuance, and contribute to the production of those beliefs.[58] It does not position interdisciplinarity as a smooth co-mingling or happy interaction between distinct disciplines: the intersection of art and medicine need not be seamless, smooth, or easy. As the main images driving the chapters make evident, their intersection was more fraught than fluid.[59] These images are fascinating precisely because they are *problematic*: confounding, ambiguous, and downright odd. Resistant to interpretation, resistant to their intended function (as 'documents' for dissemination, as 'evidence'), the images require close looking, critical analysis, and much contextualisation.

Like the history of photography, the history of light therapy is marked by frustrated attempts to harness and master the light. 'Volatile and unpredictable', according to Melissa Miles, light's destructive force is perpetually written out of, yet always leaking through, photography's history.[60] Light therapy's contradictions and injurious effects are hidden away in the primary literature and yet underpin its nascent development. In asking the question, 'What do pictures want?' W. J. T. Mitchell explained that, 'We need to reckon with not just the meaning of images but their silence, their reticence, their wildness and nonsensical obduracy.'[61] Wily and stubborn, the images I analyse are powerful because they refuse to 'clarify' or 'illuminate' (words describing light as a source of knowledge and revelation, Miles notes) what light therapy was in a uniform, intelligible way.

I am certainly not the first to privilege the use, meaning, or materiality of 'things' to analyse the past. Carter viewed bottles of sunscreen as social, cultural, and technological artefacts that actively mediated how British bodies interacted with sunlight, as relevant as any medical text.[62] And Mitchell stated,

> Images matter in more than one sense. That is, they make a difference, are important, and make demands. But they are themselves matter, in the sense that they are always embodied in material objects, in things, whether stone, or metal, or canvas, or celluloid, or in the labyrinth of the lived body and its memories, fantasies, and experiences.[63]

Inasmuch as I write of 'images', I recognise they might more appropriately be described as material remnants, as *objects*, often damaged or hidden away in archival boxes. Alongside these objects and guided by studies in material culture, I also discuss light-therapy lamps and goggles, including how they were ambivalently represented in advertisements. Ellen Lupton, in *Mechanical Brides* (1993), stated that,

> the material remnants of everyday life ... do not have a stable meaning, decreed by their makers and frozen in their formal structure (materials, style, technique). Instead, meaning emerges through social practices, including an object's representation in various media, its connection to shared customs, and its significance to the people who own or operate it.[64]

Once considered invaluable to public health, since the late twentieth century ultraviolet lamps – now in the form of sunbeds – have been perceived by many to be dangerous devices for purely cosmetic ends. Yet they also live on in the form of lamps for Seasonal Affective Disorder (SAD), daylight alarm clocks, and contemporary phototherapy lamps for dermatological conditions. Gracing this book's cover is a 1936 advertisement for the 'Vi-tan' mercury vapour lamp, manufactured by the Thermal Syndicate (see also Plate 1). As I discuss in Chapter 4, the 'Vi-tan' was promoted as a technologically advanced substitute for natural sunlight, even surpassing the sun's powers by offering higher quantities of ultraviolet radiation. Historically, these devices 'harnessed bodies to the sun' (see epigraph) – their users encouraged to climb aboard Apollo's golden chariot, with great aspirations for perfect health. However, as objects, their modern design, shiny components, and intended use in the home did not sway or comfort practitioners unanimously, as Russ's warnings above make clear. Public cases of burns, electrocution, and even death roused considerable concern, suggesting that these objects simultaneously signified the hope of health and the possibility of peril.

Like Joel Howell's study of X-ray machines, my interest in light therapy's technology (its devices, practices, and user knowledge) is a useful avenue into examining practitioners' desires to see it as systematic.[65] Seeking to become a legitimate form of medicine – a science and not 'merely' an art – light therapy relied on the latest technological apparatus, attempted to standardise dosages and exposure methods, and produced qualified experts to operate and administer them. Amidst the chaotic jumble of competing views over the optimum light source, duration of treatment, intensity of exposure or skin reaction, these experts fought to present light therapy at its most 'scientific', modern, and effective.

Surely we might consider that this chaos, this messiness, be conceptualised as productive in so far as it led to more research, more discussion, and more imagery. It continues to do so today, with seasonal rounds of medical and popular articles on light's benefits during the winter, which emphasise its use for SAD, and its dangers during the summer, driven by the promotional use of sunscreens. The history of vitamins presents important similarities. Rima Apple argued that the perpetual puzzlement over the necessity of vitamin supplementation only led to further dependence upon science's 'ambiguous authority'.[66] Since their discovery in the 1910s, vitamins have excited and confounded pharmacists, physicians, and the public. Apple explained that 'Increasingly sophisticated studies produced more questions than they answered', so that the scientific evidence has been, and remains, 'inconsistent and in dispute'.[67] She perceptively observed that such ambiguity propels more and more scientific input. Pharmaceutical companies use science to promote their vitamin products, newspapers discuss the worth and worthlessness of taking vitamins to the public by quoting from scientific authorities, while laboratories conduct endless studies and trials to ascertain (in)conclusive results.

Bodily exposure to light, whether for therapeutic or aesthetic ends, likewise persists as a contested subject to this day: does it kill or cure? Yet the tenuous place light exposure occupies, both within the medical community and in the imagination of the general public, is not a new phenomenon.

Vers la lumière

My interest in the history and visual culture of light therapy began through my art-historical research on the Côte d'Azur, one of the earliest locations of heliotherapy. There, ill modern artists such as the Impressionist Pierre-Auguste Renoir (1841–1919) and the Neo-Impressionist Henri-Edmond Cross (1856–1910) spent their last years painting and alleviating their bodily pain in the southern sunshine.[68] Maurice Denis (1870–1943), in his heartfelt obituary for Cross in 1910, described the artist's journey to the coast as both an aesthetic and therapeutic quest for light: a new palette and a '*cure de soleil*' for his chronic degenerative arthritis.[69] Only two kilometres away from Cross's remote home in Saint-Clair was a sanatorium at La Fossette offering '*cures de soleil et d'air*'. One of Cross's most well-known paintings, *La Plage ombragée* (1902), was based on the beach of La Fossette.[70] The sanatorium was not an isolated example. Heliotherapy was rapidly adopted and institutionalised at sanatoria along the Côte d'Azur by the first decade of the twentieth century. In fact, there are references to sunlight as therapeutic in French medical dissertations from as early as 1799.[71] By the 1910s, the therapy held tremendous significance for the French nation amidst fears of degeneration and international war.[72]

No history of light therapy is complete without reference to its development in Switzerland and its most famous practitioners, Drs Oskar Bernhard (1861–1939) and Auguste Rollier (1874–1954).[73] At Samaden, Bernhard began using sunlight to treat wounds from 1902, and Rollier opened his first sanatorium in Leysin a year later, the first of thirty-six. Both studied under the well-known surgeon and Nobel laureate Theodor Kocher (1841–1917).[74] Indeed, Bernhard and Rollier came close to being Nobel laureates themselves; between 1920 and 1933, the former was nominated five times, the latter three, for their work with heliotherapy.[75]

Alongside Tegner's Finsen monument, the photographs of Rollier and Bernhard present light therapy at its most aesthetically polished (though see also Chapter 6 for contemporary images of light therapy by Danish photographer, Nicolai Howalt, b. 1970, Fig. 6.1).[76] Their heavily illustrated publications provide an impressive visual archive of heliotherapy patients (Figs. 5.7, 5.15–5.16). As early as 1912, Rollier's photographs were receiving press in the *BMJ*. A special correspondent, attending a paper given by one of Rollier's staff, perceptively remarked on their aesthetic qualities, while still being convinced by the 'striking' effect:

> Dr. F. Morin (Leysin) made a short but excellent communication on the treatment of tuberculosis of glands, joints, bones, and skin by exposure to sunlight. It was illustrated by lantern slides, and a large number of photographs. In most cases the treatment extended over months, even years, but there was no question that the improvement was great. A most striking photograph was that of a young patient with arrested disease of the tibia ski-ing [sic] stark naked over Alpine snow [...] Here the effects of the light treatment were shown, but it was curious that while all photographs of the patient before the treatment were printed on bright, glossy paper, whereby details were accentuated, the after-results were invariably printed on dull matt paper, no doubt for artistic effect.[77]

It was not the last occasion Rollier employed strategic aesthetic tactics to disseminate light therapy as simultaneously an art and a science. He photographed his patients well into the 1940s.[78] Rollier considered his before and after photographs 'more eloquent than words' in demonstrating the regenerative powers of sunlight.[79] Their persuasive power moved influential British physicians, including Sir Alfred Fripp (1865–1930, Guy's), surgeon to King Edward VI and King George V (the latter receiving treatment for pleurisy in 1928 with mercury vapour lamps).[80] Fripp was convinced of the necessity of using sunlight to treat tuberculous children after viewing these photographs in 1921, which 'persuaded and delighted him on the spot'.[81] Fripp later attended the opening of Britain's first public sunlight clinic, in St Pancras in 1925, and was an honorary consultant to the London Light Clinic.[82] So great was Rollier's fame that the London County Council discussed the merits of sending soldiers and convalescents to his facilities in Leysin at their own cost.[83]

Thus, while this book concentrates on the British development of light therapy, it necessarily references other nations. British practitioners were keenly aware of the work and imagery of foreign physicians, citing them, visiting their facilities, and translating their key publications into English. As is apparent from the *Times* supplement, the British public were also kept informed of a range of international interests in therapeutic light through words and images, from Finsen's Light Institute in Denmark to Rollier's famous sanatoria in the Swiss mountains, from the fashionable beaches of the Côte d'Azur to Hans Surén's (1885–1972) *Nachtkultur* (Naked Culture) movement in Germany (Fig. 1.1, central image). Light therapy developed globally, used throughout Continental Europe, North America, North Africa, Russia, India, and New Zealand.[84] In these varied locations the political meaning and value of bodily exposure to light also varied considerably, Paul Overy explaining:

> The concerns with sunshine and the open air which had been a major feature of the social-democratic lifestyle of the 1920s and early 1930s also played an important role in the *Wohnkultur* of Nazi Germany, as they had earlier in fascist Italy, and in the ideology of the Soviet Union.[85]

Individual and national investments in light, therefore, were not apolitical – they did not transcend competing politics – but rather were readily absorbed into them. In Britain, bodily exposure to light was promoted by members of Labour and Conservative governments throughout the early twentieth century and taken up by social reformers like the eugenicist and campaigner Dr Caleb Saleeby (1878–1940), social elites such as Nobel laureate and playwright George Bernard Shaw (1856–1950), and social outcasts, not least nudists (Chapter 5).[86]

'British' light therapy

In contrast to other nations during the same time period, Britain's heavy investment in light therapy was marked by conflicting, even confounding, views towards its benefits and risks. Unlike in France, Switzerland, and the United States, for example, Britain's relationship with light was (and remains) particularly fickle.

There are early references to sunlight's curative value in nineteenth-century British medical literature. In 1830, the surgeon and writer James Johnson (1777–1845) wrote of sun-deprived patients as akin to etiolated celery – blanched and lifeless – necessitating a change of air.[87] In the 1850s, nursing legend Florence Nightingale (1820–1910) noted that the sun cured bodies physically and mentally with the skill of an artist, impressing its effects upon the human form much as it did onto photographic film:

> It is the unqualified result of all my experience with the sick, that second only to their need of fresh air is their need of light; that, after a close room, what hurts them most is a dark room. And that it is not only light but direct sunlight they want [...] People think the effect is upon the spirits only. This is by no means the case. The sun is not only a painter but a sculptor. You admit that he does the photograph. Without going into any scientific exposition we much admit that light has quite as real and tangible effects upon the human body.[88]

Nightingale's poetic depiction is but one of many representations of the sun's painterly, sculptural, and photographic effects on the beauty, contours, and skin of patients' bodies.

In 1877, the chemist Thomas Blunt (1842–1929) and physician (later Sir) Arthur Downes (1851–1938) demonstrated that sunlight is bactericidal, publishing their findings in the proceedings of the Royal Society of Medicine.[89] Several years later, in 1890, the medical missionary Dr Theobald Palm (1848–1928) argued that rickets was the result of lack of sunlight. He advocated sunbaths as a routine preventive and curative practice for mothers and children and later became a vice-president to Saleeby's Sunlight League.[90]

When, in the mid-1890s, Niels Finsen began experimenting with light in Copenhagen, British medical practitioners were already primed and open to thinking about light as a powerful, natural therapeutic. Like his international contemporaries, Finsen was well aware of the bactericidal and irritating properties of actinic light, in particular the blue, violet, and ultraviolet rays, and he experimented with both natural and artificial light. His 'Finsen lamp', a modified carbon-arc lamp, had telescopic arms and quartz glass lenses that filtered light down onto the infected lesions of lupus vulgaris patients (Fig. 2.6). Targeting lesions one by one, his lamps destroyed the tubercle bacilli and enabled smooth scarring on patients' skin. So effective was the treatment – which he proved, as Rollier would, by means of powerful before and after photographs (Fig. 2.4) – that Finsen became internationally renowned, and by 1896 he opened an institute in Copenhagen that was privately and state funded.[91] He and his Finsen Institute won a number of awards, including a Grand Prix at the Art Nouveau *Exposition Universelle* of 1900, which also showcased escalators and talking films for the first time to the public.[92] Most prestigiously his development of phototherapy earned him a Nobel Prize in Medicine in 1903, the same year the Curies and Henri Becquerel won their joint Prize in Physics for the discovery of radioactivity (Chapter 4).

Finsen's publications were translated into German, French, and English, enabling global dissemination. And the world took notice. By 1900, Britain imported phototherapy into its best hospitals, primarily through the intervention of fellow Dane, Queen Alexandra (1844–1925), then Princess of Wales.[93] Having visited the Finsen Institute in 1899, the princess was so impressed that she purchased a Finsen lamp and donated it to the London Hospital, effectively creating its light department. The department's regular appearance in the press was due in no small part to the hospital's chairman, Sydney Holland, who doggedly appealed for more and more funds to cover its significant running costs. As founder of the *Daily Mail* (1896) and owner of *The Times* (1908–22), Alfred Harmsworth (Lord Northcliffe, 1865–1922) had a major part to play in the public awareness of the hospital's phototherapy facilities as well; the newspaper magnate was one of their main benefactors, having donated the department's second Finsen lamp.[94] Anne Jamieson argued that greater attention should also be paid to public demand in driving the dissemination of phototherapy:

> When the Light Department at the London Hospital first opened, they were inundated by an 'endless stream' of [lupus vulgaris] sufferers and, within a few days, the waiting list was more than two years. Would-be patients came from around the country and from the colonies too, as far afield as New Zealand and Newfoundland.[95]

Following Finsen's lead, the light department's medical officer, dermatologist James Sequeira (1865–1948), ensured that patients were photographed before, during and after treatment, with case records still extant in the hospital's archives.

The London Hospital treated lupus patients initially with natural sunlight, setting up Finsen's focusing lenses on the tennis grounds (Fig. 2.9).[96] But heliotherapy did not initially have quite the same impact that phototherapy did, despite Finsen using both at his institute. The *BMJ* and the *Lancet* followed developments in heliotherapy early on, with sporadic reports from the 1890s to the 1910s. Some held it in high esteem and predicted its bright future.[97] Sir Henry Gauvain claimed he began using heliotherapy at Treloar Hospital from its opening in 1908, influenced by the *hélio-marin* (sun and sea) treatment at Berck under Drs François Calot (1861–1944), Jacques Calvé (1875–1954), and Henri Cazin (1836–91).[98] Later on he championed Rollier's method in Britain, and, along with Saleeby, wrote a foreword for Rollier's English publication, *Heliotherapy* (1923).

Though enthusiastic about natural sunlight's therapeutic charms, British practitioners expressed uncertainty that they could access and harness it on home soil. A recurring theme throughout the British history of light therapy is a lamentation towards the island's regrettable climate and consequent envy for the ready, unobstructed sunshine of France's southern coast and Switzerland's mountains. *The Times*' medical correspondent bemoaned in the 1928 supplement that, 'From October till March Great Britain is a sunless country.'[99] Some doubted heliotherapy could be practised in Britain at all. The physicians Eleanor H. Russell and William K. Russell wrote in 1925 that,

> it is very difficult and almost impossible to practise heliotherapy in this country, owing to its low altitudes and its climatic conditions. The moisture-laden atmosphere and the smoky air filter out practically all the therapeutic rays of the sun, particularly in our large cities, and especially in winter, so that the sunlight we get is almost free from these rays.[100]

For the Russells, reliance on artificial sources was a necessity, and certainly the primary medical literature and visual material attest to Britain's enthusiastic employment of phototherapy. The sheer speed at which it entered into hospitals, including the London Hospital, Guy's, St Thomas', and the Manchester and Salford Hospital for Skin Diseases, indicates Britain's medical profession was ready and willing to welcome phototherapy's technologically impressive paraphernalia.[101]

Other practitioners argued that there were excellent opportunities to practise heliotherapy in the country, particularly during the spring and summer in the south of England, where, Gauvain attested, 'abundant sunshine for therapeutic purposes is available, sometimes largely in excess of the patient's needs'.[102] Saleeby's book, *Sunlight and Health*, was advertised in *The Times*' 1928 supplement, declaring that 'our English sunlight is good enough if used aright', while that same year Hill stated more emphatically that, 'It is noteworthy that on clear days readings of ultra-violet in England may be as high as in the tropics.'[103] This was not a case of heliotherapy being in rivalry with phototherapy, even if some practitioners expressed preference for natural over artificial sources or vice versa: Gauvain, Saleeby, and Hill promoted and employed both in clinical practice and for the public, and entrepreneurs fostered public access to both.[104] In Poole, for example, the Branksome Chine Solarium functioned as a solarium during the summer with the aid of 'Vita' glass in the lounge, while one of its halls provided phototherapy during the winter.[105] In the *Times* supplement, readers encountered a mix of images of natural and artificial exposures, with little sense that one was necessarily better than the other (Figs. 1.1–1.4). It makes for complicated (visual) reading and resists the temptation of writing what Jordanova called a 'seductive' and 'glamorised' narrative.[106] Her choice of words is fitting, since the history of bodily exposure to light is bound up with both sex and fashion.

Off the beaten (narrative) path

The history of bodily exposure to light is enmeshed with the history of leisure. With images such as Fig. 1.2, it is not surprising to see why: beaches, gardens, and open fields were ideal locations for heliotherapy; nudity was encouraged since the skin needed unfettered exposure to light; and physicians were convinced of the light's psychological benefits, making the sight of smiles at sanatoria commonplace. Yet historians consistently overlook the early medical history of using light to treat diseases, instead following a well-worn narrative path on popular sunbathing that begins in the 1920s with the glamorous fashionista Coco Chanel (1883–1971). Physicians, stumbling with eagerness in her wake, are positioned as providing the much-needed 'justification' for an already-prevalent 'fad'. Sally Dunne Romano stated, for instance:

> In the early twentieth century, as the idea gained widespread popular acceptance, the medical profession played an important, though supporting role in promoting the connection between sunlight and good health. Medical and scientific theories and opinions reinforced and gave 'expert' backing to popular ideas about sunlight, health and tanned skin.[107]

Previous to the 1920s, we are told, tanning was associated only with the lower classes, especially manual labourers stuck outdoors all day roasting in the sun. Carter fleshed out this narrative by discussing the intertwined nineteenth-century histories of class, race, and travel – of skin colour and colonial conquest.[108] He also explained how beliefs about the beauty of pale skin and of tanned skin coexisted by the turn of the century, the former eventually outmoded as an 'aristocratic code of beauty' associated with sickliness and vice by 'an emerging aesthetics of middle-class bodily health and beauty'.[109] I tackle the subject of skin colour and race in Chapter 5, and throughout the book I add further context to light therapy's emergence by bringing in the histories of light chemistry, photography, electricity, and radiation.

Instead of positioning medical understandings of light as something separate from public ones – of viewing medicine and leisure as operating at opposite ends of a spectrum – I make the following three assertions:

First, that during the nineteenth and early twentieth centuries the former enabled the latter. Having been established by the nineteenth century in specific medical institutions, the therapeutic use of light predated and subsequently drove widespread public use during the twentieth century.

Second, that by the 1920s medical perceptions effectively naturalised the concept of light as fundamental to well-being, health, and happiness. Martin Edwards stated that by the 1930s and 1940s light therapy fizzled out.[110] But primary evidence makes it clear that going to light clinics, using home-use lamps, and sunbathing were still popular practices, encouraged through national fitness campaigns as well as during the Second World War (see Chapter 5).[111] I argue it was less a fizzling out than a *soaking in*, the increasingly familiar sight of bodies exposed to the sun or sophisticated lamps absorbed into the public consciousness like sunlight on skin.

Third, that this was less a 'trickle down' process, from authoritative physician to naive public, than a messy intersection of, and active struggle between, competing practitioners, patients, and members of the public, complicated additionally by image makers, manufacturers, and the popular press.[112] As individuals took on responsibility for (and pleasure in) their own exposures, medical practitioners fought even harder to retain their authority as experts on therapeutic light, to warn the public (as Russ would do), and to emphasise that, however beneficial, light equally was dangerous and mysterious. This was fundamentally an issue of control. Indeed, as I show in the chapters that follow, throughout its history light therapy has been perpetually 'out of control', a medical practice struggling to fix dosage standards, visualise its methods, prove its efficacy, and define itself. As I stated earlier, whether light therapy really worked is not my concern here. Instead, it is imperative to understand that the widespread interest in light's therapeutic potential at this time produced a myriad of theories, practices, images, and technological paraphernalia, whether mainstream, popular, commercial, or 'quack', and that unravelling their messy intersection to produce an easily digestible narrative is beside the point: light therapy's tensions, complexities, and failures communicate far more about its past – and present – than its successes.[113]

My three assertions are in keeping with both Carter's argument that physicians (and especially dermatologists) continue to act as keen mediators between bodies and sunlight, and Apple's argument that the history of vitamins is similarly marked by a self-perpetuating cycle of enduring deference to scientific authority – a back-and-forth game of 'benefits' versus 'risks' that only creates more and more competing and contradictory documentation, without ever presenting a satisfactory resolution one way or the other.

It is not just secondary literature that follows prescriptive narrative patterns in telling light therapy's 'story'. The primary literature played a major part in shaping its history through legitimising tactics that, consciously or not, were employed to make light therapy 'durable', to quote Carter.[114] These included locating the therapy's origins in ancient history while also making it modern and scientific, as well as establishing a hagiography of its 'pioneers'.

The therapy's proponents waxed lyrical about its illustrious heritage in ancient Egypt, Greece, and Rome, and even further back in human history. Bernhard opened his 1926 translation, *Light Treatment in Surgery*, by declaring:

> The beneficial properties of sunlight, the increased metabolism to which it conduces, and its vitalizing influence on body and mind have been known by instinct to the inhabitants of the earth from the oldest times [...] The sight of the sun has awakened religious sentiments in all peoples. Out of these

> sentiments grew the idea of a personal Sun God, and from this idea again sun-worship has developed. This was really the first religion.[115]

Practitioners such as Bernhard provided a 'natural' and logical justification for the use of heliotherapy, grounded in the medical wisdom, religions, and instincts of ancient civilisations. This is exemplified by the consistent, if not formulaic, structure of primary texts, which almost invariably began with a chapter on history featuring sun deities Ra and Apollo as well as Graeco-Roman enthusiasts Hippocrates, Celsus, and Galen. It was, of course, also produced through dramatic visual representations of figures worshipping the sun (Figs. 1.1, 1.7). This narrative pattern is so 'durable' it can still be found in secondary sources introducing the subject.[116]

At the same time, and particularly with early twentieth-century medical texts about phototherapy, there are introductions on the nature of light and electromagnetic forces, citing the work of contemporaries Wilhelm Röntgen (1845–1923), Sir Oliver Lodge (1851–1940), and William Thomson (Lord Kelvin, 1824–1907).[117] For practitioners, the 'primitive' uses of therapeutic light were not antithetical to modern, 'scientific' ones. By 'folding' the time of the ancients onto that of scientific progress, Carter argued that the therapy 'could simultaneously point both to the past and to the future'.[118] Lastly, they located 'modern' light therapy in 1890s Denmark, building its modern hagiography on the genius of Finsen. Finsen did not just 'invent' or 'discover' phototherapy, he positively unearthed it from the dark, smoky oblivion of the Industrial Revolution.[119] Jamieson argued that Finsen's influence was so great that his institute successfully perpetuated a Finsen 'brand': a Finsen technique, Finsen standards, and Finsen equipment.[120]

The major players and the big leagues

After Finsen came Bernhard and Rollier, then in Britain Sequeira, Gauvain, Hill, and Saleeby.[121] These were British light therapy's leading actors, and they fought to make it scientific, progressive, and 'systematic' (Chapter 2, and see Chapter 6 on its overlooked *others*, its 'invisibles': nurses, patients, and artists). Together they formed a tight circle and constantly cited each other's work and visited each other's facilities.[122]

Gauvain's sanatoria in Hampshire specialised in treating children with external forms of tuberculosis, especially of the bones and joints (Fig. 1.8). For this reason, Treloar Hospital (Alton) was known as a 'Cripples' hospital, later college, and provided work opportunities for those who, because of their physical disability, could not undertake normal paid work into adulthood.[123] In 1919, a branch was opened on Hayling Island to provide sea-bathing treatments as aids to the light and open air (Fig. 1.9). In 1920, Gauvain received a knighthood for his work with ill children at Treloar's, and he was considered Britain's leading heliotherapist. Hill was a physiologist specialising in the circulatory and respiratory systems, and in 1914 became

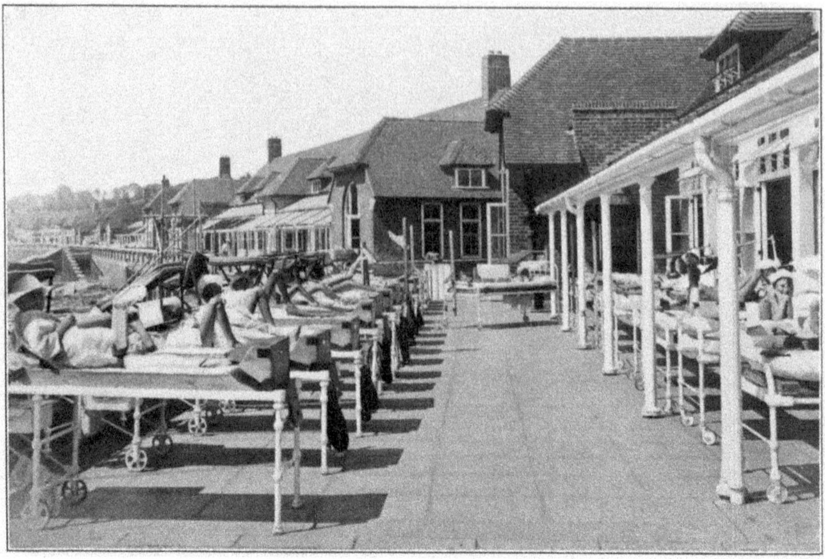

Figure 1.8 'Out on the terrace', Treloar Hospital, undated.
In *Alton 1908–1929–1937* (London: Treloar Hospital, 1937), p. 13. Wellcome Library, London.

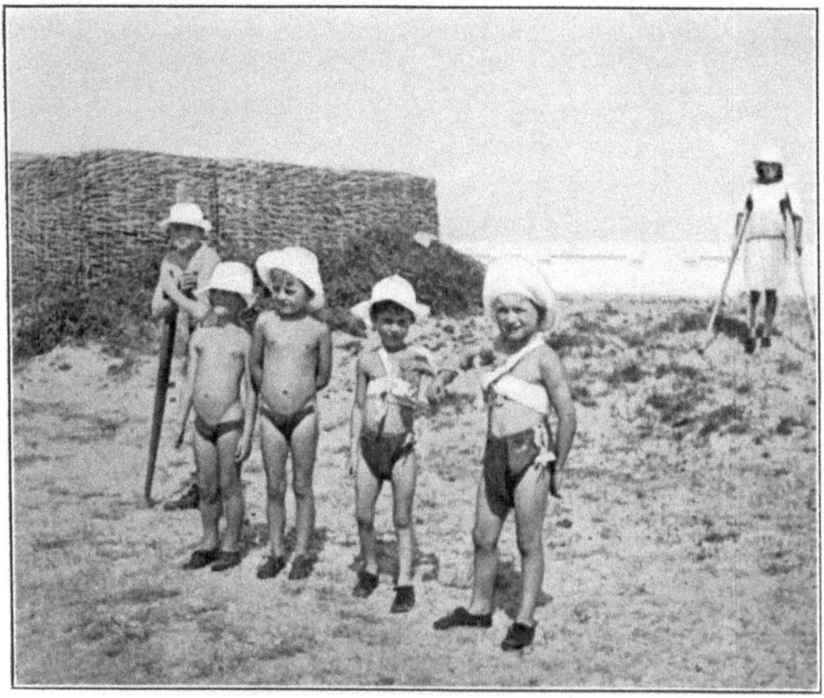

Figure 1.9 'A glimpse of Hayling', Treloar Hospital's seaside branch on Hayling Island, undated.
In *Alton 1908–1929–1937* (London: Treloar Hospital, 1937), p. 15. Wellcome Library, London.

head of the applied physiology department at the NIMR, run by the MRC. He was knighted in 1930.[124]

Gauvain and Hill were members of the MRC's CBAL, and, along with Saleeby, they helped found the People's League of Health (in 1917). The league campaigned for issues such as housing and sanitary reform, better nutrition, open-air living, and sunbathing, and was succeeded by the New Health Society (f. 1925) of William Arbuthnot Lane (1856–1943). Combatting the perceived degeneration of the British 'race', the leagues, John Stanislav Sadar explained,

> promoted the primitiveness of naturism and extant nineteenth-century practices of holidays, sport and leisure, sun-tanning and open-air living, looser and less clothing, hygiene, vegetarianism and temperance. They also advocated the new consumer products appearing under the guise of particular health claims, such as vitamin pills, artificial sunlamps and irradiated foodstuffs, as possible antidotes to a needy body. The membership propagating the needy body was its various antidotes included those at the forefront of British public life: prime ministers Asquith (1908–16), Lloyd George (1916–22), and Chamberlain (1937–40); Medical Research Council Tuberculosis Committee Chairman Charles John Bond; industrialist Henry Wellcome; zoologist Julian Huxley; and the progeny of Charles Darwin.[125]

Saleeby, initially involved in the Eugenics Education Society (f. 1907), acted as chairman for the National Birthrate Commission during the First World War and created the Sunlight League in 1924 under the patronage of Queen Alexandra.[126] Saleeby's aim was to banish what he termed the 'diseases of darkness' – rickets, tuberculosis, alcoholism, depression, and suicide – primarily through smoke abatement laws. For Saleeby, the smog of coal fumes rendered the sunlight's therapeutic and visualising powers inert; it sullied the lungs, blocked off ultraviolet radiation to needy citizens, and obscured the light authorities needed to monitor them.[127] Beyond the clinic, laboratory, and hospital, then, these physicians engaged directly with the government and the public to encourage the consumption of therapeutic light. In addition to giving public talks, Saleeby published under the pseudonym of 'Lens' in a regular column in the *Statesman*, while Hill frequently provided ultraviolet radiation readings for *The Times*.

The Sunlight League published the journal, *Sunlight* (f. 1924), and organised the opening of several light clinics in London, the first in St Pancras in 1925. It was overseen by Dr William Beaumont (d. 1967), who by 1930 became the medical director of the Institute of Ray Therapy in Camden. The institute offered phototherapy free to the poor and charged other patients according to their income and number of dependents.[128] The London Light Clinic opened in 1925, expanded in 1927, and was run by the British Humane Association.[129] Its medical superintendent was Dr Edward Deck (see epigraph) and its general supervisor Hill. The London Light Clinic ran along similar lines to the Institute for Ray Therapy and in 1932 professed to have 120,000 patients. Both clinics also acted as training centres for practitioners wishing to specialise in the subject, the examinations overseen by the Chartered Society of Massage and Medical Gymnastics from the 1920s.[130]

Another well-known light clinic was run by the Bermondsey Borough Council, having opened already by 1924. It expanded in 1936, a pamphlet by the major lamp manufacturer, Hanovia, explaining that the clinic now had facilities to treat fifty patients at once, providing 1,600 treatments per day. Hanovia supplied the lamps, as it did to many other clinics, hospitals, health centres, factories, to the public directly, and even to the National Gallery to examine artworks.[131] But two health centres took the lead in terms of integrating the latest light-therapy facilities with innovative architectural design: the Peckham Health Centre (Peckham Experiment, 1935), designed by British modern architect Sir Owen Williams (1890–1969), and the Finsbury Health Centre (1938), designed by socialist Russian émigré Berthold Lubetkin (1901–90). The centres were at the forefront of preventive care for the working and poorer classes, incorporating light therapy as part of a larger health programme that included swimming, dancing, and physical culture.[132] Overy has characterised modernist architecture of the interwar period as marked by a fascination for 'light, air and openness', heavily influenced by sanatoria design.[133] Le Corbusier (1887–1965) is repeatedly mentioned for his preoccupation with sunlight, as is British architect Edwin Maxwell Fry (1899–1987), who built his 'Sun House' in 1935 and designed an open-air school for tuberculous children at Papworth (Cambridge) with Bauhaus founder Walter Gropius (1883–1969).[134]

The most public expression of this Art Deco love of the sun, however, was surely the lido. Standing in for the beach within the urban sprawl of the city, the lido provided an open space mixing genders, classes, and ages, united in their bodily exposure to the sunlight, air, and water. The Serpentine Lido ('Lansbury's Lido', 1930), in particular, was built following the urging of the Sunlight League to radical politician George Lansbury (1859–1940).[135] It was one of the League's many campaigns, a product of its aim to be 'above party, class or creed'.[136] The sight of sunbathers was encountered high and low by the 1930s, in the visual arts and in popular media; 'sunbathers were everywhere', Christopher Wilk stated, 'shown in mass-circulation magazines and in newsreels, in design publications, in art galleries and in public exhibition spaces'.[137] The desire for fit and healthy bodies became a national imperative, in Britain and elsewhere. As I explain in Chapter 5, the individual who consumed light was performing no less than an act of citizenship.

Exposing children

Problematically, such ennobling acts by individual citizens were not necessarily voluntary. Here we arrive at a difficult topic, that of exposing children, the therapy's main target group. Many thousands of children received heliotherapy and phototherapy during the early twentieth century, in Britain and abroad. They were used to treat a variety of childhood illnesses and conditions, chief among them anaemia, malnourishment, and rickets. The discovery that ultraviolet light could stimulate vitamin D production and hence cure rickets had a profound effect on child health provision. Saleeby declared in 1929 that half of all three-year-olds in the country suffered from rickets.[138] Little wonder public authorities and physicians placed such faith in light's beneficial powers, with the photographic material showing such remarkable recoveries (Figs. 1.5–1.6, 5.7). Russ, in a public radio broadcast of 1928, stated that 'it is no exaggeration to say that the children are literally nourished by sunlight'.[139] Dr Katherine Gamgee, specialising in maternal and child health, explained it was the duty of local health and education authorities to provide children with suitable access to light, as 'Such a clinic as a Light Department taps very widely the child population of any area, and, if it prove successful, it will be found that very soon all the feeblest and illest children in the neighbourhood will flock to it.'[140] Parents, especially mothers, were encouraged to bring their children to these clinics, on referral by their general practitioner or medical officer of health, as well as to expose them independently under a watchful eye (Fig. 1.1).

As this book's reproduced images show, many children were photographed receiving treatment, or before and after it, to disseminate light therapy's methods and results. The identities of these children remain unknown – they are very rarely mentioned in archives, and often further anonymised by having their names appear only as initials in case studies or their faces obscured by wearing goggles in the images. In a time before formalised patient consent laws, it is doubtful they gave their consent to receive exposures or to be photographed doing so (or, furthermore, for those photographs to be distributed), which I find both professionally and personally distressing.

'Exposing' is an apt choice of word, calling to mind the act of irradiating itself (treating the patient) but also the acts of subjecting (endangering), opening to the light (photographing), uncovering (laying bare), and displaying (exhibiting). Therefore, by discussing the exposing of children I mean putting vulnerable children in front of or under light sources, capturing their likenesses onto the photosensitive film of the camera, showing their nude bodies to receptive medical and public audiences, and reproducing such images once again throughout this book (and online, no less, through the Open Access version). These exposures – to the light of the lamp, to the camera, and to the gazes of primary and secondary audiences – deserve critical contextualisation, ethical considerations, and sensitivity.[141] I cannot control the life of the photographs any more than their original producers, even with restrictive licensing laws, and how viewers choose to react to these images remains uncertain.[142] That many of the images represent anonymous, vulnerable, nude children makes my position all the more precarious. Being in this position, however distressing, presents me with an opportunity, as well as a responsibility, to be ever mindful of the power of images.[143]

The Treloar archives, held at the Hampshire Record Office in Winchester, make an ideal case in point. Treloar's medical superintendent, Gauvain, published images and films of his child patients in various medical and popular venues (Figs. 1.7–1.8). As a result, Treloar's was well known to the general public and to the social elite, the latter pictured frequently as benevolent donators and privileged visitors on its annual founder's day. In photographs and films, wealthy patrons draped in furs mix uneasily with nude child patients, both on public display to various ends. In these representations, the institution was conveyed both as a space of modern, scientific medicine and intimate, loving care (Figs. 1.8, 1.10). Constantly monitored and intensely observed, some patients were involved in long-term controlled trials at the sanatorium, for example concerning ultraviolet light's effects on mental retardation (Chapter 5).[144] This is but one example of many experiments involving child patients as 'guinea pigs' for light therapy research and forms part of a larger history involving children as research subjects as Susan Lederer has shown.[145]

Figure 1.10 'In the hay', Treloar Hospital, undated. In *Alton 1908–1929–1937* (London: Treloar Hospital, 1937), p. 7. Wellcome Library, London.

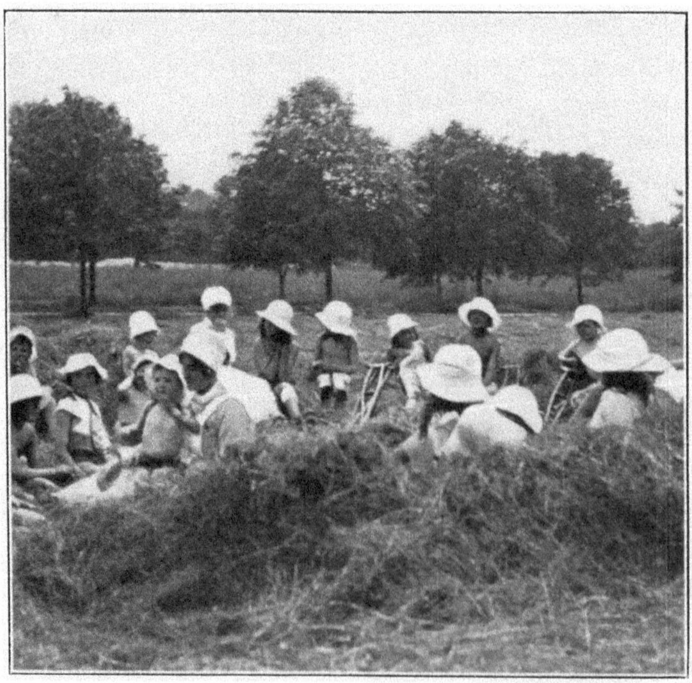

Now carefully closed to public view, Treloar's archival photographs, illustrated publications, and case records remain hidden to all but 'bonafide medical researchers'. The images of Treloar Hospital reproduced here are from alternative sources. Permission requests to reproduce images from the Treloar archive have been ignored or denied to me by their current rights-holder.[146] Its reasoning for doing so has not been explained, but I suspect the matter rests with the subject of exposing children, revolving around issues of patient consent and anonymity, child nudity, and the ethics of display. Though I have viewed its archive in person, the photographs remain invisible in this book.

The silent, resistant nature of these representations retains their power and exemplifies ambivalent and contentious perceptions – already in place at the time of their making – towards exposing (photo)sensitive patients to actinic light among the medical community and the popular press. These two kinds of 'exposure', concerning not only the irradiating of the children but their requisite bare flesh recorded and displayed via photography, are inextricably intertwined and have made the choice whether or not to reproduce images of these child patients a difficult task.[147] At the same time, it is not my place to celebrate or denigrate the use of light therapy, in the past or today, or portray its practitioners as either saviours or villains. Its patients, similarly, cannot categorically be viewed as victims, even its most vulnerable and powerless patients. The complexity of this subject matter is embedded within its very representation, and the images in this book allow, if not demand, us to think through the complexities of light therapy as a medical practice, their own rich meanings and manner of production providing a unique entry point into the therapy's contentious history.

The chapters

Soaking Up the Rays contains four main chapters, each driven by an image, or set of images and objects, that leads a discussion on a specific theme in light therapy's history. Just like *The Times*' supplement, a variety of representations of light therapy, both visual and textual, is encountered throughout the book.

Chapter 2 tracks the ambivalent role of sunburn in the dosage standardisation of ultraviolet light through documentary photographs of *c.* 1893–1940. These photographs are particularly difficult to read ('illegible'), both literally and figuratively, beginning with a photograph of Finsen's irradiated, sunburnt forearm (Fig. 2.1). It is one of the earliest images, if not the first, of modern light therapy. This now lost, poorly reproduced photograph presents the results of Finsen's self-experimentation with a carbon arc lamp. Assessing ultraviolet light's impact upon the body, Finsen concluded that one's own skin acted as a registration device for dosing therapeutic light. Significantly, he relied on another light-sensitive registration device, namely photography, to communicate his findings and to legitimise phototherapy to an international medical community. This chapter questions British physicians' conflicting perceptions towards sunburn (solar erythema) in the therapeutic process, as a physiological marker at once feared and desired during the cure. Both the visual sign of damage *and* therapeutic success, the solar erythema's value was hotly contested among practitioners. British physicians and researchers came to convey enormous conceptual weight onto the visual production of solar erythema, a phenomenon known to be visibly transient, latent, and variable according to the individual, and thus a particularly uncooperative visual anchor on which to standardise exposures. The chapter argues that the very desire to 'fix' sunburn (to photographically record it and to pin it down according to measurable qualitative and quantitative data) betrays deep-seated anxieties on the part of practitioners to wrestle control over light therapy as a purportedly 'systematic' form of medicine. It deals with the troublesome nature of visual evidence, especially photographs, through a focused study of light therapy's clinical history.

Chapter 3 takes the relationship between light therapy and its photographic representation further by thinking through the complexities of these intertwined 'light technologies'. Practitioners made frequent analogies between photographs and skin, and they looked to photographic processes and larger developments in photochemistry in order to understand how and why light therapy worked on patients. But what began as a natural alliance between photography and light therapy soon became an uneasy, incestuous relationship between the visualising and therapeutic powers of light. Damaged and overexposed photographs offer poignant examples of this uneasy relationship, especially those attempting to capture a particularly difficult subject: open arc light therapy in process, which splayed blinding, excessive actinic light onto any and all exposed to it. By contrast is an unusually 'good', if obscure, photographic negative of a session taking place at the South London Hospital for Women and Children (Fig. 3.1). It was taken by the émigré photographer Edith Tudor-Hart, who produced many photographic representations of light therapy during her intriguing and secretive career. Counterpoints to Tudor-Hart's photograph are damaged attempts, marked by lens flare and 'solarisation'. Chapter 3 argues that light therapy was encountered and represented photographically as an *obscure* practice, in which these light technologies do not so much converge as collide.

Through particularly striking advertisements, Chapter 4 focuses on risk, damage, and injury through the art of visualising the penetrating rays of invisible light. It situates ultraviolet lamps and their advertisements as modern objects communicating ambivalent messages about risk and safety. The chapter argues that manufacturers and practitioners relied heavily on montage as an adept, vanguard medium for representing the emanating invisible rays of natural and artificial light (Plate 1). Manufacturers encouraged British consumers to expose their bodies to lamps designed for independent use and self-surveillance during which the individual became simultaneously operator and patient. Sunburn and suntan were both desirable outcomes of these vitalising exposures to ultraviolet radiation, represented in advertisements with 'radiant' bodies. The advertising of these lamps intensified during the 1920s and 1930s, despite growing awareness of ultraviolet light's carcinogenic properties. Chapter 4 contextualises physicians' use of infrared and ultraviolet rays in relation to the contemporaneous development of radiotherapy, including X rays and the beta, alpha, and gamma rays of radium. Burns, lesions, and skin cancers from all of these rays are investigated, as well as the similar ways in which these risky, invisible rays were visualised, ingested, and marketed. The complex relationship between these different wavelengths – sometimes perceived as allies, sometimes enemies – in the therapeutic process elucidates surprising tensions in light therapy's past, connecting the tanning lamp to the atom bomb.

Through colour advertisements that convey the glowing tans of healthy mothers, thriving babies, and virile men, Chapter 5 discusses the politics and aesthetics of suntan (Plate 3). It analyses practitioners' perceptions of the suntan as the external sign of stored solar energy in the body, of the body visualised as literally 'photogenic' (light-generating). Practitioners, government officials, and eugenicists greatly desired tanned flesh for the British public, and lamp manufacturers and tourist companies offered light for consumption in the battle against 'sun starvation'. Rich and poor alike received therapeutic exposures of light in hospitals, clinics, and at home, and, as they internalised and consumed the penetrative rays of light, their bodies were perceived to gain unparalleled vitality and regenerative force for the benefit of individual and nation. Sunlight and artificial light were directed onto nursing mothers' breasts, 'backwards' children, and injured soldiers. In the regeneration of these highly valued subjects, physicians and politicians perceived light as an aid to national salvation. Yet in encouraging citizens to emulate the dark skins of 'primitive' races, they conveyed ambivalent attitudes towards the merits of suntanned skin. Through dramatic colour representations of suntanned bodies, Chapter 5 investigates suntan as simultaneously a visual marker of recharged health and a troubling act of racial transgression during a period of heightened eugenic fervour in Britain and Europe.

By way of conclusion, Chapter 6 discusses the concept of the 'dead point' in light therapeutic practice. For some physicians, too deep a suntan could inhibit further curative effect, a 'dead point' or plateau during treatment. From this point, treatment would stop, and the patient's skin would be allowed time to rest and recover. Once the skin lost its tan, the treatment would start again, creating cycles of 'dead points' and recoveries. As an initial inhibitor to progressing forward, the 'dead point' finds resonance with light therapy's numerous historical dead ends. Contained within the closed stores of the Wellcome Library, for example, is an unusual painting about light therapy, made by a now-obscure British artist, Beatrice Langdon (Plate 8). In

1938, she painted the light department of the Royal London Hospital, a work commemorating the impact of the Finsen lamp in the battle against lupus vulgaris. The exact reasons for Langdon's painting are, however, unknown, and Chapter 6 leads off from the mysteries and loose threads surrounding the work to discuss the many other silences, absences, and dead ends in the history of light therapy.

I view such dead points/ends as opportunities to ask different kinds of questions, to use different kinds of approaches (especially visual), and, therefore, to acquire different kinds of knowledge about medicine's past. The key images discussed in each chapter could be viewed as 'failures' or 'dead points' – as being unable to legibly communicate light therapy as a progressive treatment in an easily digestible, visual form. Yet, by failing to do so, they succeed in communicating the deep-seated anxieties, confounding perceptions, and ambivalent socio-political investment of practitioners and enthusiasts in 'harnessing' British bodies to natural and artificial light.

Notes

1 Edward J. Deck, *The Sun and How to Use It* (London: The Sunlight League, 1926), p. 3.

2 *The Orientation of Buildings* (London: Royal Institute of British Architects, 1933), p. 3. My thanks to Simon Carter for this reference.

3 In factories, miners could receive artificial sunlight after a shift. On farms, vegetables and animals were irradiated to increase crop growth, milk supply, and egg production, see *Sunlight*, 1:8 (1929), 30. Early examples of heliotherapy and phototherapy available in hotels and sanatoria include: Nordrach-on-Dee (near Balmoral), advertised in *British Medical Journal* (hereafter *BMJ*), 30 December 1911, p. 42; Glan Ely sanatorium (near Cardiff) by 1915, see 'A Combined Attack against Tuberculosis in Wales', *BMJ*, 14 August 1915, p. 263; and Peebles Hotel-Hydropathic, see the archives at Scottish Borders Council Archive and Local History Service, Hawick. It was also available at spas, see 'Where the Sun Is on Tap: Five Shillingsworth of Artificial Sunshine at Harrogate', *Yorkshire Evening Post*, 17 March 1925, p. 7. Local councils provided both too, by funding clinics and designating open spaces for sunbathing. Hastings even published printed instructions for sunbathers, see *Sunlight*, 2:3 (1930), p. 120; in 1932, it had a medical offer on the beach to give advice to sunbathers, reported in *Sunlight*, 2:6 (1932), p. 188. The opening of sunlight clinics was frequently remarked upon in local and national presses, often accompanied by photographs. See, for example, 'Artificial Sunlight at Plymouth: Amenities of Cornwall Resort', *Western Morning News*, 24 February 1926, p. 1; and 'Burnley Children to Have Artificial Sunlight Treatment', *Burnley Express and Advertiser*, 25 February 1928, p. 11. There were privately run centres offering phototherapy too: see 'Gloucester's "Sun-Ray" Centre', *Cheltenham Chronicle and Gloucestershire Graphic*, 28 April 1928, unpaginated, and an advertisement for the Midlands Sun Ray Clinic in *Nottingham Evening Post*, 20 August 1927, p. 4. One centre could cater to different classes and clientele: centres in the borough of Greenwich treated maternity and child welfare patients, patients referred from the tuberculosis dispensary, fee-paying adults in the evening, and secondary school students; see M. Macdonald, 'Artificial Sunlight Treatment in Greenwich', *Sunlight*, 2:11 (1934), 295–6.

4 'Sunlight: Extensive Use by Public Authorities', *The Times*, 16 May 1928, p. 13, as cited in Anne Kinloch Jamieson, 'An Intolerable Affliction: A History of Lupus Vulgaris in Late Nineteenth- and Early Twentieth-Century Britain' (Ph.D. dissertation, University of Leeds, 2010), p. 132.
5 'A New Science', *The Times*, 'Sunlight and Health' special supplement, 22 May 1928 (hereafter *Times* supplement), p. x.
6 'A New Science', *Times* supplement, p. x.
7 On Celanese fabric see the advertisement for British Celanese Ltd (London), *Times* supplement, p. xxxv. On 'Vita' glass, see John Stanislav Sadar, 'Unpacking the Latent Bodies of Interwar Ultraviolet Health Glass' (Ph.D. dissertation, University of Pennsylvania, 2010) and *Through the Healing Glass: Shaping the Modern Body through Glass Architecture, 1925–35* (London and New York: Routledge, 2016).
8 Allen and Hanburys Ltd (London) advertisement, *Times* supplement, p. vii.
9 'A New Science', *Times* supplement, p. x.
10 'The Coming of the Sunlight: Influence on the Nation's Health', *Times* supplement, pp. x–xi, at p. x.
11 'A New Science', *Times* supplement, p. x.
12 A. Webster, 'Ergosterol: Parent Substance of Vitamin D', *Times* supplement, p. xi.
13 Sidney Russ, 'The Story of the Rays: The Magnetic Theory of Light', *Times* supplement, p. xix.
14 Quoted in 'Light Treatment in Hospitals', *Times* supplement, pp. xxxi–ii, at p. xxxii.
15 Quoted in P. H. Oakley Williams, 'A Day's Work at "The London"', *Pall Mall Magazine*, May 1903, pp. 68–78, at p. 73. See also Sir Henry Gauvain, 'Organisation and Work of a Light Department in a Hospital for Surgical Tuberculosis', *Lancet*, 4 July 1925, pp. 10–16, at p. 11.
16 See, for example: 'Spreading Fame of the Leeds "Sun Ray" Centre', *Yorkshire Evening Post*, 27 October 1927, p. 8; Leonard Hill, G. B. Dixon, and Dora C. Colebrook, 'Discussion on Influence of Sunlight and Artificial Light on Health', *BMJ*, 12 September 1925, pp. 470–7, at p. 477; and Martin Edwards, *Control and the Therapeutic Trial: Rhetoric and Experimentation in Britain, 1918–48* (Amsterdam and New York: Rodopi, 2007), p. 76.
17 Quoted in 'Light Treatment in Hospitals', *Times* supplement, p. xxxii.
18 Edwards, *Control*, p. 74.
19 Though the *Times* supplement titled its lead article 'A New Science', Gauvain stated in 1934, 'In the present state of our knowledge heliotherapy is an art rather than an exact science.' Sir Henry Gauvain, 'Reflections on Sun Treatment: the Theory of Varying Stimuli and Varying Response', *The Practitioner*, 132 (February 1934), pp. 1–12, at p. 6.
20 Light apparatus was frequently housed with X-ray equipment, including at the London Hospital. See G. Allpress Simmons, 'The Constitution and Organization of the X-Ray Department of a General Hospital', *BMJ*, 27 August 1910, pp. 535–7; and Anne Kinloch Jamieson, 'More than Meets the Eye: Revealing the Therapeutic Potential of Light, 1896–1910', *Social History of Medicine*, 26:4 (2013), 715–37.
21 Hanovia advertisement, *Times* supplement, p. xxxiii.
22 See the advertisements for the 'Uvral' Junior twin carbon arc lamp, available via Bower Electric Ltd (London), *Times* supplement, p. xxxvii, and the Marion therapeutical multi carbon arc lamp, by the Amalgamated Photographic Manufacturers Ltd (London), p. xxxviii.
23 The conversion was used with the following website: www.thisismoney.co.uk/money/bills/article-1633409/Historic-inflation-calculator-value-money-changed-1900.html (accessed 17 February 2016).

24 Raymond Williams, 'Advertising: The Magic System', in *Problems of Materialism and Culture: Selected Essays* (London and New York: Verso, 1997), pp. 170–95, at p. 182. Katy Price explained this shift is termed the 'Northcliffe revolution', after Lord Northcliffe (Alfred Harmsworth); Katy Price, *Loving Faster than Light: Romance and Readers in Einstein's Universe* (Chicago, Ill.: University of Chicago Press, 2012), p. 6; and Ernest Turner, *The Shocking History of Advertising* (Harmondsworth: Penguin, 1965), p. 140.

25 Lupus vulgaris is not the 'lupus' we are more familiar with today, systemic lupus erythematosus.

26 Edwards, *Control*, p. 70.

27 See, for example, Albert Eidinow, 'Observations on Some of the Principles of Artificial Sun Treatment', *British Journal of Tuberculosis*, 19:3 (1925), 113–26, at p. 114; Myrtle Vaughan-Cowell, *Artificial Sunlight: Its Use and Application* (London: H. Edgar Smithers, 1928), pp. 17–18; and *Actinotherapy Technique* (Slough: Sollux, 1943), pp. 21–2. See also Richard Hobday, *The Healing Sun: Sunlight and Health in the 21st Century* (Forres: Findhorn Press, 1999), p. 15.

28 Erythemata, beyond solar erythema, have been used historically to diagnose, visualise, and reveal symptoms, brought out at the visible level of the surface/exterior of the body. They have acted as 'registers' in Charcot's 'skin writing' (hysterical dermography), in allergy scratch tests, tuberculosis tests, and even product testing on the inner forearm. My thanks to Mary Hunter for this.

29 'Sunlight and the Skin', *Times* supplement, p. xiii. See also Martyn Evans, 'Wonderful Treatment', in Pekka Louhiala, Iona Heath, and John Saunders (eds), *Medical Humanities Companion*, vol. III: *Treatment* (London: Radcliffe, 2013), pp. 17–32, at p. 18.

30 Hugo Bach, *Irradiation with the Alpine Sun Quartz Lamp*, ed. R. King Brown (Slough: Sollux, 1931), p. 36.

31 Vaughan-Cowell, *Artificial Sunlight*, pp. 17–18; and Auguste Rollier, *Le Pansement solaire: héliothérapie de certaines affections chirurgicales et des blessures de guerre* (Lausanne and Paris: Librairie Payot & Cie., 1916), pp. 67–8.

32 See Sir Henry Gauvain, 'The General Principles of Treatment in Tuberculous Disease of the Bones and Joints in Children', *BMJ*, 26 November 1921, pp. 876–84, at p. 881; Niels R. Finsen, *Phototherapy*, trans. J. H. Sequeira (London: Edward Arnold, 1901), pp. 54–5; and *Times* supplement, p. xii.

33 Edwards, *Control*, p. 16.

34 This will be no revelation to scholars of art history and visual culture. Howell points out, along these lines, 'A danger of writing for many audiences is that what is seen as radical by one may be seen as obvious by another.' Joel D. Howell, *Technology in the Hospital: Transforming Patient Care in the Early Twentieth Century* (Baltimore, Md.: Johns Hopkins University Press, 1996), p. 9.

35 See the articles in *Medical Humanities*, special issue, 'Patient Portraits', 39:1 (2013).

36 See Caroline A. Jones and Peter Galison (eds), *Picturing Science, Producing Art* (London and New York: Routledge, 1998), pp. 1–23, at p. 6.

37 Eidinow, 'Observations on Some of the Principles', p. 126.

38 The only comparable case is that of X rays, which could be used to diagnose a cancerous tumour, for example, and also treat that tumour by continued exposure.

39 'A New Science', *Times* supplement, p. x.

40 I thank Natasha Ruiz-Gómez and Mike Sappol for prompting me to think of the images in these different ways.

41 Carolyn Thomas de la Peña, *The Body Electric: How Strange Machines Built the Modern American* (New York: New York University Press, 2003), p. 138.
42 Simon Carter, *Rise and Shine: Sunlight, Technology and Health* (New York and Oxford: Berg, 2007), p. 8.
43 See Elizabeth Knowles, *Laura Knight in the Open Air* (Bristol: Sansom & Co., 2012).
44 Catherine Wallace, *Catching the Light: The Art and Life of Henry Scott Tuke, 1858–1929* (Edinburgh: Atelier Books, 2008); and Michael Hatt, 'A Great Sight: Henry Scott Tuke and His Models', in Jane Desmarais, Martin Postle, and William Vaughan (eds), *Model and Supermodel: The Artist's Model in British Art and Culture* (Manchester: Manchester University Press, 2006), pp. 89–104.
45 Frances Spalding, *British Art since 1900* (London: Thames & Hudson, 1989), p. 20.
46 See Linda Dalrymple Henderson, 'X Rays and the Quest for Invisible Reality in the Art of Kupka, Duchamp, and the Cubists', *Art Journal*, 47:4 (1988), 323–40; Linda Dalrymple Henderson, *Duchamp in Context: Science and Technology in the* Large Glass *and Related Works* (Princeton, NJ: Princeton University Press, 2005); and Linda Dalrymple Henderson, 'Francis Picabia, Radiometers, and X-Rays in 1913', *The Art Bulletin*, 71:1 (1989), 114–23; Gavin Parkinson, *Surrealism, Art and Modern Science: Relativity, Quantum Mechanics, Epistemology* (New Haven, Conn.: Yale University Press, 2008); Edward Juler, *Grown but Not Made: British Modernist Sculpture and the New Biology* (Manchester: Manchester University Press, 2015); Pascal Rousseau, 'Radiation: Metabolising the "New Rays"', in Angela Lampe and Clément Chéroux (eds), *Edvard Munch: The Modern Eye* (London: Tate Publishing, 2012), pp. 161–9.
47 See Tania Woloshyn, 'Regenerative Tanning: Pigmentation, Neo-Lamarckian Eugenics and the Visual Culture of the *Cure de Soleil*', in Fae Brauer and Serena Keshavjee (eds), *Picturing Evolution and Extinction: Regeneration and Degeneration in Modern Visual Culture* (Newcastle upon Tyne: Cambridge Scholars Publishing, 2015), pp. 193–216. An image of *Solrosen* by Ebbe (1868–1941) features on the cover of Jørgen Peter Müller, *My Sun-Bathing and Fresh-Air System* (London: Athletic Publications, 1927).
48 My thanks to Nicolai Howalt for informing me about this phrase. For a discussion of the multiple meanings of 'towards the light' in a French context, see my thesis: '*Vers la lumière*: Painters and Patients on the Côte d'Azur, *c.* 1887–1910' (Ph.D. dissertation, University of Nottingham, 2008).
49 This is common in the visual cultures of science and medicine, Hentschel remarking that, 'The establishment of scientific photography notwithstanding, astronomers, chemists, physicists, and spectroscopists alike depended on others to get their drawings or photographs into print. And these too often completely obscure artists are indeed historiographic aliens.' Klaus Hentschel, *Mapping the Spectrum: Techniques of Visual Representation in Research and Teaching* (Oxford: Oxford University Press, 2002), p. 8.
50 Jennifer Tucker, 'The Historian, the Picture, and the Archive', *Isis*, 97:1 (2006), 111–20, at p. 114.
51 Similarly, Ellenbogen argued that Marey's chronophotographic data enabled the study of human kinetics; without photography, such a study could never have existed: Josh Ellenbogen, *Reasoned and Unreasoned Images: The Photography of Bertillon, Galton, and Marey* (University Park, Pa.: Pennsylvania State University Press, 2012).
52 Ludmilla Jordanova, *History in Practice* (London: Arnold, 2000), p. 1.
53 Carter, *Rise and Shine*, p. 11.

54 See Carter, *Rise and Shine*, pp. 9, 39, 46, in which Carter positions medical authority as following the public interest in sunlight, an afterthought to justify the public's 'independent' interests, and an establishment that needed to be 'enrolled' to legitimise light therapy.

55 Roger Cooter and John Pickstone (eds), *Medicine in the Twentieth Century* (Amsterdam: Harwood Academic Publishers, 2000), pp. xiii–xix, at p. xiii.

56 See Kerry Segrave, *Suntanning in 20th Century America* (Jefferson, NC: McFarland & Co., 2005); Daniel Freund, *American Sunshine: Diseases of Darkness and the Quest for Natural Light* (Chicago, Ill.: University of Chicago Press, 2012); John Stanislav Sadar, '"Vita" Glass and the Discourse of Modern Culture', in Grace Lees-Maffei (ed.), *Writing Design: Words and Objects* (London and New York: Berg, 2012), pp. 103–17; Sally Dunne Romano, 'The Dark Side of the Sun: Skin Cancer, Sunscreen and Risk in Twentieth-Century America' (Ph.D. dissertation, Yale University, 2006); and Ina Zweiniger-Bargielowska, *Managing the Body: Beauty, Health, and Fitness in Britain, 1880–1939* (Oxford: Oxford University Press, 2010). Exceptions include Meghan Crnic, 'Seeking the Salubrious Sea: The Health and Environments of Urban American Families, 1870–1930' (Ph.D. dissertation, University of Pennsylvania, 2013); and Jamieson, 'An Intolerable Affliction'. Jamieson's Ph.D. dissertation devoted two chapters to light therapy for the treatment of lupus vulgaris in late-nineteenth- and early twentieth-century Britain. In her examination of the early literature, Jamieson discovered that the British medical profession was strongly invested in phototherapy, becoming pivotal to dermatology's development.

57 These include Anthea Callen, Ludmilla Jordanova, Tanya Sheehan, Kelley Wilder, Mary Hunter, Mechtild Fend, Fae Brauer, Keren Hammerschlag, and Natasha Ruiz-Gómez.

58 Jordanova, *History in Practice*, pp. 189–90. See also Kirsten Ostherr, *Medical Visions: Producing the Patient through Film, Television, and Imaging Technologies* (Oxford: Oxford University Press, 2013), p. 17; and José van Dijck, *The Transparent Body: A Cultural Analysis of Medical Imaging* (Seattle, Wash.: University of Washington Press, 2005), p. 11.

59 My thanks to Keren Hammerschlag for the wonderful phrase, 'more fraught than fluid'.

60 See Melissa Miles, *The Burning Mirror: Photography in an Ambivalent Light* (North Melbourne: Australian Scholarly Publishing, 2008).

61 W. J. T. Mitchell, *What Do Pictures Want? The Lives and Loves of Images* (Chicago, Ill.: University of Chicago Press, 2005), p. 10.

62 Carter, *Rise and Shine*, pp. 1–2, 6.

63 Mitchell, *What Do Pictures Want?* p. 108.

64 Ellen Lupton, *Mechanical Brides: Women and Machines from Home to Office* (New York: Cooper-Hewitt National Museum of Design, Smithsonian Institute, and Princeton Architectural Press, 1993), p. 10. See also Margarete Sandelowski, *Devices and Desires: Gender, Technology, and American Nursing* (Chapel Hill, NC: University of North Carolina Press, 2000), pp. 29, 31, 42.

65 Howell defines 'technology' in three ways: as physical artefact (e.g., machine), as an activity, and as a form of knowledge (Howell, *Technology in the Hospital*, p. 8).

66 Rima Apple, *Vitamania: Vitamins in American Culture* (New Brunswick: Rutgers University Press, 1996), p. 3.

67 Apple, *Vitamania*, p. 179.

68 Tania Woloshyn, 'Health and Consolation in Renoir's Late Southern Works, *c.* 1895–1919' (MA dissertation, Queen's University, 2004); and Tania Woloshyn, '*Vers la lumière*'. See

also Tania Woloshyn, 'Aesthetic and Therapeutic Imprints: Artists and Invalids on the Côte d'Azur, *c.* 1890–1910', *Nineteenth-Century Art Worldwide*, 11:1 (2012).

69 Maurice Denis, 'Henri-Edmond Cross [1910]', in *Théories, 1890–1910: Du Symbolisme et de Gauguin vers un nouvel ordre classique* (Paris: Bibliothèque de *L'Occident*, 1912), pp. 156–60, at p. 157.

70 Paul Joanne, *Les Stations d'hiver de la Méditerranée* (Paris: Librairie Hachette et Cie, 1906), p. 47; Isabelle Compin, *H. E. Cross* (Paris: Quatre Chemins – Editart, 1964), p. 194.

71 Michel Bertrand, *Essai touchant l'influence de la lumière sur les êtres organisés, sur l'atmosphère, et sur différens composés chimiques* (Paris: HY, 1799).

72 Tania Woloshyn, '*Le Pays du soleil*: The Art of Heliotherapy on the Côte d'Azur', *Social History of Medicine*, 26:1 (2013), 74–93.

73 Bernhard's key publication, *Sonnenlichtbehandlung in der Chirurgie* (Stuttgart: Ferdinand Enke, 1917) was translated and published as *Light Treatment in Surgery* (London: Edward Arnold, 1926). Rollier's was *La Cure de soleil* (Lausanne and Paris: Baillière & Fils and Constant Tarin, 1914), translated and published as *Heliotherapy* (London: Henry Frowde and Hodder & Stoughton, 1923). Earlier, in Switzerland, Germany, and Austria, proponents of natural therapies, such as Arnold Rikli (1823–1906), Sebastian Kneipp (1821–97), and Vincent Priessnitz (1799–1851), had been advocating the healing benefits of bodily exposure to light and air since the early nineteenth century.

74 Hobday, *The Healing Sun*, p. 99.

75 Christopher Wilk, 'The Healthy Body Culture', in Christopher Wilk (ed.), *Modernism: Designing a New World, 1914–1939* (London: Victoria and Albert, 2006), pp. 248–67, at p. 253; and Sadar, 'Unpacking', p. 76.

76 Perhaps this is not surprising considering their associations with the art world. Rollier employed the dancer Margaret Morris at Leysin and treated Adolf Loos' partner, the dancer Bessie Bruce. Bernhard knew the artist Giovanni Segantini. Likewise, the photographer Jacob A. Riis wrote a tribute to Niels Finsen upon his death (1904), Caleb Saleeby's mother-in-law was the poet Alice Meynell, and Sir Leonard Hill moonlighted as an artist and was the first president of the Medical Art Society. On Rollier's photographic archive, see Tania Woloshyn, 'Patients Rebuilt: Dr Auguste Rollier's Heliotherapeutic Portraits, *c.* 1903–1944', *Medical Humanities*, 39:1 (2013), 38–46.

77 'The International Tuberculosis Congress at Rome (Continued)', *BMJ*, 27 April 1912, pp. 960–3, at p. 962.

78 See Auguste Rollier, *Quarante ans d'héliothérapie* (Lausanne: F. Rouge & Cie, 1944).

79 Rollier, *Heliotherapy*, pp. 6–7.

80 Edwards, *Control*, p. 67.

81 Caleb Saleeby, 'The late Sir Alfred Fripp, KCVO', *Sunlight*, 2:1 (1930), pp. 38–9, at p. 38. See also Guy Hinsdale, 'The Sun, Health and Heliotherapy', *Scientific Monthly*, 9:3 (1919), pp. 253–62, at p. 260; and Auguste Rollier, 'The Share of the Sun in the Prevention and Treatment of Tuberculosis', *BMJ*, 21 October 1922, pp. 741–5.

82 *The Times*, 22 May 1928, p. 5; Carter, *Rise and Shine*, p. 44.

83 London Metropolitan Archives, LCC/PH/GEN/04/141, 'Treatment in Switzerland, Leysin and Davos Platz Sanatorium, General Question of Sunlight Treatment, London County Council, 1921–48'.

84 This is not specific to light therapy: 'No technology in the twentieth century has evolved in national isolation. Ideas and skilled minds moved with the great migrations and carried new

technologies across national borders.' Bettyann Holtzmann Kevles, *Naked to the Bone: Medical Imagine in the Twentieth Century* (Reading: Helix Books, 1998), p. 6. On the international use of light therapy, see 'The Present Position of the Light Treatment of Lupus', *BMJ*, 4 January 1902, pp. 44–7.

85 Paul Overy, *Light, Air and Openness: Modern Architecture between the Wars* (London: Thames & Hudson, 2007), p. 116.

86 On Shaw, see Freund, *American Sunshine*, p. 107; Richard Hobday, *The Healing Sun*, p. 128; and Richard Hobday, *The Light Revolution: Health, Architecture and the Sun* (Forres: Findhorn Press, 2006), p. 3.

87 James Johnson, *Change of Air; or, The Pursuit of Health and Recreation* (London: S. Highley, 1837), p. 7.

88 Florence Nightingale, *Notes on Nursing: What It Is, and What It Is Not* (London: Harrison, 1859), pp. 47–8. See also Nightingale, *Notes on Hospitals* (London: Longman, Green, Longman, Roberts, & Green, 1863), pp. 18–19. Saleeby similarly described the sun as a sculptor, vitamin D its chisel, 'which works from within, and builds not lifeless forms of marble but the living, breathing and sentient bodies of children and men and women'. Caleb Saleeby, 'Mother and Baby Week', *Sunlight*, 1:9 (1929), pp. 12–16, at p. 14. Photographers also described the sun as an artist, see Miles, *Burning Mirror*, p. 84.

89 Arthur Downes and Thomas P. Blunt, 'Researches on the Effect of Light upon Bacteria and Other Organisms', *Proceedings of the Royal Society of Medicine*, 26 (1877), 488–500. Koch demonstrated that sunlight could kill the tuberculosis bacilli in 1890: Robert Koch, *Ueber bakteriologische Forschung* (Berlin: Hirschwald, 1890), cited in Philip E. Hockberger, 'A History of Ultraviolet Photobiology for Humans, Animals and Microorganisms', *Photochemistry and Photobiology*, 76:6 (2002), 561–79, at p. 577. See also Hobday, *The Healing Sun*, p. 91.

90 Theobald A. Palm, 'The Geographical Distribution and Aetiology of Rickets', *Practitioner*, 45:4 (1890), 270–9 and 45:5, 321–42, at p. 342; and Jadesola Ekpe, 'The Chemistry of Light: The Life and Work of Theobald Adrian Palm (1848–1928)', *Journal of Medical Biography*, 17 (August 2009), 155–60. See also Carter, *Rise and Shine*, pp. 40–1; and Hobday, *Light Revolution*, p. 52.

91 Finsen, *Phototherapy*, p. iv; and Georg Bröchner, 'An Apostle of Light: Professor Finsen at Home', *Pall Mall Magazine* (June 1904), 202–8, at p. 204.

92 Jamieson, 'An Intolerable Affliction', p. 97.

93 Jamieson provides details on the introduction of Finsen lamp into particular hospitals throughout the UK, see 'An Intolerable Affliction', pp. 119–21. In her research she has uncovered evidence suggesting that the London Hospital was not, in fact, the first to employ phototherapy in Britain: St Thomas' Arthur Barry Blacker and internationally renowned dermatologist (later Sir) Malcolm Morris both claimed to have been used phototherapy earlier.

94 Jamieson, 'An Intolerable Affliction', p. 158.

95 Jamieson, 'An Intolerable Affliction', pp. 122–3.

96 'The "Light Treatment" at the London Hospital', *BMJ*, 30 June 1900, pp. 1595–7, at p. 1596.

97 'The Fifteenth International Congress of Medicine', *Lancet*, 5 May 1906, pp. 1267–74, at p. 1268.

98 See the letters exchanged between Gauvain and Treloar about travelling to Berck in 1908, Treloar Archives, Winchester, 8A11/1. See also G. S. E. Moynihan, *The Lord Mayor Treloar Hospital and College* (Southampton: Paul Cave, 1988), p. 18.

99 'The Coming of the Sunlight', *Times* supplement, pp. x–xi, at p. x. See also W. Annandale Troup, *Therapeutic Uses of Infra-red Rays* (London: Actinic Press, 1936), p. 74; Eleanor H. Russell and William K. Russell, *Ultra-violet Radiation and Actinotherapy* (Edinburgh:

E. & S. Livingstone, 1925), pp. 40–1, 44; Victor Dane, *The Sunlight Cure: How to Use the Ultra-violet Rays* (London: Athletic, 1929), p. 11. It continues today, see Hobday, *Healing Sun*, pp. 18–19.

100 Russell and Russell, *Ultra-violet Radiation*, p. 44.

101 Manchester and Salford Hospital for Skin Diseases Archive, John Rylands Library Special Collections, University of Manchester, MMC/9/18.

102 Gauvain, 'Reflections on Sun Treatment', p. 8. See also Müller, *Sun-Bathing*, p. 78.

103 Advertisement for Saleeby's *Sunlight and Health* in *The Times*, 22 May 1928, p. 10; Leonard Hill, 'Sunlight and Sunburn', *The Times*, 14 July 1928, p. 15.

104 Gauvain, 'Organisation and Work of a Light Department', pp. 10–16; Saleeby in Hanovia, *Get Back in the Sun with a 'Homesun'*, pamphlet, 1940, p. 7; on Hill, see Chapter 2.

105 See *Sunlight*, 2:6 (1932), p. 188.

106 'The use of familiar, seductive narratives becomes an issue for historians if, in writing up their research, they seek to trade on or reconstruct stories uncritically. However delicious, they should not be glamorised, or used as substitutes for analysis.' Jordanova, *History in Practice*, p. 187.

107 Dunne Romano, 'The Dark Side of the Sun', pp. 51–2. See also Freund, *American Sunshine*, p. 37; Mary Blume, *Côte d'Azur: Inventing the French Riviera* (London: Thames & Hudson, 1992), p. 74; David B. Morris, 'Light as Environment: Medicine, Health, and Values', *Journal of Medical Humanities*, 23:1 (2002), 7–29, at p. 9; and Carolyn J. Heckman and Sharon L. Manne (eds), *Shedding Light on Indoor Tanning* (London and New York: Springer, 2012).

108 Carter, *Rise and Shine*, pp. 11–12. See also Charlotte Mathieson, '"A Brown Sunburnt Gentleman": Masculinity and the Travelling Body in Dickens's *Bleak House*', *Nineteenth-Century Contexts*, 36:4 (2014), 323–34.

109 Carter, *Rise and Shine*, p. 31.

110 Edwards, *Control*, p. 84.

111 See Zweiniger-Bargielowska, *Managing the Body*; and Ken Worpole, *Here Comes the Sun: Architecture and Public Space in Twentieth-Century European Culture* (London: Reaktion, 2000), p. 47.

112 On public appropriations of medical concepts, see Matthew Lavine, *The First Atomic Age: Scientists, Radiations, and the American Public, 1895–1945* (New York: Palgrave Macmillan, 2013), pp. 7, 9; and Nancy Tomes, *The Gospel of Germs: Men, Women, and the Microbe in American Life* (Cambridge, Mass.: Harvard University Press, 1998), p. 13.

113 See Thomas de la Peña, *The Body Electric*, p. xv.

114 Carter, *Rise and Shine*, pp. 39, 43.

115 Bernhard, *Light Treatment*, p. 1.

116 See, for example, Freund, *American Sunshine*, pp. 1–2; and Edwards, *Control*, p. 68.

117 See Russell and Russell, *Ultra-violet Radiation*, Chapter 2, 'Radiant Energy', pp. 27–39.

118 Carter, *Rise and Shine*, pp. 58, 64–5.

119 See Hobday, *Healing Sun*, p. 92; and Hobday, *Light Revolution*, pp. 75–6. The history of radiotherapy presents similarities. Lavine explained 'in newspapers and textbook hagiographies alike, [Marie Curie] did not so much isolate radium as give birth to it, labor in a chilly shack standing in rhetorically for labor pains'. Lavine, *First Atomic Age*, p. 55.

120 Jamieson, 'An Intolerable Affliction', p. 134.

121 'Heliotherapy: Disease Treatment by Sunlight', *Times* supplement, p. xii; Franz Thedering, *Sunlight as Healer: A Popular Treatise* (Slough: Sollux, 1926), p. 5. In a US history of light therapy, Augustus James Pleasonton and John Harvey Kellogg would be included, see Dunne

Romano, 'The Dark Side of the Sun', pp. 57–8. In Denmark, Axel Reyn continued Finsen's work at the Institute, while Louis Lortet, Philibert Genoud, Jean Saidman, Hubert Jausion, Paul Armand-Delille, Paul Carton, Alexandre Aimes, and Charles Brody were important figures in France.

122 Hill wrote the preface to Bernhard's *Light Treatment in Surgery*, Reyn and Sequeira began incorporating full-body phototherapy on lupus patients after Rollier (Jamieson, 'An Intolerable Affliction', p. 132). Gauvain refitted his phototherapy rooms at Treloar's after visits to the Finsen Institute and Sequeira's success at the London Hospital (Jamieson, 'An Intolerable Affliction', p. 134) but was also heavily influenced by Rollier's methods.

123 Roger Cooter, 'The Disabled Body', in Roger Cooter and John Pickstone (eds), *Medicine in the Twentieth Century* (Amsterdam: Harwood Academic Publishers, 2000), pp. 367–83, at p. 371; and Roger Cooter, *Surgery and Society in Peace and War: Orthopaedics and the Organization of Modern Medicine, 1880–1948* (Basingstoke: Macmillan, 1993). See also Seth Koven, 'Remembering and Dismemberment: Crippled Children, Wounded Soldiers, and the Great War in Great Britain', *American Historical Review*, 99:4 (1994), 1167–1202.

124 H. H. Dale, 'Hill, Sir Leonard Erskine (1866–1952)', *Oxford Dictionary of National Biography*, http://dx.doi.org/10.1093/ref:odnb/33872 (accessed 18 January 2016).

125 Sadar, '"Vita" Glass', p. 108.

126 G. R. Searle, 'Saleeby, Caleb Williams Elijah (1878–1940)', *Oxford Dictionary of National Biography*, http://dx.doi.org/10.1093/ref:odnb/47854 (accessed 18 January 2016).

127 See Carter, *Rise and Shine*, pp. 67–76; Sadar, '"Vita" Glass', pp. 107–8; and, more generally, Zweiniger-Bargielowska, *Managing the Body*; Dan Stone, *Breeding Superman: Nietzsche, Race and Eugenics in Edwardian and Interwar Britain* (Liverpool: Liverpool University Press, 2002); and Chris Otter, *The Victorian Eye: A Political History of Light and Vision in Britain, 1800–1910* (Chicago, Ill.: University of Chicago Press, 2008).

128 See William Beaumont, *Fundamental Principles of Ray Therapy* (London: H. K. Lewis & Co. Ltd, 1931), pp. 7, 106; William Beaumont, 'An Institute of Ray Therapy: A Voluntary "Light" Clinic for London', *BMJ*, 25 January 1930, pp. 163–4, at p. 163. The institute commissioned the artist Frank Brangwyn (1867–1956) to design their insignia, included on their stationery. See London Metropolitan Archives, A/KE/463.

129 See *The Times*, 22 May 1928, p. 5; 'London Light Clinic', *The Times*, 5 April 1932, p. 16; 'The London Clinic', *Sunlight*, 1:10 (1929), 32.

130 Beaumont, *Fundamental Principles*, p. vii; Vaughan-Cowell, *Artificial Sunlight*, pp. 98–9.

131 Hanovia, *The New Light Treatment Department (Solarium) in the Public Health Centre, Bermondsey* (Slough: Hanovia, 1936), p. 19. My thanks to Justin De Syllas for this reference. On the National Gallery's use of Hanovia lamps, see 'X-ray Test for Pictures', *The Times*, 29 June 1935, p. 8. On the Bermondsey Borough Council, see the Wellcome Collection's exhibition, *Here Comes Good Health*, 2012. Hanovia still exists, continuing to provide ultraviolet radiation apparatus to disinfect water sources.

132 Carter, *Rise and Shine*, pp. 90–1; Worpole, *Here Comes the Sun*, pp. 57–9, 64–5; and Esyllt Jones, 'Nothing Too Good for the People: Local Labour and London's Interwar Health Centre Movement', *Social History of Medicine*, 25:1 (2012), 84–102.

133 Overy, *Light, Air and Openness*, p. 29.

134 Hobday, *Light Revolution*, pp. 96–7, 104. Earlier examples include Port Sunlight, the garden-city movement, and the Papworth Village Settlement; see Carter, *Rise and Shine*, pp. 85–9. Carter also noted that Hill and Gauvain were involved in RIBA's committee on building orientation during the early 1930s, *Rise and Shine*, pp. 91–2.

135 On lidos see Carter, *Rise and Shine*, pp. 93–4; and Worpole, *Here Comes the Sun*, pp. 113–15. On the Serpentine Lido, see *Sunlight*, 1:9 (1929), 17.

136 Stated on the inner back page of each *Sunlight*.

137 Wilk, 'The Healthy Body Culture', p. 250. Vanguard depictions include, for example, Alexander Rodchenko, *Sun-Lovers*, 1932, gelatin silver print, private collection.

138 Editorial Foreword, *Sunlight*, 1:8 (1929), 3.

139 Sidney Russ, 'A Broadcast Talk on the Ultra-violet Rays', *Lancet*, 10 November 1928, pp. 1006–7, at p. 1007.

140 Katherine Gamgee, *The Artificial Light Treatment of Children* (London: H. K. Lewis & Co. Ltd, 1927), p. 86.

141 These issues were explored in the symposium, 'The Ethics of Display: Exhibiting Vulnerable Bodies', University of Warwick, 21 March 2016; and the Florence Nightingale Museum exhibition, *The Kiss of Light: Nursing and Light Therapy in Twentieth-Century Britain*, May–November 2015. Van Dijck has pertinently written, 'In a culture that increasingly concedes private grounds to public cameras, medical-ethical issues are media-ethical concerns as well; the ethics of representation, therefore, are part and parcel of the aesthetics of display.' Van Dijck, *The Transparent Body*, p. 14.

142 This is all the more distressing in the recent wake of the Jimmy Savile child sexual abuse scandal in the UK (2012 onwards) and ongoing justifiable concerns about online child pornography. See also the American photographer Sally Mann's autobiography, *Hold Still: A Memoir with Photographs* (New York: Little Brown & Company, 2015), in which she discusses the paedophilic responses and accusations her family portraits of her young, nude children received and even the experience of a stalker.

143 See Mieneke te Hennepe, 'Private Portraits or Suffering on Stage: Curating Clinical Photographic Collections in the Museum Context', *Science Museum Group Journal* (spring 2016), http://dx.doi.org/10.15180/160503 (accessed 18 September 2016).

144 'Light as Brain Food', *The Times*, 29 May 1925, p. 5; and Gauvain, 'Organisation and Work of a Light Department', p. 13.

145 Susan E. Lederer, *Subjected to Science: Human Experimentation in America before the Second World War* (Baltimore, Md.: Johns Hopkins University Press, 1995).

146 We were similarly denied use in the *Kiss of Light* exhibition, the museum's director, Natasha McEnroe, explaining that the rights-holder wished to remain 'whiter than white' when it came to avoiding potential upset to viewers, the original patients, or their heirs. It is a curious and meaningful phrase, since the act of exposure intentionally and conscientiously made (primarily) white children turn brown. See Chapter 5 for a discussion on tanning in relation to dirt, race, and the 'infectability of being black'.

147 Relatedly, see Marguerite S. Shaffer, 'On the Environmental Nude', *Environmental History*, 13:1 (2008), 126–39. The editor, Neil M. Maher, pointed out in a note that one of the nudist photographs, of a family camping in the 1950s, was cropped to exclude a front-facing young girl, 'because of her age and her positioning in the photograph' (p. 126).

2

Dosing sunburn

> Though light treatment has been extensively scientifically investigated, especially during the last few years, it should be remembered that it owes its origin to shrewd clinical observation and its justification to clinical experience. Fascinating as are theories endeavouring to explain the biological action of light, they still remain incomplete, are sometimes contradictory, and are frequently confusing. Many and wide gaps in our knowledge still remain and I recognise fully that the scientific principles of light therapy still rest on an incomplete and not too stable basis.[1]
>
> (Henry Gauvain, 1925)

> With all the extravagant claims that have been made for ray therapy as a curative agent on the one hand, and its disparagement as a useless means of self-deception and auto-suggestion on the other, the question of dosage requires serious consideration.[2]
>
> (William Beaumont, 1931)

Out of darkness and mist emerges a ghostly disembodied arm, marked by strange, illegible shapes and letters (Fig. 2.1). At first glance, it recalls the photographing of spirits more than medical subjects. Is this photographed forearm the product of a medical experiment gone wrong, or one its researcher got right?

Figure 2.1 is an odd and eerie photograph. It dates to *c.* 1893, now lost and only existing through poor reproductions. It represents the irradiated forearm of Dr Niels Finsen, the Danish researcher, Nobel laureate, and inventor of phototherapy. While not British, this photograph was reproduced and discussed by light-therapy practitioners internationally, and it provides a point of origin for the British images I analyse in this chapter. From its amateurish quality, especially those misty areas that are likely the result of clumsy 'fixing' during the development process, one might simply describe it as a bad photograph. Its illegibility, however, is of the utmost significance.

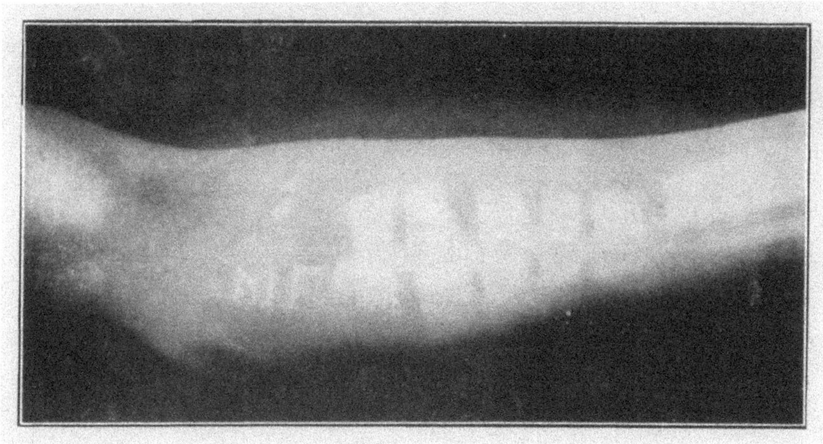

Figure 2.1 'Finsen's forearm, the day after its exposure for 20 minutes … by irradiation from a carbon arc [light].' In Axel Reyn, 'Histoire de l'actinothérapie', in Charles Brody (ed.), *Traité d'hélio- et d'actinologie* (Paris: Maloine, 1938), vol. I, p. 41. Author's collection.

The successes and failures of photography, as a light technology, to represent light therapy's methods, effects, and values are paramount to the book's central argument: from its inception light therapy was, and remains, an unstable, varied, and confounding medical practice.

Figure 2.1 presents, to my knowledge, the earliest image of modern light therapy or 'scientific light treatment', representing a rarely depicted but crucial component: the solar erythema ('sunburn').[3] Shifting and shifty, physicians' attitudes towards solar erythema as simultaneously dangerous and desirable persist throughout light therapy's history. Historically, 'sunburn' was variously defined as erythema caloricum (heat erythema), photoelectricum (the electric effects of light), dermatitis solaris (dermatitis due to the sun), eczema solare (eczema due to the sun), as well as erythema solare (inflammation due to the sun).[4] Such confusion centred on understandings of inflammation (erythema) resulting from the sun's light as distinct from its heat. As early as 1858, the famous French neurologist Dr Jean-Martin Charcot suggested that solar erythema was generated by the blue, violet, and ultraviolet end of the spectrum, not by the infrared and red (heat) rays.[5] Despite this differentiation becoming commonly understood by the 1890s, practitioners were still at pains to spell out the differences between these kinds of 'burns' well into the 1920s, distinguishing them not according to any visual referents but rather to timing: a heat erythema manifested immediately; a light (solar) erythema was characterised by its latent appearance.[6]

Yet, as an acute inflammation of the skin, accompanied by redness, pain, a burning or stinging sensation, and sometimes blisters, the word 'sun*burn*' persisted throughout the nineteenth and twentieth centuries, and it persists today. For the sake of clarity I employ the term 'solar erythema' to mean the reddening of the skin in response to actinic light, particularly ultraviolet light, as was its typical meaning by light-therapy practitioners. However, this is not to ignore or let slip an awareness of the unstable, multivalent meanings of the word 'sunburn'. They heavily inform my reading of the primary literature and visual material on the benefits and risks of 'dosing' light. In this chapter, I argue that such instability of definition in the texts, analogous to the illegibility and paucity of the images, can be a productive rather than limiting way into an analysis of light therapy's history. I want us to remain aware throughout the chapter of the powerful status of images as 'evidence' or 'documentation', particularly when it comes to evidencing medical practices and success.

In Section I of this chapter, I show that, as the initial visible sign of the skin's reaction to light treatment, the solar erythema was closely scrutinised and discussed by practitioners of both natural sunlight therapy (heliotherapy) and artificial light therapy (phototherapy). Patients' photosensitivities were monitored closely to gauge whether the treatment would be successful or not, but the degree and kind of reaction produced to determine 'success' varied enormously among practitioners, in Britain and abroad. As I discuss in Chapter 5, pigmentation ('suntan') had a related role to play, many practitioners desiring greatly to see bronzed flesh as a marker of healing over red, blistered, and peeling skin. But others did not. Some of Britain's leading practitioners, including Sir Leonard Hill and his colleague Dr Albert Eidinow of the MRC's NIMR, actively sought red flesh, not brown, as the sign of the cure under way.

The relationship between erythema and pigmentation – as distinct physiological phenomena, as sequential processes in a single reaction, or as one and the same thing – consequently emerges as extraordinarily complicated within the primary literature and imagery.[7] Black-and-white photography, the major medium of light therapy's visual culture, epitomises the ambiguity when we consider how difficult it is to differentiate between the hues of erythema (red) and pigmentation (brown) when presented in tones of grey. Take the photograph of Finsen's forearm, for example (Fig. 2.1): our only clue as to whether this is a representation of erythema or of pigmentation is in the written description by Finsen's successor, Dr Axel Reyn, who explained that the photograph was taken the day after the arm was exposed to a carbon arc lamp, and thus too soon for pigmentation to have developed. This chapter concentrates on the many textual and few visual representations of solar erythema, of what it was, how it functioned in the therapeutic process, and its contentious role in the development and legitimisation of light therapy.

From modern light therapy's inception in the 1890s to its widespread use by the 1930s, the solar erythema took a leading role in practitioners' attempts to present the therapy as scientifically standardised and systematic – or, conversely, as holistically tailored to the individual patient. This is the focus of Section II. Despite being latent, variable, and unique to each patient, practitioners spent enormous time and energy trying to standardise erythema production so as to 'dose' ultraviolet radiation safely and effectively. This tension between standardisation and individualisation, the hallmarks of biomedicine and holism respectively, lay at the heart of a struggle to control and legitimise light therapy during its nascent growth and widespread appeal, *c.* 1890–1940. The MRC was not merely caught up in this struggle, which by the late 1920s had reached new heights; it facilitated both sides of it, to the confusion and anxiety of light therapy's professional and lay proponents. Conceptualised as the anchor that would stabilise a raft of conflicting theories about dosing light, the solar erythema was invested with a tremendous amount of authoritative weight. Intriguingly, this was a role that it constantly resisted and undermined.

Photographs by British light therapists that depict solar erythema on patients' skin (Figs. 2.2, 2.3) are no more legible than Finsen's (Fig. 2.1). In Section II, I approach the solar erythema and its visual and written representations as resistant, unfixed, and uncooperative. Whether a risky product of excessive or mismanaged exposure,

Figure 2.2 'Photograph showing erythema produced by graduated exposure of forearms to ultra-violet rays.' In Eleanor H. Russell and William K. Russell, *Ultra-violet Radiation and Actinotherapy* (Edinburgh: E. & S. Livingstone, 1925), Figure 53, p. 153. Author's collection.

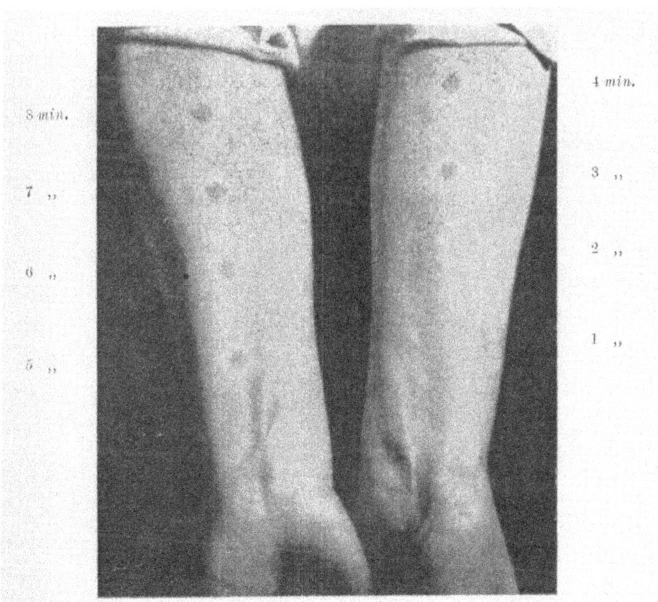

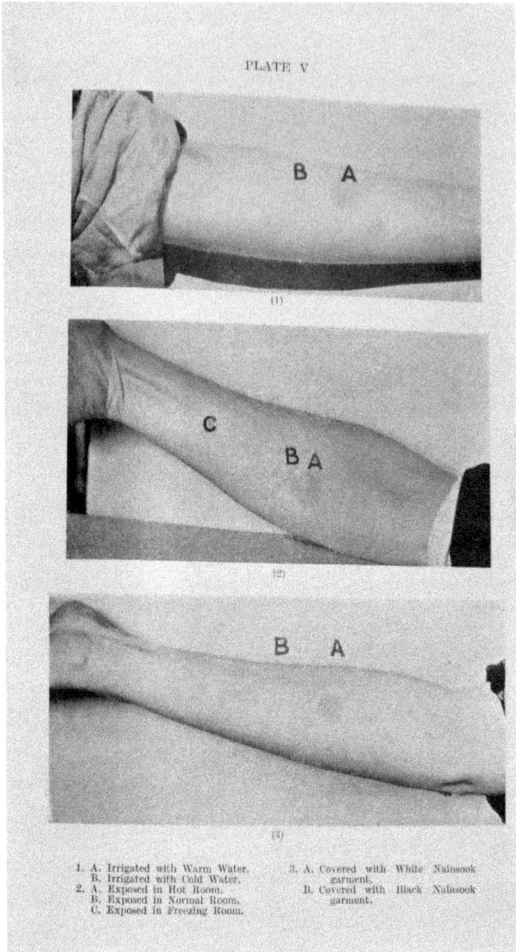

Figure 2.3 'Exposure of arm to mercury vapour lamp for ten minutes.' In Leonard Hill, *Sunshine and Open Air: Their Influence on Health, with Special Reference to the Alpine Climate* (London: Edward Arnold, 1925), Plate V, opposite p. 80. Author's collection.

or the 'delicious burning' that marked the path to health, the solar erythema was an ambiguous sight in twentieth-century medicine and public health.[8] I want to explore this ambiguity, with Finsen's photographed forearm leading the way.

I Setting standards

Niels Finsen is credited with the invention of phototherapy, which he employed primarily to treat lupus vulgaris (tuberculosis of the skin, Fig. 2.4). This was a particularly disfiguring disease with no known cure and most often attacked the face like the sexually transmitted disease, syphilis, with which it was often confused. Consequently, it forced sufferers to hide away from the public eye. By the end of the

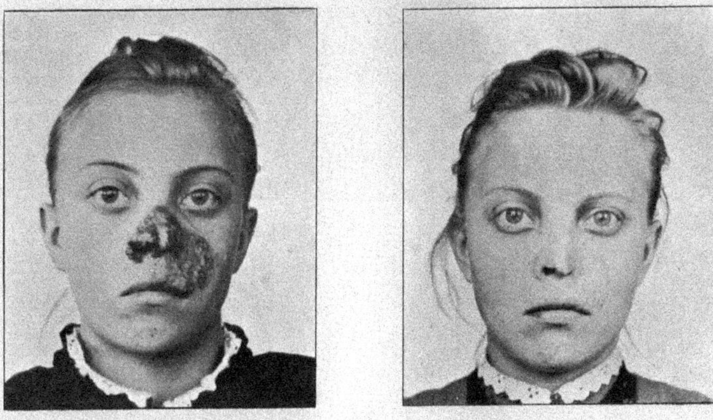

Figure 2.4 Before and after photographs of a patient suffering from lupus vulgaris. In Niels R. Finsen, *Die Bekämpfung des Lupus Vulgaris* (Jena: Gustav Fischer, 1903), unpaginated. Author's collection.

nineteenth century, as Anne Jamieson explained, it was generally agreed to be a form of external tuberculosis and bacterial in origin.[9] Finsen was one of several international physicians and scientists experimenting with light to kill bacteria or to cauterise wounds during the nineteenth century, if not earlier.[10] The light's ability to burn lesions had been controlled and concentrated with lenses, but this was primarily due to its heating action. What made Finsen's method different was his exclusive use of the blue, violet, and ultraviolet rays, what he called the 'chemical' or 'actinic' rays, by filtering and cooling the rays of sunlight through coated lenses and, later, those of artificial light generated from carbon arc lamps. Following new scientific evidence disseminated during the late 1870s and 1880s that ultraviolet light was bactericidal, he directed the actinic rays onto tubercular lesions to destroy the bacteria.[11]

Finsen became aware of actinic light's destructive powers by conducting experiments with sunlight in 1893, using himself as a test subject. In his first experiment he exposed his bare forearm to direct sunlight for three straight hours, including a two-inch band painted in India ink that he described as 'blackened' to 'imitate the colour of the negro's skin'.[12] (For more on colour and race, see Chapter 5.) The area protected by the ink, he stated, was unmarked after exposure, while the rest of his forearm showed 'After some hours a very well-marked erythema, accompanied by pain and slight swelling', which lasted for several days.[13] Once healed and pigmented, he exposed his arm again, without painting the skin, noting that the previously covered portion that had remained white suffered badly this time from erythema. By contrast, the pigmented areas had naturally protected his skin. When he described the solar erythema, he explicitly understood it as an 'eruption' manifested from the 'harmful influence of the chemical rays'.[14] Finsen described solar erythema and pigmentation as sequential cutaneous reactions to this light using the language of disease: the first was an 'acute' manifestation and the second a 'chronic' one.[15]

In Finsen's second experiment he exposed his forearm again to actinic light, but instead of sunlight he held it close to a carbon arc lamp for twenty minutes (Figs. 2.1, 2.5). Figure 2.5 presents the before and after photographs of the experiment, again poorly reproduced, here via the American physicist and lighting designer for General Electric, Matthew Luckiesh, with August John Pacini, in their 1926 book *Light and Health*. Luckiesh and Pacini offered details of the second experiment:

> *Finsen* a quarter of a century ago studied the influence of light on the skin. He made few and simple experiments, but they were devised, performed and interpreted with an unerring instinct rightly termed genius. In one of his experiments he exposed his white and unpigmented forearm to the light from a 40,000 candle-power arc-lamp at a distance of 50 centimeters for ten minutes. At this distance the heat became disagreeable, so he exposed the arm ten minutes longer at 75 centimeters. He had glued on his arm a disc of quartz and a series of glass plates – red, yellow, blue and clear. He also painted the initials N F and other figures with India ink.[16]

In the experiment, Finsen tested the transparencies of these different materials to the actinic rays, specifically seeking to understand which mediums would allow ultraviolet light to pass through them and which would not. The solar erythema that appeared three hours later, photographed the following day, was a cutaneous reaction he was counting on.[17] Unlike the first experiment, he was not measuring his own skin's sensitivity to actinic light or ascertaining the protective role of pigment. Rather in this second experiment his arm became a testing ground, a registration device akin to a sensitive photographic plate used contemporaneously in spectroscopy, for revealing the materials' transmitting properties. By doing so, he used his own arm as a light register, a subject I explore in detail in Chapter 3. Finsen noted that solar erythema developed on the uncovered portions of his forearm and through the quartz glass, save for the bits of glue, but not on the skin covered by the coloured or clear ordinary glass plates and India ink. He concluded that quartz glass allows the actinic rays of light to pass through it, whereas ordinary glass does not.

As already noted, Finsen was not the first to distinguish between solar and heat erythema, nor was he the first to experiment on himself using an electric arc lamp.[18] He was, however, the first to apply this knowledge to the therapeutic use

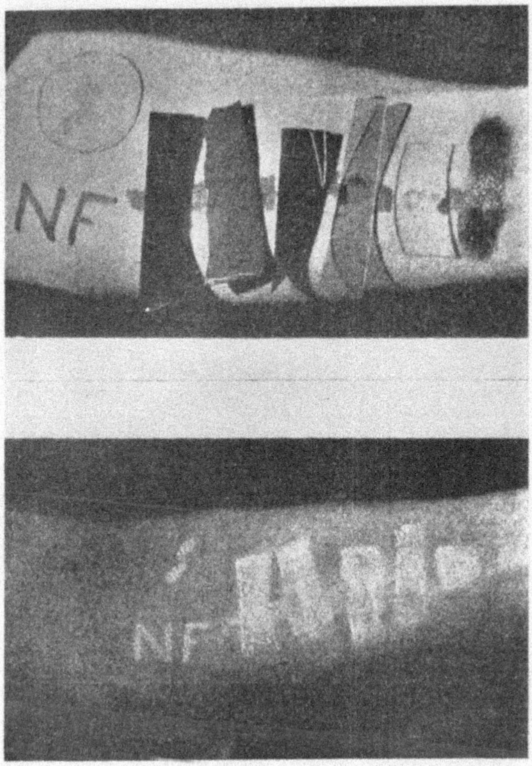

Figure 2.5 'Copies of original illustrations published by Finsen. Above are indicated the pieces of various media which he glued to his forearm. Below are the results of solar radiation illustrated. Much detail has been lost in reproduction.' In M. Luckiesh and A. J. Pacini, *Light and Health* (Baltimore, Md.: The Williams & Wilkins Company, 1926), Figure 7, opposite p. 98. Wellcome Library, London CC BY-NC 4.0.

of ultraviolet radiation and translate his experiments into a systematised treatment, which he called 'phototherapy'. Following his exactitude and scientific methods, the Finsen Institute (f. 1896) integrated the clinic and the laboratory, providing a space for the direct observation and treatment of patients as well as experimentation with ultraviolet, X, and gamma rays.

Finsen's initial experiments were followed by his novel modification of the carbon arc lamp, already used in street and theatre lighting, welding, and as searchlights, which became famously known as the 'Finsen light' or 'Finsen lamp' (Fig. 2.6). The modifications included shielding the arc of light and redirecting the emitting rays into telescopic arms, which filtered the light through a series of expensive quartz lenses (instead of ordinary glass lenses). The infrared and red rays were absorbed along the way, so as to avoid heat erythema, by colour filters and water flowing between the lenses. The lamp's arms were pressed against the patients' diseased skin by skilled nurses. An additional water-cooled lens was strapped directly to the patient's face, compressing the skin and draining blood from the area to facilitate the light's penetration (Fig. 2.7). By this method, the light directly targeted each lesion, requiring

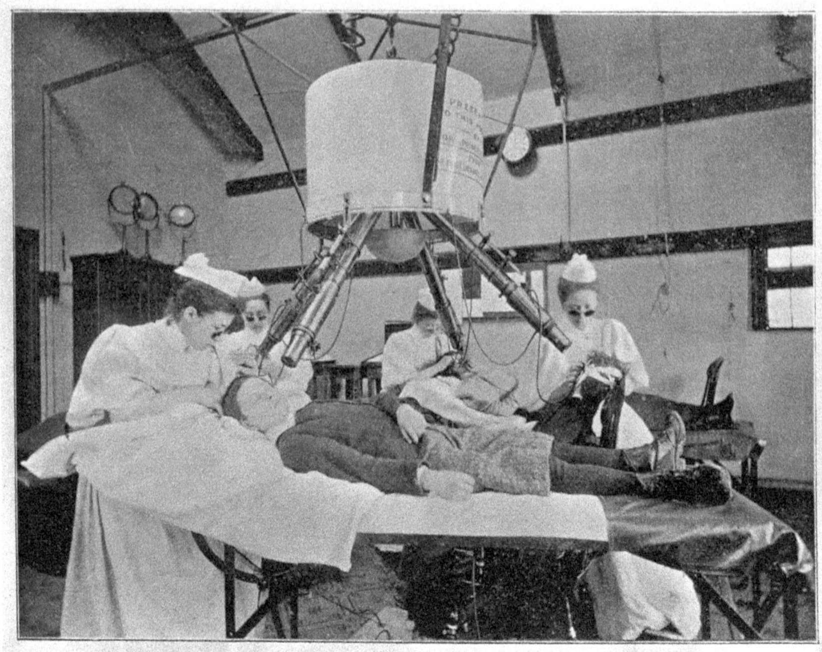

Figure 2.6 'The treatment by the electric light', at the [Royal] London Hospital, *c.* 1900.
Wellcome Library, London CC BY-NC 4.0.

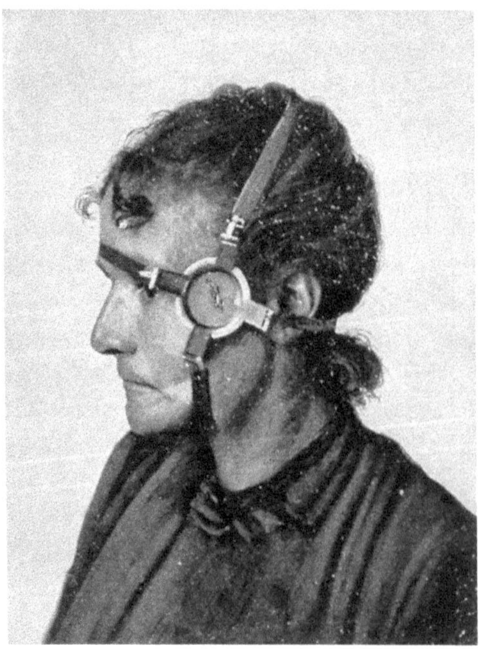

Figure 2.7 Photograph of patient with compressor.
In Niels R. Finsen, *Phototherapy*, trans. J. H. Sequeira (London: Arnold, 1901), Figure 6, opposite p. 70. Wellcome Library, London.

one to two hours of this localised treatment per area. Finsen's laboratory assistant at the institute, Valdemar Bie, specified that, 'In this manner an area of skin of about 1½ centimetre in diameter is treated for one hour every day. The treated skin reddens and swells, a bulla may appear, but necrosis has never been observed.'[19] Others, like the medical superintendent of the Treloar Hospital for Crippled Children (Hampshire), Sir Henry Gauvain, reported using the Finsen lamp for up to two hours per lesion in 1925.[20]

For Finsen, actinic light had similar properties to other kinds of chemicals by cauterising and irritating tissues; he complemented phototherapy with iodine and pyrogallic and boric acids on the lesions.[21] Those who used his method asserted that it was painless for patients, despite noting the irritants used and the erythematic reactions following local treatment.[22] As Jamieson pointed out, however, what constituted 'painless' must be understood in relation to the other methods for treating lupus vulgaris at the time, such as scraping and cutting the skin.[23] By comparison, phototherapy seemed tame for a disease that was notoriously difficult to treat. It was equally praised for its cosmetic results, the scar tissue perceived as soft, supple, and even.[24]

While Finsen stated that exposing the patient's entire body to actinic light could be beneficial (known as 'full body' or 'general' treatment), it is evident from phototherapy's inception – used by Finsen primarily as a lesion-specific ('local') treatment – that ultraviolet light was prized precisely because of its damaging, bactericidal abilities. It is also clear from his early personal experiments that solar erythema played a weighty role: it was the anchor securing his claims that light, and especially ultraviolet light, could be used to great therapeutic effect.

Finsen was known throughout the world for his work with phototherapy, and Britain was no exception. He became internationally renowned for the treatment's success and in 1903 won the Nobel Prize in Medicine. Through the intervention of Queen Alexandra (then Princess of Wales), Finsen's methods and equipment were imported to the (Royal) London Hospital in 1899, where they instigated the birth of the 'Light Department', headed by Stephen Mackenzie and James Sequeira, in May 1900 (Fig. 2.8). The department employed phototherapy with carbon arc lamps and, to a lesser extent, heliotherapy using Finsen's glass lenses (Fig. 2.9). One month after opening to patients, a report in the *BMJ* outlined its principles of light treatment:

1. That the chemical [blue, violet, and ultraviolet] rays of the sun or of the electric light can produce an inflammation of the skin.
2. That they can produce an effect through the skin.
3. That they can kill microbes on, in, or close under the skin.[25]

Again, note that local phototherapy, employed especially for dermatological diseases, was defined by its power to do damage, both in its lethal action on bacteria and its

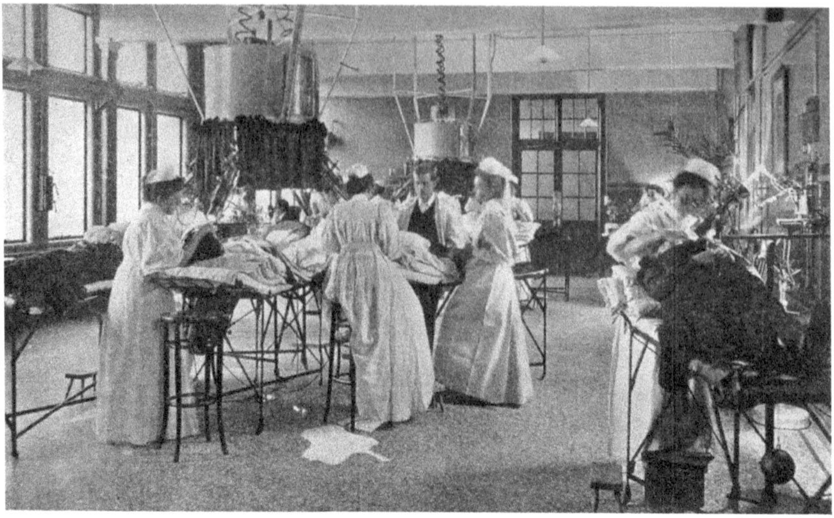

Figure 2.8 'The Light Department, London Hospital, showing patients being treated with Finsen lamps for lupus.'
In William Beaumont, *Fundamental Principles of Ray Therapy* (London: H. K. Lewis & Co., 1931), p. 3. Author's collection.

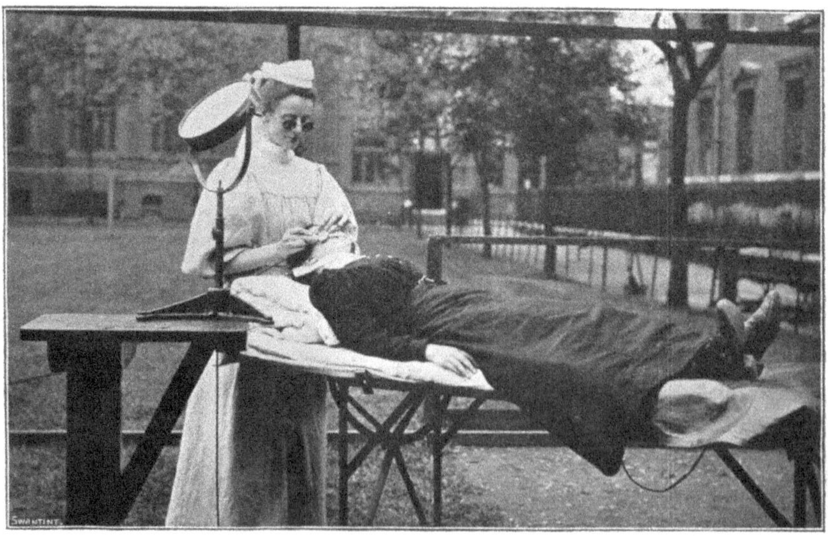

Figure 2.9 [Ernest Harnack], 'Finsen's apparatus for concentrating the sun's rays', courtyard of the [Royal] London Hospital, *c.* 1900.
In Ettie Sayer, *Medical Electricity and Light* (London: Scientific Press, 1913), p. 85. Thackray Medical Museum, Leeds.

inflammatory capacities on the skin. For this reason, early references to the blue, violet, and ultraviolet rays not only as 'chemical' or 'actinic' but also as 'injurious' occur frequently in light-therapy literature.[26] I return to this point at the end of the chapter, and again in Chapter 4, when discussing historic and contemporary perceptions about ultraviolet radiation and bodily damage.

Exposure methods

Exposure methods varied widely among practitioners when it came to general treatment by actinic light, frequently described as a light 'bath' in either natural or artificial form. Differing perceptions about the roles of solar erythema and pigmentation were at the heart of these. Suffering from Pick's Disease, Finsen died in 1904, but his institute in Copenhagen continued to flourish after his death. While it specialised in treating lupus vulgaris by local phototherapy, the physicians there also used general phototherapy and heliotherapy. Finsen discussed the potentials of general light baths already by 1895, and the institute employed them as a complement to local treatment from as early as 1900.[27] Combining the destructive action of local applications and the stimulating action of general applications, the Finsen Institute and, soon afterwards, the London Hospital, reported greatly increased rates of successful cures among lupus vulgaris patients.[28]

The Finsen Institute's Medical Superintendent, Axel Reyn, explained in 1923 that its method was to use artificial light for long general exposures on patients and to purposefully provoke a 'pronounced erythema' during the initial stages of treatment:

> Consequently, the first light bath which a patient gets is of thirty to forty minutes' duration; then we generally give the patient light baths every other day, increasing the time as we go on, so that after a fortnight's treatment fully two and a half hours are reached, but this time is seldom exceeded.
>
> [...]
>
> With the mercury light [a mercury vapour lamp, which produced more ultraviolet radiation than the carbon arc lamp] we begin with five to ten minutes, increasing slowly, for the erythema brought about by this light is extremely painful. During the irradiation the patients have to turn their bodies round, so that all parts of the body are irradiated.[29]

Reyn declared this method was in contradistinction to that used by the Swiss heliotherapist, Dr Auguste Rollier, who had employed heliotherapy from 1903 and who was arguably the most famous of light therapists (see Chapter 1).[30] Rollier avoided producing solar erythema in patients and favoured pigmentation. He claimed to have 'systematised' heliotherapy by his methods, gained through clinical experience and by his documentation, not least through the visual.[31] Rollier began by carefully acclimating the patient to the sunlight of the Swiss Alps, in Leysin, by exposing body parts in short doses until deep pigmentation was acquired (Fig. 2.10). In his acclimation chart, Rollier segmented the patient's body into regions of increasing photosensitivity, a visual device through which his heliotherapeutic practice emerged as standardised, minutely observed, and strictly managed. He first exposed the patient's feet, then calves, thighs and so on at five-minute intervals per day. By this slow, graduated method of bodily exposure he avoided erythema production. But, like Reyn, and indeed many other light therapists, Rollier believed in long exposures to actinic light following the acclimation period, lasting several hours a day (in some cases every day for months or years), in order for his patients to derive full therapeutic benefit. As discussed in Chapter 5, pigmentation was conceptualised as a natural form of skin protection, a filter or 'screen' that could facilitate treatment – or hinder it. For Rollier, the suntan was a visual sign that the treatment was working. Those patients who bronzed well were perceived to be on the road to recovery, while those whose skin developed only a severe solar erythema were regarded ominously as lost causes. As the French heliotherapist Dr François Chiaïs put it, in 1907: 'If pigmentation does not develop, the prognosis is most dire.'[32]

Figure 2.10 'Our diagram of insolation. Progression according to which the sick [patient] is exposed to the sun.'
In Auguste Rollier, *La Cure de soleil* (Paris: Baillière & Fils; Lausanne: Constant Tarin, 1914), Figure 8, p. 65. Martine Gagnebin and author's collection.

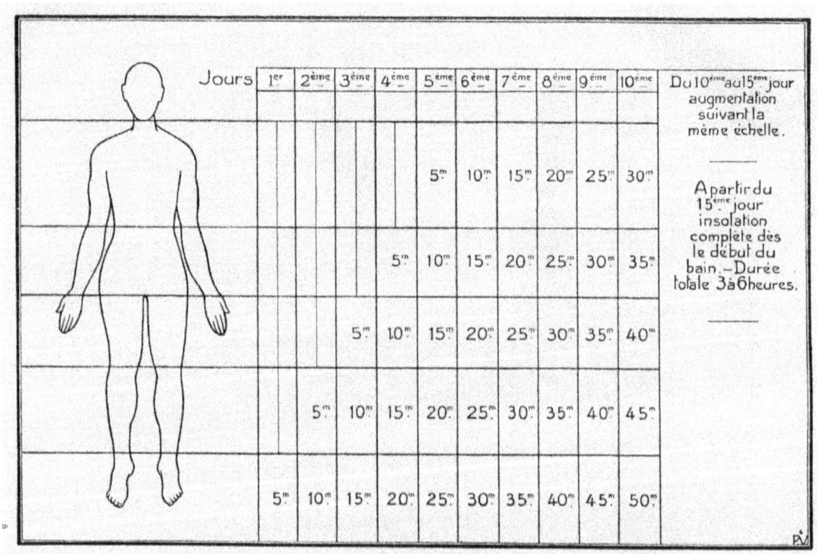

Fig. 8.
Notre schéma d'insolation. — Progression suivant laquelle le malade est exposé au soleil.

The exposure methods of the Finsen Institute in Denmark (referred to as the 'Copenhagen technique'[33]) and the 'Rollier method' in Switzerland were far from unanimously celebrated. British practitioners varied widely in their attitudes towards these methods, though great deference was shown to both. Heavy praise was given to the results and meticulousness of the Finsen Institute's procedures. Indeed, Jamieson convincingly argued that, though difficult to replicate, the techniques, exactitude, and equipment of the institute contributed towards the production of a powerful 'Finsen brand'.[34] Gauvain, who visited the institute on multiple occasions and modelled his own extended light department (1924) at Treloar's on its layout, procedures, and equipment, imitated Reyn's long exposure methods when using carbon arc lamps for general exposure.[35] So did many other British practitioners.[36] Yet Gauvain equally imitated the acclimation method of Rollier, favouring pigmentation and declaring that 'sunburn' was an undesirable reaction with dangerous consequences:

> Sun-burning may contribute to the onset of sunstroke or heat-stroke by making the subject ill through absorption of the product of damaged tissues. The blister which results in extreme cases of sunburn may leave an open sore which in turn may become infected and is thus a source of danger. Sunburn should always be avoided [...] By carefully graduated exposure such sores may be avoided; they do not occur when the skin has gradually become well pigmented and chocolate-coloured.[37]

Others, including the highly respected British researchers Sir Leonard Hill and Albert Eidinow (NIMR), were particularly aware of the conflicting methods of Reyn and Rollier. They were equally critical of both. Hill and Eidinow faulted the Copenhagen technique for using light sources weak in ultraviolet radiation but abundant in heat rays for hours at a time, during which patients were confined to poorly ventilated rooms and sweated copiously.[38] They also disapproved of lengthy general exposures to the whole body whether by heliotherapy or phototherapy, because the development of pigmentation during these extended periods necessitated progressively higher, longer doses to provoke the desired solar erythema (which, unlike Rollier, they viewed as essential to the cure). As Eidinow put it, by this method the skin became 'rapidly light-tolerant and immune', where the natural protection that pigmentation afforded became an inhibitor to treatment because it desensitised the skin to ultraviolet radiation.[39] They viewed the goal of exposure to be the production of solar erythema without subsequent pigmentation, and, as such, distinguished their method from both the methods of the Danish and the Swiss.

Hill and his colleagues at the NIMR advocated short, intense exposures to ultraviolet light with quartz mercury vapour and carbon arc lamps. They devised a method of exposing areas of patients' skin to lamps for only a few minutes at a time, every other day, 'dosed' according to what they called the 'minimal perceptible erythema' (MPE).[40] Hill and Eidinow defined the MPE as lasting less than forty-eight hours, potentially followed by peeling and not resulting in pigmentation. Their constant for determining MPE production was, in their words, 'normal' or 'average' white skin.[41] In the many reports and articles they presented throughout the 1920s, they maintained that this kept the patient's skin in a constant 'light-sensitive' state and was much cheaper in terms of electricity consumption.[42] William Beaumont, medical director of the Institute of Ray Therapy in Camden, observed that shorter doses were also less 'exhausting' for patients, especially children.[43] Hill and Eidinow's greatest criticism of the methods of Rollier as well as of the Finsen Institute was that, 'No importance is attached to the biological response of the skin after radiation.'[44] By orientating light treatment entirely around the solar erythema, Eidinow and Hill claimed to have, like Finsen and Rollier before them, invented a 'simple systematic technique' to guide phototherapeutic practice.[45]

Wrestling control

Eidinow stated that any lamp emitting ultraviolet rays would work with their method, and though they developed it for phototherapy he stated it could potentially guide heliotherapy as well.[46] Importantly, they also viewed it as a step towards standardising light therapy, Hill stating in 1925:

> One clinician uses lamps weak in ultra-violet rays and strong in heating effect, and gives very long exposures five days a week. Another uses lamps powerful in ultra-violet rays, and gives very short exposures once or twice a week; one believes in doses which produce a mild erythema [MPE], another avoids the production of erythema; one thinks the production of pigment hastens the curative effect, another believes it screens off the radiation and should be avoided. Varied and unstandardized as are at present the methods of treatment, yet all claim that they secure equally good curative effects. The need of the moment, then, is to standardize the lamps for treatment and find out the most economical methods of exposure.[47]

Their compulsion to systematise and standardise light therapy according to qualifiable and quantifiable phenomena was indicative of a larger push by this time towards standardisation and controlled organisation, in medicine and science as well as in industry. Like radiologists, who were similarly struggling at the same moment to gain legitimacy as a group of specialised practitioners, light therapists turned to standardisation as a way to wrestle control over their equipment, their patients, and their reputation. Increasing dependence upon patient attendance records, budget ledgers, and dosage units are evidence of a shared experience among these ray technicians.[48]

As employees of the MRC, Hill and Eidinow were also under the direction of its secretary, Walter Morley Fletcher, a man who privileged scientific research over the empiricism of clinical practice.[49] As key members of the MRC's CBAL, Hill and Eidinow conducted a series of laboratory-based experiments on animal and human subjects with ultraviolet light. Significantly, this committee had existed since 1922, indicating an early interest by the MRC to ascertain scientific data about actinic light's actions. In its report for 1923–24, it spoke of light therapy giving 'new hopes ... of a wide-spread diminution of disease and a great future improvement in the health, stature and beauty of the people in this country', particularly with regard to its use for rickets.[50]

Further pressured from the mid-1920s by the minister of health, who was receiving frequent requests to fund light clinics, the MRC needed to prove conclusively and scientifically that light therapy was truly effective.[51] Dr Dora Colebrook, who acted as secretary of the CBAL and was already familiar with light therapy from her time at the North Islington Infant Welfare Centre, took on the task from 1926 to 1928. In his book, *Control and the Therapeutic Trial*, Martin Edwards argued that light therapy suffered its first major 'scandal' in 1929, when the MRC published the results of Colebrook's randomised controlled trials. Colebrook conducted two trials, the first involving adults, treated by local phototherapy for varicose ulcers, and the second on schoolchildren, who were treated by general phototherapy to assess changes to their general health.[52] In both trials her results indicated that the therapy had little medical value, with no perceptible improvement on patients' conditions. The 1929 report presenting her findings shocked the medical community and was discussed not only in journals such as the *BMJ* and the *Lancet* but also in national and local newspapers.

Experienced clinicians took particular offence to Colebrook's trials and were equally disturbed by the MRC's sudden volte-face, having previously published favourable results and having among its members the highly respected practitioners Sequeira, Gauvain, and Hill. Crucially, for these practitioners the negative findings could be accounted for by incorrect technique and dosage. For instance, a passionate diatribe by Dr Maurice Weinbren, a light-therapy practitioner and radiologist with experience at Mount Vernon, Middlesex, and Queen's Hospitals, pointed out the various faults of Colebrook's studies and its 'misleading' results. He stated that Colebrook, in her 'intensive' study (sarcastically commented), only administered sub-erythemal doses on the varicose ulcers and only one to two times a week. Improperly dosed, the results, unsurprisingly for Weinbren, were poor.[53] As is clear, the visible production of solar erythema through local phototherapy was requisite in Weinbren's mind. No redness, no effect. More vehemently, Dr F. W. Alexander (once medical officer of health for

Poplar), was quoted in the *Yorkshire Post* as exclaiming, 'I don't understand what this report of the Medical Research Council is driving at. It seems utterly absurd. Nor do I know how they have given the treatment. Given properly, I know of no more powerful therapeutic treatment. Such criticism seems absolutely ridiculous.'[54] Manufacturers of light-therapy lamps also protested loudly, concerned about the knock-on effects to their sales. Gathering at a London meeting to discuss the 'ultra-violet ray controversy' and its 'death blow at their industry', the manufacturers pointed out that their distress was considerable and understandable: the industry employed 10,000 people, and they reported 30,000 medical practitioners in Britain were using light therapy.[55] The manufacturers, like many practitioners, called for more sufficient scientific trials to be done. In its defence, the MRC employed a 'rhetoric of control' to assert that Colebrook's scientific test methods were systematically and rigorously undertaken according to Edwards, who viewed them as foundational to the use of randomised control trials.

Edwards' argument presumed that light therapy, by being widely employed and popularly discussed among the medical community and the popular press, was, by 1929, already legitimate and established as 'mainstream medicine' – hence the 'scandal'.[56] On the one hand, Finsen's Nobel Prize (1903), Gauvain's knighthood (1920), and ongoing royal sanctioning indicates that it was a legitimate medical therapy by this time. On the other hand, light therapy's zealous use and popularity caused the MRC considerable distress from the early 1920s onwards, as Edwards himself showed, because few standardised guidelines about its application and methods existed. From the early 1920s, the MRC struggled to legitimise the therapy through various scientific and 'controlled' studies, yet that control was forever out of its grasp. There was tension even within its CBAL, the clinicians Sequeira and Gauvain indifferent and apparently unhelpful to Colebrook in her scientific trials.[57] Edwards positioned the 1929 'scandal' as a major setback in the therapy's history, concluding that by the 1930s it was already fizzling out in popularity.[58]

Primary evidence suggests otherwise, as we will see throughout this book. But what of the effect of Colebrook's results? For practitioners and manufacturers, light therapy's reputation could be restored by more trials, more data, and thus more investment in it, presenting important similarities with the history of vitamins (see Chapter 1).[59] According to one journalist, the MRC report did little to diminish interest in the therapy, noting interestingly that following its publication the number of institutions offering light therapy *increased*:

> Since the Medical Research Council administered their cold douche on the subject of violet-ray treatment, there has been much less heard about heliotherapy, writes a correspondent. But I gather that the Ministry of Health is one of many authorities who refuse to accept the M.R.C.'s verdict as final or conclusive. It is even doubtful whether the M.R.C. intended that it should

> be so regarded. Last year there were 135 institutions where heliotherapy is practised as against only 97 the year before, and the number is steadily growing. The official attitude is, however, that strict care must be exercised in the use of violet-ray treatment, both as to its handling and application.[60]

Failures and errors when administering light were explained as the result of faulty technique, improper dosage, and lack of skill. Dr Allan Hamilton, of the Poplar Light Clinic, could not account for his poor results, and in his confusion he was equally sceptical of his own skill and his peers' extravagant claims. He stated, rather poetically:

> Any new form of treatment has its enthusiasts, and they have not been wanting here. So far I have not been able to achieve all that has been claimed for this new method, and I have asked myself whether this is due to lack of skill and experience on my part, or whether some of the pioneers may not have painted their pictures with ultra-violet hues.[61]

Jamieson explained that the same poor results occurred when using the Finsen lamp for lupus vulgaris patients, with failure attributed to bad technique, lack of attention to detail, the wrong equipment, and unskilled operators.[62] In other words, it was not that the light was perceived as ineffective or that the therapy as a whole was to blame. Rather, blame lay with individual practitioners – Colebrook being an exemplary case. If Colebrook's trials achieved anything, it was to confer even more attention onto light's 'handling and application', centred on the issue of dosage.

II 'Fixing' doses

As is clear from the opening article of *The Times*' special 1928 'Sunlight and Health' supplement, dosage standardisation preoccupied practitioners well before the MRC's 1929 report: 'Every year [from 1920 onwards], indeed, has brought with it, in addition to new observations and deductions, new doubts and difficulties. There is, as yet, no certain knowledge of the remote effects of artificial sunlight. There is no certain knowledge about the correct doses of artificial sunlight.'[63] Earlier, in a 1925 article in the *Lancet*, Eidinow expressed his anxiety over the lack of standards in measuring and regulating ultraviolet dosage:

> Up to the present very little attention has been given to the question of dosage of ultra-violet light sources, and many workers consider this superfluous. The individual variations in sensibility to light *make it impossible to fix a standard dose*, even with a standard source of light. From this point of view it is indeed very difficult to determine the most suitable method for administration of

> light treatment, and further to decide if any harmful effects can take place from excessive dosage with light.[64]

For Eidinow, the sheer variety of lamps in use, emitting different wavelength ranges and intensities, negated the possibility of accurately comparing patient records from different hospitals and clinics. The same could be argued for sites around Britain using heliotherapy, since climatic and topographical differences (quite aside from seasonal variations) affected patients' exposure to the sun's ultraviolet radiation. As with other drugs, light rays – especially ultraviolet rays – produced different effects on the patient according to quantity, Beaumont clarifying by analogy with opium:

> It is well to bear in mind that the effect of big doses is not the same as that of small doses. In this respect ray therapy is no different from other forms of treatment. The effects of opium illustrate this. Small doses of opium render a patient excitable, large doses drowsy. It is the same drug, but the dose is different.[65]

Here Beaumont neglected to mention the dangers of an overdose, a matter that clearly concerned Eidinow as the above quote indicates.

What fascinates me is that Eidinow, along with his colleagues at the NIMR, devoted themselves to the very thing he described as impossible: the task of 'fixing' a standard therapeutic dose of ultraviolet radiation. The various meanings of the verb 'to fix' are significant when we consider its applications in science, medicine, and art: to fix a scientific principle or standard is 'to secure' it or 'to make (it) permanent'; to fix a broken leg is 'to mend' it, 'to set (it) right' or 'to secure (its) position'; to fix an image is 'to make (it) permanent' or 'to secure' it. The very invention of photography depended upon this matter of 'fixing'; the ability not to simply record impressions onto surfaces but to keep them there marked the official beginnings of photography in the 1830s. Ironically, the very source that produced those impressions, namely light, could erase them by means of prolonged exposure. In her book, *The Burning Mirror*, Melissa Miles has discussed the frustrations experienced by early photographers in experimenting with light, revolving around the issue of control: 'The desire to develop an agent that would "fix" photographs, and thereby exert "a protecting power" against the sun's rays, can … be understood as a struggle to stabilise this troubling ambivalence and construct light as a productive origin for photographic image-making.'[66] Unless they could be made permanent, producing images with light had little value in disseminating information.

The struggle to make permanent or stabilise the light's imprint on the photosensitive emulsion, requisite to legitimising photography as a recording medium, finds important correlations with light therapy's problematic investment in dosage standardisation as a means to legitimisation. Finsen's photographed forearm presents a convergence of photography's and light therapy's drive to 'fix' (Figs. 2.1, 2.5). Its fuzzy contours and misty patches are evidence of insufficient fixing in the taking and developing of the photograph, obscuring the legibility of the solar erythema manifest on Finsen's skin. In the version in Figure 2.5, underexposure in the reproduction process has created so much loss of contour and so much darkness as to literally obscure clear reading of the 'after' photograph. Even the authors, Luckiesh and Pacini, point out this problem in the image caption: 'Much detail has been lost in reproduction.'

When it came to the 'impossible' task of fixing a standard dose of light, Hill and Eidinow undertook several experiments at the NIMR, under the auspices of the MRC. Different methods for measuring ultraviolet light included chemical and 'biological' tests, by bleaching coloured solutions and irradiating test subjects to determine standard units of measurement. The most successful measurement in the end was according to erythema production on the skin, as Finsen had done.[67] Eidinow took it as a given that erythema production signalled ultraviolet radiation's consequent therapeutic 'value', a reference to its medical worth but one ironically residing in ambiguous, unfixed gradations of light and dark in photographic representation (Figs. 2.1–2.3).[68] For the test, they covered the skin with fabric, save for three circular flaps that would be opened at succeeding intervals. Hill explained that the first exposure was five minutes, the second ten minutes, and so on.[69] Black-and-white photographs indicate this testing method was performed according to different numbers of openings, different times of exposure, and different environmental conditions (Figs. 2.2–2.3).

Contemporaneous British images of MPE testing also include hand-drawn illustrations (Fig. 2.11).[70] In Figure 2.11, a drawing from Dr Hugh Morris's *Physiotherapy in Medical Practice* of 1939 presents the test set-up, including placement of black paper on the patient's forearm and indications to cover the rest of the skin with towels. This proved to be the cheapest and easiest of methods for testing, with materials easy to hand and hygienically discarded, just as sheets of dark paper came to be used to shield patients' eyes instead of expensive goggles.[71]

Hill and Eidinow, working with bacteriologist Dr Leonard Colebrook (Dora Colebrook's brother), further correlated erythema production with the blood's increased bactericidal powers, and this is a major reason they privileged short doses that produced solar erythema without subsequent pigmentation. But even here they cautioned that standardising ultraviolet dosage according to blood testing required more time and resources than MPE testing, and it was complicated by the fact that human blood was already normally high in bactericidal properties. Worryingly, their tests had shown that an *overdose* of ultraviolet light could actually *lower* the blood's ability to kill bacteria, putting the sick patient even more at risk.[72] In the end, the

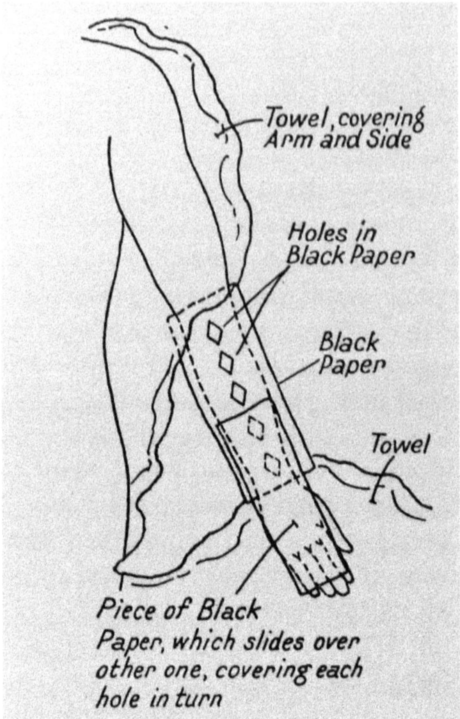

Figure 2.11 'To illustrate method of testing the sensitivity of a patient to ultraviolet radiation.' In Hugh Morris, *Physiotherapy in Medical Practice* (London: Edward Arnold, 1939), Figure 92, p. 188. Author's collection.

researchers' choice was clear: 'The treatment should be controlled by the erythema produced.'[73]

Eidinow invented his own equipment for the purpose (known as the 'Eidinow test-dosage armlet'), likely used for the erythema test in a photograph provided by Drs Eleanor H. Russell and William K. Russell (Fig. 2.2).[74] As with Figure 2.1, the Russells' photograph obscures the subtle gradations ('values') of erythema production on the forearms, which have been used together in this instance as registers for eight sequential one-minute exposures. Similarly, in his 1925 *Sunshine and Open Air*, Hill included photographs presenting the results of forearms irradiated through armlets while under various surrounding temperatures or through interposing materials (Fig. 2.3). Much like Finsen's photographed forearm, the arms register the effects of ultraviolet light through cold versus warm water (photograph 1), during hot, normal, or freezing temperatures (photograph 2), as well as through black-and-white coloured fabric (photograph 3). Both Finsen's and Hill's experiments tested materials mediating contact between ultraviolet light and the body, acting as either aids or hindrances, and these practitioners interpreted their findings by perceiving solar erythemata as explicit visual referents.

Aside from Eidinow's armlet, other erythema test kits were invented for determining dosage. The most elaborate device was invented by the influential French practitioner Dr Jean Saidman, creator of the equally elaborate 'Turning Solarium' (Aix-les-Bain, Vallauris, Jamnagar) and Gauvain's associate. Saidman's 'sensitometric test' or the 'Saidman Sensitometer' (Figs. 2.12–2.13), patented in 1927, incorporated a clockwork shutter to expose areas of the patient's abdomen or thigh by eighteen one-minute intervals, imprinting onto the skin its intricate design of shapes and numbers in the form of solar erythema. By this means Saidman determined the individual patient's '*seuil d'érythème*' – their erythemal threshold.[75] Yet once again, when we defer to the visual records, the subtle values of erythema intensities elude photographic representation (Fig. 2.13). Some of the shapes appear more faded than others, suggesting possibly that these indicate lower doses, but the fading could equally have been produced in the process of taking, developing, or reproducing the photograph.

These scientific investigators looked to photography as a medium to record and disseminate their findings. This in itself is certainly not surprising, as photography held tremendous authority for 'objectively' recording and disseminating science and medicine as Lorraine Daston and Peter Galison make clear.[76] But photography's relationship with light therapy was made fascinatingly tangled and uneasy by virtue of the fact that they were both, in Tanya Sheehan's words, 'technologies of light'.[77] The

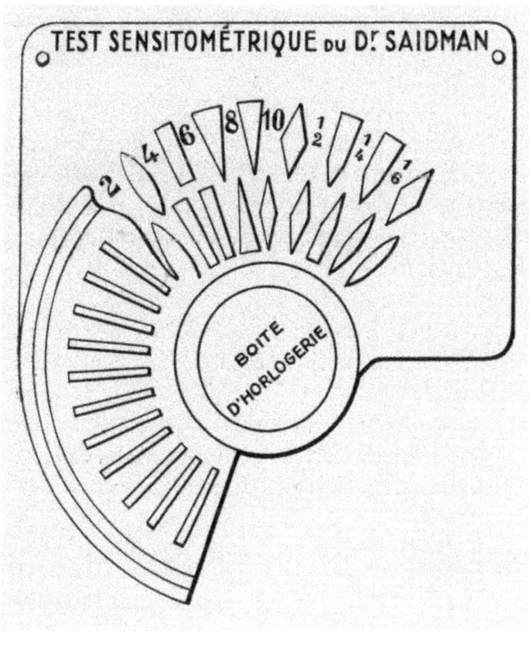

Figure 2.12 'Sensitometric test of Dr Saidman' (illustration of device). In Dr Stoïanoff, 'Actinométrie, héliométrie', in Charles Brody (ed.), *Traité d'hélio- et d'actinologie* (Paris: Maloine, 1938), vol. I, Figure 211, p. 392. Author's collection.

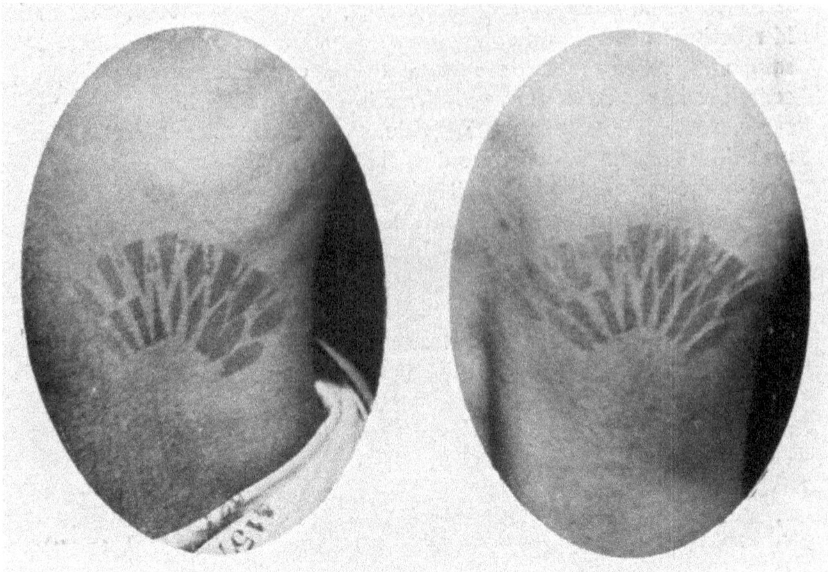

Figure 2.13 'Sensitometric test of Saidman' (before and after photographs).
In Hubert Jausion, 'L'Héliodynamothérapie des alopécies', in Charles Brody (ed.), *Traité d'hélio- et d'actinologie* (Paris: Maloine, 1938), vol. II, Figures 577–8, p. 1185. Author's collection.

poor legibility of the solar erythema in these photographs (Figs. 2.1–2.3, 2.5, 2.13) can be accounted for by some very difficult and specific conditions.

One relates to photographic processes, particularly difficulties achieving correct lighting and focusing, proper developing, and reproduction, which are all affected by the skill and available equipment of the producers. These are, of course, the challenges of producing and reproducing any analogue photograph, then as now, but photographing light therapy presented extraordinarily tricky circumstances, especially when the lamps were turned on as they produced overexposed and damaged negatives, as I discuss in Chapter 3.

Another condition, with respect to photographing solar erythema specifically, relates to the difficulties of capturing an elusive and uncooperative subject. In photographs, practitioners' audiences were presumably meant to encounter visual evidence of the efficacy of these erythema-centred tests. This was their intended function. But what is represented instead is evidence of a physiological phenomenon resistant to legible visual (re)presentation, to being clearly 'fixed'. In the photographic evidence, the subtly varied values, if not the very presence, of solar erythema remain illegible. Which of the hazy marks is the 'just perceptible' MPE in these photographs? *Could* it be represented photographically?

In Figure 2.2, the four-minute mark looks darker and more defined than the five- and six-minute marks, when logically it should appear fainter, lighter, and less distinct. Such photographs therefore act as records, yes, but not of the solar erythema clearly measured, defined, and standardised. Rather, they record practitioners' desperation to secure the solar erythema as a visual anchor, one that could legitimise the therapy yet refused to do so – it refused its authoritative role, refused to be weighed down. The *drive* to 'fix' the solar erythema, in visual and written form, says much about practitioners' ambitions to make light therapy appear as a modern, scientific, and systematic treatment.[78]

The erythema materialised

Quantifying, qualifying, and visually analysing solar erythema preoccupied British practitioners, far more so than pigmentation ever did.[79] Many followed Hill and Eidinow's test methods, and by 1927 the 'spot test' was already being described as well known.[80] In the first (1933) edition of the *Actinotherapy Technique* handbook, produced by the major lamp manufacturer Hanovia (Slough), the editors explicitly noted that lamps emitting any quantity of ultraviolet light, and indeed the very 'technique

Figure 2.14 'Erythema chart (for first exposure).' In *Actinotherapy Technique* (Slough: Sollux, 1933), pp. 42–3. Author's collection.

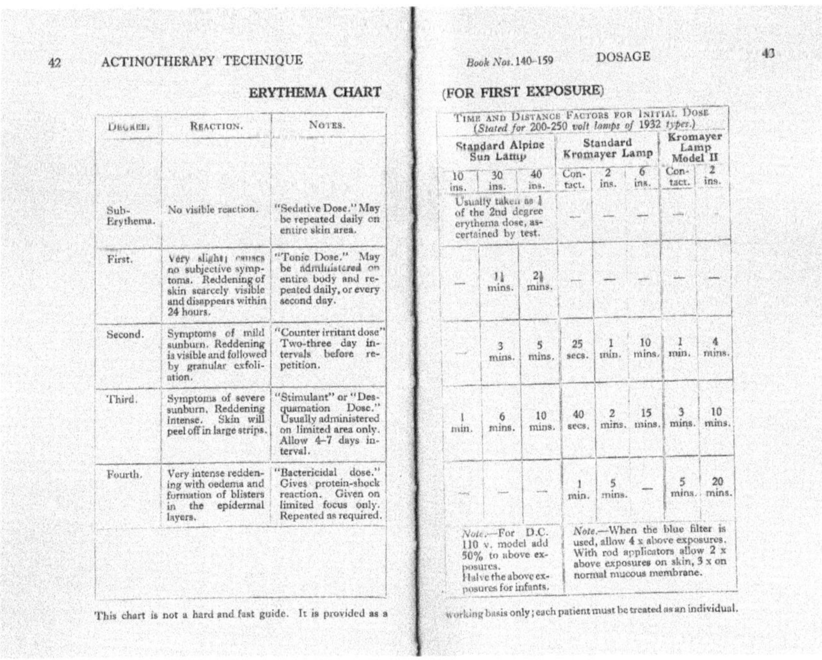

42 ACTINOTHERAPY TECHNIQUE

Book Nos. 140-159 DOSAGE 43

ERYTHEMA CHART (FOR FIRST EXPOSURE)

Degree.	Reaction.	Notes.	Time and Distance Factors for Initial Dose (Stated for 200-250 volt lamps of 1932 types.)							
			Standard Alpine Sun Lamp			Standard Kromayer Lamp			Kromayer Lamp Model II	
			10 ins.	30 ins.	40 ins.	Contact.	2 ins.	6 ins.	Contact.	2 ins.
Sub-Erythema.	No visible reaction.	"Sedative Dose." May be repeated daily on entire skin area.	Usually taken as ¼ of the 2nd degree erythema dose, ascertained by test.			—	—	—	—	—
First.	Very slight; causes no subjective symptoms. Reddening of skin scarcely visible and disappears within 24 hours.	"Tonic Dose." May be administered on entire body and repeated daily, or every second day.	—	1½ mins.	2½ mins.	—	—	—	—	—
Second.	Symptoms of mild sunburn. Reddening is visible and followed by granular exfoliation.	"Counter irritant dose" Two-three day intervals before repetition.	—	3 mins.	5 mins.	25 secs.	1 min.	10 mins.	1 min.	4 mins.
Third.	Symptoms of severe sunburn. Reddening intense. Skin will peel off in large strips.	"Stimulant" or "Desquamation Dose." Usually administered on limited area only. Allow 4–7 days interval.	1 min.	6 mins.	10 mins.	40 secs.	2 mins.	15 mins.	3 mins.	10 mins.
Fourth.	Very intense reddening with oedema and formation of blisters in the epidermal layers.	"Bactericidal dose." Gives protein-shock reaction. Given on limited focus only. Repeated as required.	—	—	—	1 min.	5 mins.	—	5 mins.	20 mins.
			Note.—For D.C. 110 v. model add 50% to above exposures. Halve the above exposures for infants.			*Note.*—When the blue filter is used, allow 4 x above exposures. With rod applicators allow 2 x above exposures on skin, 3 x on normal mucous membrane.				

This chart is not a hard and fast guide. It is provided as a working basis only; each patient must be treated as an individual.

of ultra-violet irradiation', were to be 'standardized on erythema reactions'.[81] In this edition they included a chart presenting particular degrees of solar erythema, qualified and quantified by the visual physiological referents of peeling (desquamation), blisters, and colour intensity, as well as by measurable amounts of time, including both its latent appearance and its duration (Fig. 2.14).

The information presented in Figure 2.14 is fairly consistent with other contemporaneous medical texts, with slight variations in descriptions, suggesting that the solar erythema was broadly mapped out and subdivided in this way from the mid-1920s.[82] Interestingly, the chart employs the same vocabulary as heat burns, with the third and fourth degrees of solar erythema roughly corresponding to first- and second-degree burns.[83] A mild or first-degree erythema (MPE), it explained, lasted for only twenty-four hours; the second degree resulted in fine peeling and the third degree on a larger scale, while the fourth degree produced blisters.

Practitioners explained that solar erythema was the result of 'irritation of the deep cells and nerve endings of the epidermis', capillary dilation and increased blood flow (hyperaemia), and fluid in the tissues (oedema).[84] If sufficiently intense, as we can see with the fourth degree (Fig. 2.14), it could cause blisters and even necrosis of skin cells. In some cases these were desirable reactions – it depended upon the physician's preferred method, the disease, and its specific treatment course.[85] Beaumont explained that, 'The formation of a blister is not necessarily a sign of overdosage if it results from local treatment [...] It is quite wrong, however, for blisters to be allowed to result over a large area from general irradiation.'[86] Therefore, at least for some practitioners, desirable erythema degrees were relative to local (lesion-specific) versus general (full body) exposures. The series of *Actinotherapy Technique* handbooks is organised in part by diseases, with recommended courses of treatment dependent on erythema degrees. The series indicates that erythema production went beyond its use value in the initial test to determine dosage, guiding the treatment throughout its course as an ongoing visual referent. Even Hanovia, in a 1940 user manual for the 'Homesun' lamp, advised the public to base initial and ongoing exposures according to MPE production:

> It is generally advisable to standardize the exposure which gives, on the following day, a very faint reddening of the skin, just perceptible [MPE]. This exposure is then repeated twice or three times weekly, so that the same sub-visible reddening always results without marked increase in the time of exposure.
>
> [...]
>
> If your lamp will not [sic] longer give it, or will only do so after unduly long exposures, the arc tube is getting too old to be useful. It then needs replacing.[87]

As the manual stated, erythema production also signalled the bulb's efficacy, the skin's photosensitivity acting as a natural photometer for the equipment.

It was common practice for practitioners to use their own arm as a test subject for a lamp's output, no doubt partly in deference to Finsen (Figs. 2.1, 2.5). Hill would do this, for example, and *Actinotherapy Technique* (1933) recommended self-testing as the best way to standardise one's lamp.[88] Likewise, Hamilton declared that the minimal erythema dose could be 'easily done by experimenting on yourself and your friends, and in this way you soon get a rough idea of its energy'.[89] He also reported using the lamps on the Poplar Light Clinic's nurses to test skin reactions and dosages.[90] The operator's skin therefore acted as the standard register for determining dosage. Far from being perceived as the ennobling act of the early X-ray martyrs, whose amputated limbs marked their self-sacrifice to medical progress, this was considered routine practice for assuring high standards of treatment.

In practice, dosage was administered to patients with the same standardised values in mind. Patients' positions, for instance, were highly regulated to ensure correct dosage at the correct distance, angle, and time (Figs. 2.15–2.16). Often they were encouraged to be mobile, circulating around a single lamp or placed in an area surrounded by multiple

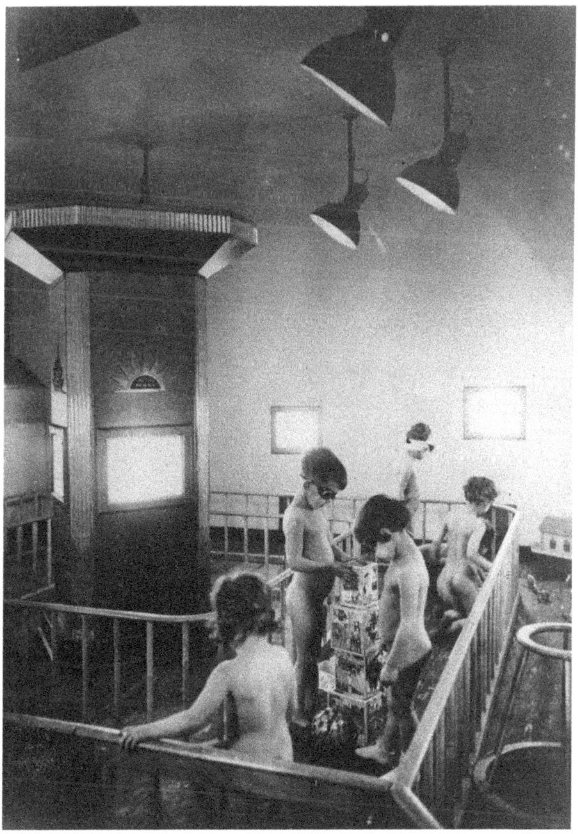

Figure 2.15 Phototherapy room with fenced ambulatory at fixed distance, Grange Road Clinic, Bermondsey, 1937. Southwark Local History Library and Archive, Wellcome Images, London CC BY-NC 4.0.

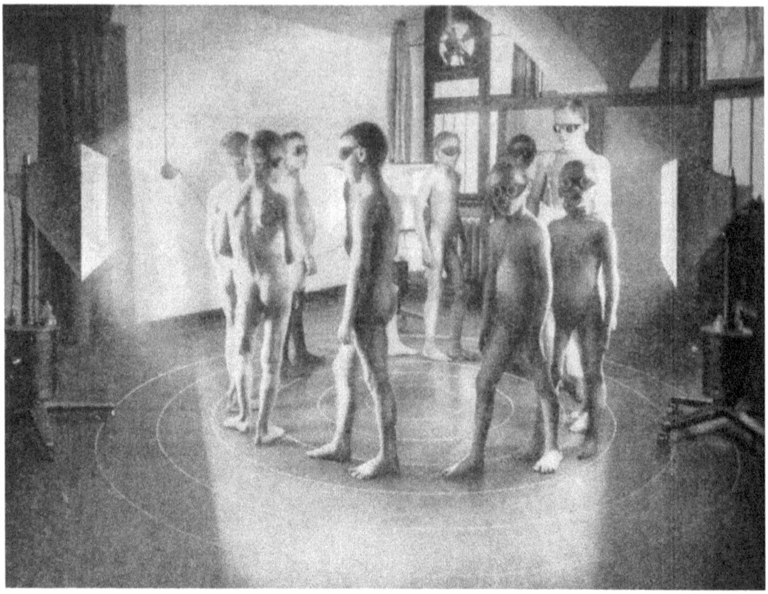

Figure 2.16 'Irradiation with Jesionek quartz mercury vapour lamp at a general hospital. (Note the dosage circles described on the floor.)' In Eleanor H. Russell and William K. Russell, *Ultra-violet Radiation and Actinotherapy* (Edinburgh: E. & S. Livingstone, 1925), Figure 48, p. 142. Author's collection.

lamps.[91] One recommended technique was to set up phototherapy treatment with multiple lamps in a circle, enclosing an area that was subdivided into concentric 'dosage circles'.[92] Patients were then treated in groups, according to height, and they walked continuously during treatment within their designated track so as to expose their bodies evenly at the correct distance. It is reminiscent of exercising prisoners, as represented by Gustave Doré in William Blanchard Jerrold's *London: A Pilgrimage* (1872).[93] The physical set-up of treatment sites and equipment acted as Foucauldian regulatory mechanisms not unlike Eidinow's 'test-dosage armlet', Saidman's 'sensitometer' or Rollier's and Hanovia's charts.[94] Together these material objects directed light-therapy practice, made it tangible ('materialised'), ordered, and standardised. Or at least they made it appear to be standardised; the unstable character of the solar erythema, on which these regulatory mechanisms depended, constantly undermined practitioners' efforts.

Sign and signature

Hanovia's chart provides vague descriptions of colour, from 'slight' to 'very intense' reddening, with no visual complement (Fig. 2.14). In the photographs of solar erythema production (Figs. 2.1–2.3, 2.5, 2.13), the limitations of black-and-white photography to define and classify this phenomenon become especially resonant. Placed alongside Hanovia's chart, is the Russells' photograph (Fig. 2.2) more or less clear in (re)presenting erythema production? Does the written word succeed where the visual fails? Would a colour chart, with varying intensities of red, instead have made the task of grading and identifying erythema values any better or easier for practitioners?[95] Perhaps not. It would have had to have accounted not only for varying intensities of red (first to fourth degrees) but also these intensities produced on varying tones of skin colour (natural or already pigmented by prior exposure), necessitating not one but multiple colour charts. The Swiss heliotherapist Oskar Bernhard stated that colour values of the solar erythema were also dependent upon the light source, without regard for the degree. A 'bluish-red erythema' was caused by the ultraviolet-rich light of the mercury vapour lamp, he stated. But a 'strong red full-blooded erythema' was produced by a carbon arc lamp, which, like sunlight, gave off plenty of heat but relatively little ultraviolet light.[96]

The overall absence of the solar erythema in visual representation might be simply explained by the limitations of various mediums: colour photography was not widely available until the mid-1930s and colour lithography was expensive. This is not to say definitively that they did not exist but that they were not *reproduced* or referenced in the primary literature, such as manuals, textbooks, trade catalogues, or dissertations. In other words, even if they did exist they were not disseminated or discussed within the field among practitioners and so logically could not have been in general use. Instead we find written charts (Fig. 2.14) or more affordable black-and white photographs (Figs. 2.2–2.3).

The solar erythema's un-'fix'-able nature, its fickleness, can be partially accounted for by the issue of latency. In addition to varying colour gradations to identify degrees, the timing for the solar erythema's appearance was not defined with any consistency in the literature. Statements by British practitioners from the 1920s and 1930s give varied descriptions about its latent appearance, ranging from 'almost immediately' to eight hours.[97] Similarly, the erythema's duration varied widely. It could disappear within twenty-four hours, as explained in the chart under the first-degree erythema (Fig. 2.14) but also persist between three days and several weeks according to other sources.[98]

Hanovia's chart presented a complicated, impressive series of numbers and categories: for different degrees of erythema, graded by differing colour intensities, extent of peeling or blistering; for different distances; for different lengths of time, by lamps of different types, models, years of manufacture, and voltage. Yet, at the bottom, it retained an important proviso: 'This chart is not a hard and fast guide. It is provided as a working basis only; each patient must be treated as an individual.'[99]

Above all, each patient reacted differently to ultraviolet radiation. Each had his or her own *unique erythematic signatures*. Recall that Eidinow declared, 'The individual variations in sensibility to light make it impossible to fix a standard dose, even with a standard source of light' (see statement above). This was not a new revelation; Finsen discussed individual variations in reactions to actinic light already by 1897.[100] It was mentioned in *The Times*' 1928 supplement and was commonly remarked upon in medical texts.[101] Some even gave up on the idea of dosage standardisation altogether, so unique were patient's erythematic reactions. Dr C. B. Heald claimed in 1929 that,

> Various methods have been devised for the measurement of the actual quantity of ultra-violet light given to a patient, but one and all, I am glad to say, have had to be given up and dosage graded as a result of clinical experience. Dosage in ultra-violet light cannot be determined by mere rule of thumb; the response of individuals to this form of energy varies so widely that only by treating the individual, and not the average, can satisfactory results be obtained.[102]

When it came to patient photosensitivity, 'No two patients are alike', the Russells declared. They added that, 'One would have a severe reaction with an exposure which would cause only the slightest reddening in another person.'[103] And yet, unlike Heald, they could not resist the impulse to generalise and categorise patient types, immediately confounding their statements by stating,

> Generally speaking, dark types can stand a longer dosage than fair, and the reddish type is the most sensitive. Children can stand about half the dose of an adult male of a similar type, and infants about half that of children. Women are as a rule more sensitive than men, and sensitiveness decreases as age increases.[104]

Patients' so-called individual variations were grouped together and classified, dependent upon factors like race (skin, eye, and hair colour), gender, and age.[105] Children, women, the fair-skinned, and the red-haired were generally, though not always, considered to be more sensitive to actinic light. Practitioners disagreed, for instance, as to whether babies' skin was more or less sensitive to ultraviolet light than adults', with diverse exposure times as a result (see Chapter 5). Such unpredictable variations and diverse opinions led Gauvain to declare, as late as 1934, that light therapy was an 'art' rather than 'an exact science'. In the same publication he even noted that patients' reactions varied throughout their lives, according to their state of health, location, and season.[106]

For George Weisz, Christopher Lawrence, and David Cantor, this focus on the individual patient characterised holism's approach to medicine, which resulted from dissatisfaction with the reductionist view of biomedicine that treated diseases, not people. According to Lawrence, standardisation in medicine was a problem holists disparaged.[107] Holists were not necessarily alternative practitioners; Lawrence and Weisz pointed out that holist approaches occurred within mainstream medicine.[108] Some practitioners of light therapy were identifiably holists, including Dr Alexander Cawadias (Physician to the St John Clinic and Institute of Physical Medicine in the 1930s), but as these historians also noted that it is difficult to slot particular practitioners into the movement.[109] Indeed, light therapy seems to have integrated the reductionism and standardisation of biomedicine, especially through dependence upon laboratory research, with the individualisation associated with holism – if not muddled the clear distinction altogether. While some historians have discussed light therapy (especially heliotherapy) in relation to holism, others have aligned it with the emergence of biomedicine in the twentieth century. Cantor, for example, wrote that,

> whereas the early modern medical practitioner tended to fit his treatment to each individual patient, his or her twentieth-century counterpart had recourse to a standard set of treatments that could be given to all patients suffering from a particular disease, and supplied by so-called 'ethical' pharmaceutical companies, or by the manufacturers of X ray and other physical equipment such as sun lamps or electrotherapy apparatus. Patient's [sic] illnesses came to be judged in part by the extent to which they responded to a standardized dose: so many physical units of radiation, or milligrams of the active principle of a drug, for example. Older ideas of regime were increasingly standardized and rationalized.[110]

Cantor's inclusion of phototherapy as part and parcel of a distinctly modern 'standard set' of therapies was certainly not an historical error. As we have seen, practitioners anxiously pushed to standardise dosages. Yet they also recognised the uniqueness of individual patient's photosensitivities, manifested through erythema production. In this sense they could simultaneously be seen as holistic in their approach to administering the treatment to their patients.

In the case of light therapy, these were not necessarily contradictory practices, expressive of a seductive narrative setting up biomedicine versus holism, standardisation versus individualisation, or the laboratory versus the clinic. Individual practitioners vacillated between these apparent poles. Gauvain welcomed an MRC-funded laboratory researcher at Treloar Hospital in 1925, only to state the same year that, 'While many important investigations on the mode of action of light have been completed in the laboratory the subject is so complex, so many factors are involved, that I believe clinical experience is still our most reliable guide.'[111] And the Swiss heliotherapist, Rollier, whose chart regimented the patient's acclimation to sunshine according to strictly monitored times and bodily locations (Fig. 2.10), stressed that 'no physiotherapeutic method demands such strict individualization as heliotherapy'.[112] For Rollier, the patient's course of exposures, in addition to sleep, diet, and exercise, could be simultaneously individualised and regimented. As Michel Foucault argued, the unique emerges from and seeps through the norm:

> the power of normalization imposes homogeneity; but it individualizes by making it possible to measure gaps, to determine levels, to fix specialties, and to render the differences useful by fitting them one to another [...] [T]he norm introduces, as a useful imperative and as a result of measurement, all the shading of individual differences.[113]

From this it seems practitioners' anxious drive to make light therapy a systematic and legitimate treatment by 'fixing' standard doses only succeeded in rocking the boat. That they chose the unique, variable, and latent solar erythema as an anchor merely destabilised their efforts even further.

Conclusion

All of the images and objects I have presented in this chapter about solar erythema point to a certain and rather fascinating tension in light therapy: between, on the one hand, recognising that patients were individuals with unique erythematic signatures and, on the other hand, attempting to force these highly variable photosensitivities to conform to a mass system. With photographs (Figs. 2.1–2.3, 2.5, 2.13), charts (Figs. 2.10, 2.14), testing devices (Figs. 2.11–2.12), and 'dosage circles' (Figs. 2.15–2.16) orientated around the production of solar erythema (or, in Rollier's case, its avoidance), practitioners invested enormous energy to standardise dosage and systematise light therapy. With these objects in mind it is evident that this drive to control was more than rhetorical, as Edwards argued: it was material.

Throughout this chapter I have not been arguing that the solar erythema, or 'sunburn', was *poorly* defined or *poorly* standardised. This would suggest a lack of effort. On the contrary, the images and texts demonstrate that, despite the repeated efforts by clinicians and laboratory researchers to pin down this transient physiological reaction, the solar erythema resisted its role, just as it remained unreadable in visual representations. Its slippery character confounded standardisation, evaded the goals intended for it, and refused to be anchored down. Well before the MRC's scandalous 1929 report of Colebrook's trials, light-therapy practitioners were desperately trying to make the solar erythema a constant in their experiments in spite of recognising its intrinsically variable character; that is, to 'fixing' something inherently unfixable. As Hanovia's chart (Fig. 2.14) makes evident, written descriptions were no clearer in pinning down the solar erythema than were images. But it is striking to note the difference in volumes of production between word and image here. The sheer amount of words dedicated to explaining, defining, and classifying solar erythema significantly outweighed the few visual representations devoted to the same tasks. The excess of the former reveals a desire to standardise not simply the solar erythema but the very practice of light therapy. The relative absence, illegibility or *silence* of the latter ironically speaks volumes about the impossibility of fulfilling that desire and the anxiety propelling it. The irradiated photographed forearms of Finsen (Fig. 2.1), the Russells (Fig. 2.2), and Hill (Fig. 2.3), obscure rather than illuminate, representing the solar erythema as unstable, resistant, and illegible. These so-called limits of the visual, then, are powerful and productive because they communicate much about light therapy's worth and aims through an aesthetics of light. Put simply, the images matter because they tell us about light therapy's medical, social, and aesthetic 'values'.

Furthermore, in this chapter I have deliberately focused on solar erythema as a physiological phenomenon perceived to be simultaneously desirable and dangerous (or 'injurious') by practitioners over some forty years, showing that this tension was at work in light therapies from their inception in the 1890s. These contentious perceptions are manifested and produced by the slippages in the terminology itself – of solar erythema and/as 'sunburn'.[114] Even within the same camp of practitioners (Hill and Eidinow) and in the same year (1925) we encounter confusing explanations of the word: Hill described sunburn as an 'excessive action of the sun' that 'floods the body' and produces tissue damage; Eidinow claimed that sunburn was indicative of ultraviolet light's therapeutic value.[115]

Already by 1940 solar erythema was described as an explicit form of bodily damage.[116] Shifting to the present (2016), we continue to encounter conflicting visual and written messages about the meaning and role of sunburn. On its website, Cancer Research UK described sunburn as 'a clear sign that ultraviolet (UV) radiation from the sun or sunbeds has damaged the genetic material in … skin cells'.[117] Suntan is described as the 'skin's response to damage from the sun'.[118] With its emphasis on visual and physiological damage, the charity characterised sunburn and suntan in ways with which we are now familiar; that is, by employing descriptors of risk and danger. Likewise, the British Association of Dermatologists listed 'sunburn' as the first 'side effect' of contemporary phototherapy, yet in its numerous leaflets it repeatedly included the phrase, 'Never let your skin burn!' to educate the public about the dangers of skin cancer.[119] Degrees of solar erythema were not explained on its website, in words or images, presenting 'sunburn' as a particularly ambiguous term. I explore burns further in Chapter 4, but for now let me emphasise that the *burn* in 'sunburn' is but one unstable referent in the slippery vocabulary of light therapy.

The weight given to the solar erythema in the drive to standardise light therapy, beginning in the 1890s, continues today. Erythema production retains its visual authority in designating light dosages. It has carried through to regulations for ultraviolet radiation dosage standards in medicine (phototherapy), public health (notably the UV Index and in determining 'phototypes') and industry (including general occupational risk assessment).[120] In spite of overt awareness that individual photosensitivities are unique and subjectively graded (as well as racially specific), the solar erythema occupies an unchallenged position by phototherapists in the dosing of ultraviolet light, complemented increasingly by sophisticated photometric devices.[121] It is true that it has been my aim to present not simply a diverse array but rather a disarray of written and visual material. But by looking carefully at the therapy's visual 'evidence' it becomes clear that focusing on the things that do not make sense in its history – the disagreements, the ambiguities, the absences, and silences – is a tremendously productive way to contextualise Britain's ongoing complicated and contentious relationship with actinic light.

Notes

1 Sir Henry Gauvain, 'Organisation and Work of a Light Department in a Hospital for Surgical Tuberculosis', *Lancet*, 4 July 1925, pp. 10–16, at p. 10.

2 William Beaumont, *Fundamental Principles of Ray Therapy* (London: H. K. Lewis & Co. Ltd, 1931), p. 90.

3 Sir Henry Gauvain, 'Popular Lecture on the Sun Cure', *BMJ*, 9 August 1924, pp. 234–6, at p. 234.

4 See Oskar Bernhard, *Light Treatment in Surgery* (London: Edward Arnold, 1926), p. 58; and Niels R. Finsen, *Phototherapy*, trans. J. H. Sequeira (London: Edward Arnold, 1901), p. 6.

5 Jean Martin Charcot, 'Erythème produit par l'action de la lumière électrique', *Comptes Rendus des Séances et Mémoires de la Société de Biologie*, 5, 2nd series (March 1858), 63–5, at p. 64. Light therapists cited even earlier references to the physicists and Alpine mountaineers Horace-Bénédict de Saussure and John Tyndall, who both noted their skin burnt badly during their expeditions in freezing conditions.

6 See, for example, Albert Eidinow, 'The Action of Ultra-violet Rays on the Skin', *British Journal of Tuberculosis*, 22:3 (1928), 136–9, at p. 139; Myrtle Vaughan-Cowell, *Artificial Sunlight: Its Use and Application* (London: H. Edgar Smithers, 1928), p. 18; and Eleanor H. Russell and William K. Russell, *Ultra-violet Radiation and Actinotherapy* (Edinburgh: E. & S. Livingstone, 1925), p. 139. The American practitioner Dr John Harvey Kellogg put it more bluntly: 'A Light Erythema Is Not a Burn', in *Light Therapeutics* (Battle Creek, Mich.: Modern Medicine, 1927), p. 36.

7 See *Actinotherapy Technique* (Slough: Sollux, 1933), pp. 22–3; Harold Blum, 'Sunlight and Cancer of the Skin', *Journal of the National Cancer Institute* (1940), 397–418, at p. 410.

8 André Gide, *The Immoralist* (1902), trans. D. Bussy (Harmondsworth: Penguin, 1981), p. 55.

9 See Anne Kinloch Jamieson, 'An Intolerable Affliction: A History of Lupus Vulgaris in Late Nineteenth- and Early Twentieth-Century Britain' (Ph.D. dissertation, University

of Leeds, 2010); and Robert Koch, 'Die aetiologie der tuberculose', *Berliner Klinische Wochenshrift*, 19 (1882), 221–30.

10 Bernhard, *Light Treatment*, p. 106.

11 See Arthur Downes and Thomas P. Blunt, 'Researches on the Effect of Light upon Bacteria and Other Organisms', *Proceedings of the Royal Society of Medicine*, 26 (1877), 488–500; Philip E. Hockberger, 'A History of Ultraviolet Photobiology for Humans, Animals and Microorganisms', *Photochemistry and Photobiology*, 76:6 (2002), 561–79, at p. 577; and Richard Hobday, *The Healing Sun: Sunlight and Health in the 21st Century* (Forres: Findhorn Press, 1999), p. 91.

12 Finsen, *Phototherapy*, p. 8.

13 Finsen, *Phototherapy*, p. 8.

14 Finsen, *Phototherapy*, p. 6.

15 Finsen, *Phototherapy*, p. 7.

16 Italics original. Matthew Luckiesh and August John Pacini, *Light and Health: A Discussion of Light and Other Radiations in Relation to Life and to Health* (Baltimore, Md.: Williams & Wilkins Company, 1926), p. 99. Finsen's experiments are also discussed in detail by Bernhard, *Light Treatment*, pp. 63–4.

17 Luckiesh and Pacini, *Light and Health*, p. 100.

18 Finsen cited the experiments of other physicians who had tested the effects of electric light on themselves, including the Russian physician Maklakoff, who exposed himself to arc lights at a smelting factory in Kolomna in 1889. See Finsen, *Phototherapy*, p. 13. The scientific experiments of Erik Johan Widmark (1850–1909), based in Stockholm, must also be mentioned, since they conclusively isolated actinic rays as the cause of solar erythema using electric light, also in 1889. These are cited in: Albert Eidinow, 'Some Observations on the Dosage of Ultra-violet Rays in Artificial Sun Treatment', *Lancet*, 15 August 1925, pp. 317–23, at p. 317; Valdemar Bie, 'Remarks on Finsen's Phototherapy', *BMJ*, 30 September 1899, pp. 825–30, at p. 825; and Hockberger, 'A History of Ultraviolet Photobiology', p. 574. Hockberger additionally cited Friedrich Hammer, *Ueber den Einfluss des Lichtes auf die Haut* (Stuttgart: Ferdinand Enke, 1891), who confirmed and extended Widmark's experiments.

19 Bie, 'Remarks on Finsen's Phototherapy', p. 827.

20 Gauvain, 'Organisation and Work of a Light Department', p. 15.

21 Bie, 'Remarks on Finsen's Phototherapy', p. 828.

22 'The "Light Treatment" at the London Hospital', *BMJ*, 30 June 1900, pp. 1595–7, at p. 1596.

23 Jamieson, 'An Intolerable Affliction', p. 104.

24 See, for example, Malcolm Morris and S. Ernest Dore, 'Further Remarks on Finsen's Light and X-Ray Treatment in Lupus and Rodent Ulcer', *BMJ*, 31 May 1902, pp. 1324–8, at p. 1325.

25 'The "Light Treatment" at the London Hospital', p. 1595.

26 See Bie, 'Remarks on Finsen's Phototherapy', p. 825; and Finsen, *Phototherapy*, pp. 1, 2, 18, 20, and 28.

27 Finsen, *Phototherapy*, pp. 54, 62; *Institut Photothérapique de M. le Professeur Finsen. Exposition Universelle de 1900* (Paris: Georges Carré et C. Naud, 1900), p. 13; Julius Moritzen, 'The "Light Cure" at Copenhagen: Professor Finsen and His Work', *American Monthly Review of Reviews*, 26 (July–December 1902), 431–5; and Gauvain, 'Organisation and Work of a Light Department', p. 12.

28 Jamieson, 'An Intolerable Affliction', pp. 131–2.

29 Axel Reyn, 'Discussion on the Artificial Light Treatment of Lupus and Other Forms of Tuberculosis', *BMJ*, 22 September 1923, pp. 499–503, at p. 502–3.

30 Reyn, 'Discussion', p. 502.

31 See Tania Woloshyn, 'Patients Rebuilt: Dr Auguste Rollier's Heliotherapeutic Portraits, c. 1903–1944', *Medical Humanities*, 39:1 (2013), 38–46. Rollier insisted, in both the English and French versions of his publications, on the words 'systematised', 'systematic', and 'scientific', as opposed to 'empirical', to describe his practice. See, for instance, Rollier, *Heliotherapy* (London: Henry Frowde and Hodder & Stoughton, 1923), pp. v–vi, 3; and Auguste Rollier, *La Cure de soleil* (Paris: Baillière & Fils; Lausanne: Constant Tarin, 1914), pp. 17–18.

32 Dr François Chiaïs, 'La cure solaire directe', in *Troisème Congrès Français de Climatothérapie et d'Hygiène Urbaine* (Cannes: n.p., 1907), p. 30.

33 Albert Eidinow, 'A Note on Phototherapy', *Lancet*, 25 September 1926, pp. 645–8, at p. 648.

34 Jamieson, 'An Intolerable Affliction', p. 134. When visiting the Medical Museion's Finsen Archive, its collections manager, Ion Meyer, also agreed with Jamieson's theory during an informal discussion we had.

35 Gauvain, 'Organisation and Work of a Light Department', p. 14.

36 See Godfrey B. Dixon in Leonard Hill, Godfrey B. Dixon, and Dora C. Colebrook, 'Discussion on Influence of Sunlight and Artificial Light on Health', *BMJ*, 12 September 1925, pp. 470–7.

37 Gauvain, 'Popular Lecture on the Sun Cure', pp. 234–5. For details on the role of nurses in light therapy, see Chapter 6.

38 Leonard Hill, in Hill et al., 'Discussion on Influence of Sunlight', pp. 471–2.

39 Eidinow, 'A Note on Phototherapy', p. 648.

40 Eidinow, 'A Note on Phototherapy', p. 647.

41 Albert Eidinow, 'Observations on Some of the Principles of Artificial Sun Treatment', *British Journal of Tuberculosis*, 19:3 (1925), 113–26, at p. 123; and Hill, in Hill et al., 'Discussion on Influence of Sunlight', p. 471.

42 Eidinow, 'A Note on Phototherapy', p. 647.

43 Beaumont, *Fundamental Principles*, p. 108.

44 Eidinow, 'A Note on Phototherapy', p. 647.

45 Eidinow, 'A Note on Phototherapy', p. 648.

46 Eidinow, 'A Note on Phototherapy', pp. 647–8.

47 Hill, in Hill et al., 'Discussion on Influence of Sunlight', p. 473.

48 Joel D. Howell, *Technology in the Hospital: Transforming Patient Care in the Early Twentieth Century* (Baltimore, Md.: Johns Hopkins University Press, 1996). Annual reports for the budgets of Treloar Hospital and the Manchester and Salford Hospital for Skin Diseases can be viewed in their respective archives: Hampshire Record Office, Treloar Archives, 47M94/A17/1–32, and John Rylands Library Special Collections, MMC/9/18. See also Lisa Cartwright, *Screening the Body: Tracing Medicine's Visual Culture* (Minneapolis, Minn.: University of Minnesota Press, 1995), p. 129.

49 Martin Edwards, *Control and the Therapeutic Trial: Rhetoric and Experimentation in Britain, 1918–48* (Amsterdam and New York: Rodopi, 2007), p. 18.

50 Cited in R. Plato Schwartz, 'The Application of Radiation in the Modern Hospital', *American Journal of Nursing*, 26:9 (1926), 691–7, at p. 696.

51 Edwards, *Control*, p. 72.

52 Edwards, *Control*, p. 74.
53 Maurice Weinbren, 'The Medical Research Council and Ultra-violet Radiation', *British Journal of Tuberculosis*, 23:3 (1929), 117–22.
54 Reported in 'Ultra-violet Ray Controversy', *Yorkshire Post*, 16 March 1929, p. 18.
55 'Ultra-violet Ray Controversy', *Yorkshire Post*, 19 March 1929, p. 12.
56 Edwards, *Control*, pp. 67–8, 85.
57 Edwards, *Control*, pp. 73–4.
58 Edwards, *Control*, p. 84.
59 Rima Apple, *Vitamania: Vitamins in American Culture* (New Brunswick: Rutgers University Press, 1996).
60 See 'Violet Ray Controversy', *Hull Daily Mail*, 18 November 1929, p. 7.
61 Allan G. Hamilton, 'Light Treatment at an Infant Welfare Centre', *Public Health* (February 1927), pp. 144–9, at p. 144.
62 Jamieson, 'An Intolerable Affliction', pp. 127, 136, 158.
63 'A New Science', *The Times*, 'Sunlight and Health' special supplement, 22 May 1928, p. x.
64 Italics mine. Eidinow, 'Some Observations', p. 318.
65 Beaumont, *Fundamental Principles*, pp. 90–1.
66 Melissa Miles, *The Burning Mirror: Photography in an Ambivalent Light* (North Melbourne: Australian Scholarly Publishing, 2008), pp. 139–40. See also Geoffrey Batchen, *Burning with Desire: The Conception of Photography* (Cambridge, Mass.: MIT Press, 1999), p. 94; Kelley Wilder, *Photography and Science* (London: Reaktion, 2009), pp. 86–7; and Jennifer Tucker, 'The Social Photographic Eye', in Corey Keller (ed.), *Brought to Light: Photography and the Invisible, 1840–1900* (New Haven, Conn.: Yale University Press with SFMOMA, 2008), pp. 37–49, at p. 45.
67 Their experiment was also based on several prior German studies, including those of Karl Wilhelm Hausser and Wilhelm Vahle. For details, see A. Webster, Leonard Hill, and Albert Eidinow, 'Measurement of Ultra-violet Light by Means of an Acetone Methylene-Blue Solution', *Lancet*, 12 April 1924, pp. 745–7, at p. 746; William Weber Coblentz, Ralph Stair, and John Meredith Hogue, *The Spectral Erythemic Reaction of the Human Skin to Ultra-violet Radiation* (Washington, DC: National Bureau of Standards, 1931), pp. 401–5, at p. 405; and Hockberger, 'A History of Ultraviolet Photobiology', p. 574.
68 Eidinow stated that 'dosage of the ultra-violet must be primarily focused on the intensity of the wave-lengths about 3000–2500 λ, since this group of rays correspond to the rays which have biological action on the skin and on the therapeutic value'. Eidinow, 'Some Observations', p. 318.
69 Hill, in Hill et al., 'Discussion on Influence of Sunlight', p. 472. See also Eidinow, 'Some Observations', p. 319.
70 The only representation I have encountered of erythemal testing in process is within a short film of *c.* 1930 about the construction and operation of Dr Jean Saidman's 'Turning Solarium' in Aix-les-Bains, which is shown as a series of film stills in Thierry Lefebvre and Cécile Raynal, *Les Solariums tournants du Dr Jean Saidman: Aix-les-Bains, Jamnagar, Vallauris* (Paris: Éditions Glyphe, 2010), pp. 235–79.
71 See Hugh Morris, *Physiotherapy in Medical Practice* (London: Edward Arnold, 1939), pp. 187–8; and Gauvain, 'Organisation and Work of a Light Department', p. 14.
72 See Leonard Hill, *Sunshine and Open Air: Their Influence on Health, with Special Reference to the Alpine Climate* (London: Edward Arnold, 1925), p. 88. See also Eidinow, 'Some Observations', p. 322; and Leonard Colebrook, 'The Influence of Sunlight upon the Bactericidal Power of Human Blood', *BMJ*, 5 July 1924, p. 11.

73 Eidinow, 'Observations on Some of the Principles', p. 124.

74 They did not directly state using the Eidinow armlet caption, but it is the only one they described, stating on the same page that it was a 'useful and convenient' way of running the test. Russell and Russell, *Ultra-violet Radiation*, p. 153.

75 See Jean Saidman, *Héliothérapie de la tuberculose: techniques nouvelles* (Paris: G. Doin et Cie, 1936); and Lefebvre and Raynal, *Les Solariums tournants*. On the Jamnagar solarium, see Jean Saidman and Pranjivan M. Mehta, *Elements of Light Therapy* (Bombay: The Popular Book Depot, 1950). The device was clearly available in Britain, though perhaps not frequently bought, being cited in Morris's book as 'suitable for high-class private practice' and described as the refined version of using simple black paper with holes (Figure 2.11). Morris, *Physiotherapy in Medical Practice*, p. 188. It is also mentioned in Alexander Cawadias, 'Ultra-violet Irradiation: Technique of Application', *British Journal of Physical Medicine*, 11:12 (1937), 225–9, at pp. 228–9.

76 Lorraine Daston and Peter Galison, *Objectivity* (New York: Zone Books, 2010). See also Wilder, *Photography and Science*, p. 50.

77 See Tanya Sheehan, '"Panes Curing Pains": Light as Medicine in the Photographic Studio', in *Doctored: The Medicine of Photography in Nineteenth-Century America* (University Park, Pa.: Pennsylvania State University Press, 2011), pp. 79–105.

78 This was not confined to Britain. In America, the physicist William Weber Coblentz began presenting reports in the early 1930s to the Bureau of National Standards in Washington on research to standardise ultraviolet dosage. In spite of his awareness of previous efforts, he declared, 'At present the physician has neither a unit of dosage nor a meter for accurately measuring the amount of ultra-violet radiation used for healing purposes.' Coblentz et al., 'The Spectral Erythemic Reaction', p. 401.

79 The degrees of colour saturation (intensities) of the suntan had different meanings entirely: unlike the solar erythema, it was not quantified, it was rarely qualified (say, by colour descriptors), and the shades/darkening of the tan had deeply embedded racial connotations. See Chapter 5.

80 Hamilton, 'Light Treatment at an Infant Welfare Centre', p. 149.

81 *Actinotherapy Technique* (1933), p. 33.

82 See, for example, Eidinow, 'Some Observations', p. 321, 'Observations on Some of the Principles', p. 124, and 'A Note on Phototherapy', p. 647; and Russell and Russell, *Ultra-violet Radiation*, pp. 153–4.

83 Jonathan Reinarz (University of Birmingham) is currently working on the medical history of burns, and I hope to discover more about the history of the classification system for burns in the future.

84 See Hill, *Sunshine and Open Air*, pp. 81, 93–4; and Russell and Russell, *Ultra-violet Radiation*, pp. 116–17.

85 As an example, the 1933 edition stated that a second-degree erythema should be produced during local treatment of bone and joint ('surgical') tuberculosis, but a first degree with general treatment, increasing dosages as the treatment progressed. *Actinotherapy Technique* (1933), p. 152.

86 Beaumont, *Fundamental Principles*, p. 100.

87 Hanovia, 'A Short Book of Instructions for Users of the "Homesun" Sunlamp', user manual, 1940, pp. 7, 9. See also *Actinotherapy Technique* (1933), p. 34.

88 See Eidinow, 'Some Observations', p. 318; and *Actinotherapy Technique* (1933), p. 33. See also John Stanislav Sadar, *Through the Healing Glass: Shaping the Modern Body through Glass*

Architecture, 1925–35 (London and New York: Routledge, 2016), Figure 1.5, p. 15, for another poorly reproduced photograph to show the testing of 'Vita' glass that bears remarkable similarity to Finsen's (Figure 2.1).

89 Hamilton, 'Light Treatment at an Infant Welfare Centre', p. 149.

90 Hamilton, 'Light Treatment at an Infant Welfare Centre', p. 148.

91 The distance between patient and lamp in phototherapy came to be regulated by a principle known as 'The Law of Inverse Squares' (Russell and Russell, *Ultra-violet Radiation*, pp. 151–2). Likewise, the angle at which ultraviolet rays struck the patient's body affected their intensity and thus erythema production, a principle called 'The Cosine Law' or 'The Angle of Incidence' (Vaughan-Cowell, *Artificial Sunlight*, p. 63). Saidman's Turning Solaria incorporated moving beds that could angle the patient to the sun at various degrees. See Saidman, *Héliothérapie de la tuberculose*, p. 13. Similarly, Sir George Bernard Shaw had a rotating shed to allow him to always face the sun.

92 Russell and Russell, *Ultra-violet Radiation*, p. 142.

93 William Blanchard Jerrold, *London: A Pilgrimage* (London: Grant, 1872). See Figure 15 via the British Library (Wf1/1856): www.bl.uk/collection-items/london-illustrations-by-gustave-dor# (accessed 1 April 2016). I am grateful to Keren Hammerschlag for this reference.

94 Charts, graphs, and standardised forms are integral to Howell's understanding of changing patient care due to medical technology: 'The standardization of forms clearly made reporting of X rays more systematic. It may have implicitly served to standardize patients as well.' Howell, *Technology in the Hospital*, p. 129. See also Martin D. Moore, 'Reorganising Chronic Disease Management: Diabetes and Bureaucratic Technologies in Post-War British General Practice', in Mark Jackson (ed.), *Routledge History of Disease* (London and New York: Routledge, 2017), pp. 420–38.

95 Colour comparison as a method for determining ultraviolet light dosage existed in the form of 'Levy-West Pastilles', discs of chemically coated card that changed tint upon different exposures to light. They too were compared against a 'standard', in this case a card of twelve varying tints supplied with the test kit. See Beaumont, *Fundamental Principles*, pp. 98–9. Hill measured ultraviolet light using a methylene blue solution exposed outside: Webster et al., 'Measurement of Ultra-violet Light'. In fact, Hill and Eidinow did initially seek out colour standards in their erythema tests; the patients' skin was checked against a Lovibond colorimeter or tintometer, a device using numbered, coloured glass pieces that was originally invented as a colour scale to grade beer in the 1880s. They found the process tedious and arbitrary, however. See Eidinow, 'Some Observations', p. 320.

96 Bernhard, *Light Treatment*, p. 113.

97 See the varying descriptions in Russell and Russell, *Ultra-violet Radiation*, p. 116; Eidinow, 'Some Observations', p. 319; and *Actinotherapy Technique* (1933), pp. 38–9.

98 Russell and Russell, *Ultra-violet Radiation*, p. 116.

99 They specified: 'It is impracticable to standardize technique in terms of minutes and inches, in view of the number of variant factors. So far as any indications for exposure are given here, e.g., on the Erythema Chart, they should be understood as referring to a patient with an average skin reaction and to a Standard Alpine Sun burner (A.C. type, or D.C. at 200–250 volts) of 1932 type which has been used not more than 100 hours.' *Actinotherapy Technique* (1933), p. 33. It was critical of the chart format in later editions, following dosage standardisation from Coblentz's studies: 'Makers of lamps sometimes provide "erythema charts" … which can be quite useful as affording an initial reference point in

dosage ... but two words of warning are needed regarding their use. Firstly, the "erythema" standard adopted must be some arbitrary physical amount; it may correspond to what will actually produce a first degree reaction on your first patient 24 hours after exposure, but is more likely to be based on the standard adopted by the Council on Physical Therapy of the American Medical Association [...] Secondly, see that any "erythema chart" you use applies actually to the make *and* the type *and* the year of manufacture for the lamp you are using. With these things in mind, you can adapt your chart to suit your cases *individually*.' Italics original. *Actinotherapy Technique* (Slough: Sollux, 1943), pp. 45–6.

100 Finsen, *Phototherapy*, pp. 62, 71.

101 'Dosage of Sunlight: Essential Moderation', *Times* supplement, p. xviii.

102 C. B. Heald, 'The Present Position of Ultra-violet Light Therapy', *BMJ*, 19 January 1929, pp. 94–7, at p. 95.

103 Italics mine. Russell and Russell, *Ultra-violet Radiation*, p. 150.

104 Russell and Russell, *Ultra-violet Radiation*, p. 150.

105 When discussing individual erythematic variations, practitioners included only those (implicitly white) patients considered 'normally' photosensitive, not those considered abnormally photosensitive. Hyper-photosensitivity could be due to a variety of causes, including albinism, vitiligo, and photo-sensitising diseases such as smallpox (variola), measles, or scarlet fever. See Beaumont, *Fundamental Principles*, p. 15.

106 Sir Henry Gauvain, 'Reflections on Sun Treatment: The Theory of Varying Stimuli and Varying Response', *Practitioner*, 132 (February 1934), 1–12, at p. 6–7.

107 Christopher Lawrence, 'Still Incommunicable: Clinical Holists and Medical Knowledge in Interwar Britain', in Christopher Lawrence and George Weisz (eds), *Greater than the Parts: Holism in Biomedicine, 1920–1950* (Oxford: Oxford University Press, 1998), pp. 94–111, at p. 105.

108 Christopher Lawrence and George Weisz, 'Introduction', in Christopher Lawrence and George Weisz (eds), *Greater than the Parts: Holism in Biomedicine, 1920–1950* (Oxford: Oxford University Press, 1998), pp. 1–22, at p. 1.

109 Lawrence and Weisz, 'Introduction', p. 4. They add, 'holism is essentially relational [...] [W]hat is holistic for one individual is frequently perceived as reductionist by another' (p. 2). On Cawadias, see David Cantor, 'The Name and the Word: Neo-Hippocratism and Language in Interwar Britain', in David Cantor (ed.), *Reinventing Hippocrates* (Aldershot: Ashgate, 2002), pp. 280–301. See also Cawadias, 'Ultra-violet Irradiation: Technique of Application', p. 225.

110 David Cantor, 'The Diseased Body', in Roger Cooter and John Pickstone (eds), *Medicine in the Twentieth Century* (Amsterdam: Harwood Academic Publishers, 2000), pp. 347–66, at p. 349. Carter, for example, has discussed heliotherapy in relation to holism, see Simon Carter, *Rise and Shine: Sunlight, Technology and Health* (New York and Oxford: Berg, 2007), pp. 65–70.

111 Gauvain, 'Organisation and Work of a Light Department', p. 13. See also Jamieson, 'An Intolerable Affliction', pp. 134–5.

112 Auguste Rollier, 'The Share of the Sun in the Prevention and Treatment of Tuberculosis', *BMJ*, 21 October 1922, pp. 741–5, at p. 742. See also Auguste Rollier, *Le Pansement solaire: héliothérapie de certaines affections chirurgicales et des blessures de guerre* (Lausanne and Paris: Librairie Payot & Cie., 1916), pp. 8, 70–1; William Palmer Lucas, 'Heliotherapy: Its General Use in Pediatrics', *Archives of Pediatrics*, April 1920, pp. 193–213, at p. 204; and Carter, *Rise and Shine*, p. 59.

113 Michel Foucault, *Discipline and Punish: The Birth of the Prison*, trans. A. Sheridan (London: Penguin, 1991), p. 184. Also cited in Jonathan Crary, *Techniques of the Observer: On Vision and Modernity in the Nineteenth Century* (Cambridge, Mass.: MIT Press, 1999), p. 147.
114 Note the conflation of 'sunburn' and 'erythema' by Hill: 'Axel Reyn is in favour of the production of erythema as a part of sun treatment, and ... Rollier and Gauvain are against any grade of sunburn.' Hill, *Sunshine and Open Air*, p. 94.
115 Hill, *Sunshine and Open Air*, p. 99; and Eidinow, 'Some Observations', p. 317.
116 See Blum, 'Sunlight and Cancer of the Skin', p. 412.
117 See the Cancer Research UK website: www.sunsmart.org.uk/advice-and-prevention/sunburn/ (accessed 24 August 2013).
118 www.cancerresearchuk.org/cancer-help/about-cancer/cancer-questions/can-a-tan-help-prevent-skin-cancer (accessed 24 August 2013).
119 www.bad.org.uk/site/1223/Default.aspx (accessed 6 November 2013); www.bad.org.uk/desktopDefault.aspx?TabId=718 (accessed 6 November 2013).
120 See Paolo Vecchia, Maila Hietanen, Bruce E. Stuck, Emilie van Deventer, and Shengli Nui, 'Protecting Workers from Ultraviolet Radiation', International Commission on Non-Ionizing Radiation Protection (ICNIRP) (with the International Labour Organziation [ILO] and the World Health Organisation [WHO]), ICNIRP 14/2007, p. 20: www.who.int/uv/publications/Protecting_Workers_UV_pub.pdf (accessed 5 August 2013).
121 I learnt this by speaking to a large group of phototherapy nurses following my paper, 'The History of Phototherapy and the "Kiss of Light" Exhibition', at the South-East of England Phototherapy Network's 21st Update Meeting, St Thomas' Hospital, 15 October 2015. During the Q&A we discussed the ongoing difficulty and subjectivity of identifying gradations of erythema production, especially in relation to different skin tones.

3

Light registers

> The existence of invisible radiation beyond the limit of the visible spectrum … came to be termed 'actinic' or 'chemical' rays, as they were supposed to be necessary before chemical reactions could take place. […] The light given out by burning magnesium (photographic 'flash powder') also causes explosive combination, as this light is very rich in actinic or short wave rays. A similar effect is produced by a mercury vapour lamp.[1]
>
> (Eleanor H. Russell and William K. Russell, 1925)

> Light is not a passive agent of revelation in photography but a variable force through which representations are made.[2]
>
> (Melissa Miles, 2008)

Of all of the elements unusual and compelling in a photograph of the South London Hospital for Women and Children (SLHWC), taken around 1934 by Austrian émigré photographer and Comintern agent Edith Tudor-Hart (née Suschitzky, 1908–73), to me the most striking is the simple fact that the photograph *exists* (Fig. 3.1). Printed for the first time from Tudor-Hart's secret archive for the recent retrospective exhibition, *Edith Tudor-Hart: In the Shadow of Tyranny* (Edinburgh, Vienna and Berlin, 2013–14), the image had only previously been an unseen and unused negative. It was one of at least two she made of the phototherapy facilities at the hospital (Fig. 3.2), part of a commission she undertook alongside fellow émigré photographer Grete Stern to illustrate the beneficent work of the institution for a 1935 fund-raising pamphlet. While Figure 3.2 was printed to be reproduced in the pamphlet and put on display at the hospital, Figure 3.1 mysteriously did not make the cut.[3]

Beautiful and eerie, the composition cleverly presents an otherwise resistant subject for the photographer: open arc phototherapy in process. The rich actinic light of a large, suspended carbon arc lamp was employed for general (full body) use on local children. Unlike the Finsen lamp, which focused and channelled the carbon arc's

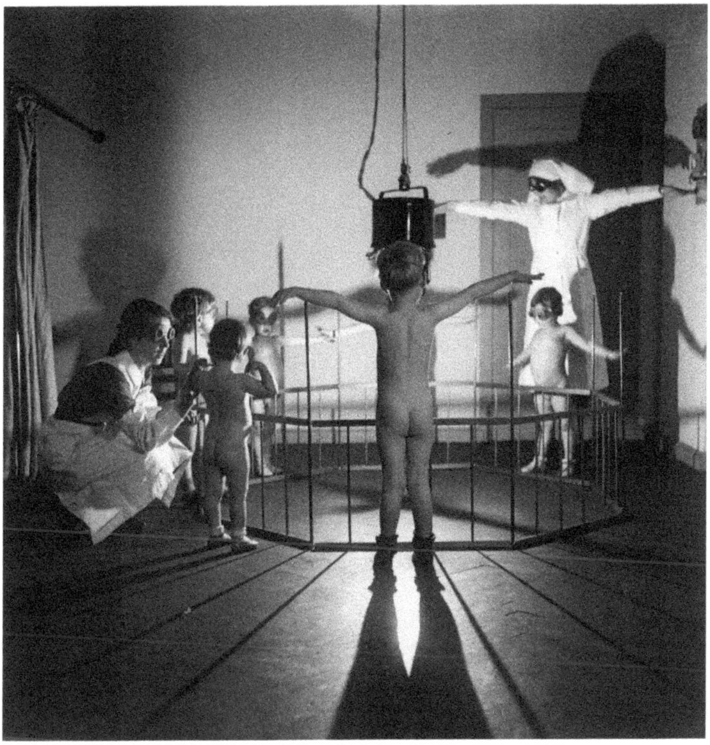

Figure 3.1 Edith Tudor-Hart, *Ultraviolet Light Treatment, South London Hospital for Women and Children*, c. 1934.
Modern silver gelatin print, 30.3 × 30.0 cm.
Wolfgang Suschitzky and Scottish National Portrait Gallery, Edinburgh. Presented by Wolfgang Suschitzky, 2004.

actinic light through telescopic arms and quartz lenses for a local (lesion-specific) exposure, this carbon arc lamp's open flame emanated unfiltered in all directions. Figure 3.1 depicts the treatment taking place, as was usual, in a darkened, enclosed interior space, the curtains and door shut and overhead lighting switched off. The children encircled the lamp behind a fixed railing, which marked off the correct distance from the lamp for the exposure, and playfully opened their arms to its actinic light. They did so guided by nurses, as much to entertain them during these exposures – which could last from several minutes up to two hours – as to maximise the surface area of their exposed skin to the lamp. The photograph presents the lamp slightly off-centre in the composition, yet the real focus is the largest of the six children undergoing ultraviolet exposure, whose arms gracefully interlace in the photograph with the shadows of the child opposite him, and whose body takes centre

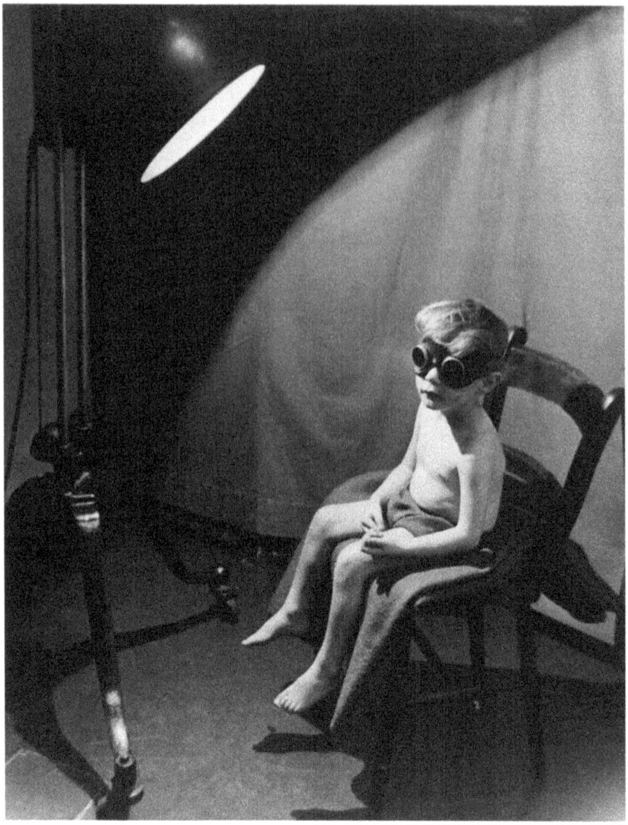

Figure 3.2 Edith Tudor-Hart, *Treatment by Ultraviolet Rays*, c. 1934.
In *The South London Hospital for Women and Children* (Birmingham: Kynoch Press, 1935), p. 16. Wolfgang Suschitzky and the London Metropolitan Archives, London.

stage. It is important that it does so, because the child acted a shield, or screen, for Tudor-Hart's camera and its photosensitive film. By positioning herself behind this child, her medium format Rolleiflex camera held at waist height, Tudor-Hart produced a legible negative under exceptionally difficult lighting circumstances.[4] A few centimetres off and the emanating actinic light of the lamp would have overexposed the film, 'injuring' the negative and thus ruining the shot.

Tudor-Hart was a professional photographer known for her technical adroitness, including her ability to control lighting.[5] But even professionals struggled to take legible photographs of phototherapy in process.[6] Her photograph is unusual in its handling of the light; while several photographs exist with this composition, where the photographer's camera was placed behind a patient-'screen', rarely are they so well lit – or so expertly printed, I suspect – without succumbing to overexposure or dramatic silhouettes (Figs. 3.3–3.4).[7] Note, for example, the back of the central child in a photograph reproduced in Victor Dane's *The Sunlight Cure* of open arc phototherapy at an unspecified London hospital (Fig. 3.3). Here the back of the child is engulfed in blackness, presenting a striking silhouette, because the only lighting in the room was produced by the arc lamp itself. We find the same in Figure 3.4, of the Institute of Ray Therapy in Camden, but whereas the photographer has managed to use one child's arm as a shield for the arc lamp on the left, the glaring actinic light of the second arc lamp has evaded its shield and burnt the sensitive film to the point of producing a 'black sun'.

By contrast, additional lighting must have been present out of shot in Tudor-Hart's version (Fig. 3.1), allowing the backs of the children in the foreground to be discernible and thus a more evenly lit overall image, whether by additional lamps or possibly through the use of a flash. However, the primary light enabling the negative to be imprinted in this dark interior – and thus for this photograph to exist at all as a

Figure 3.3 'Children receiving sunlight treatment in a London hospital.'
In Victor Dane, *The Sunlight Cure* (London: Athletic Publications, 1929), unpaginated plate. Wellcome Library, London.

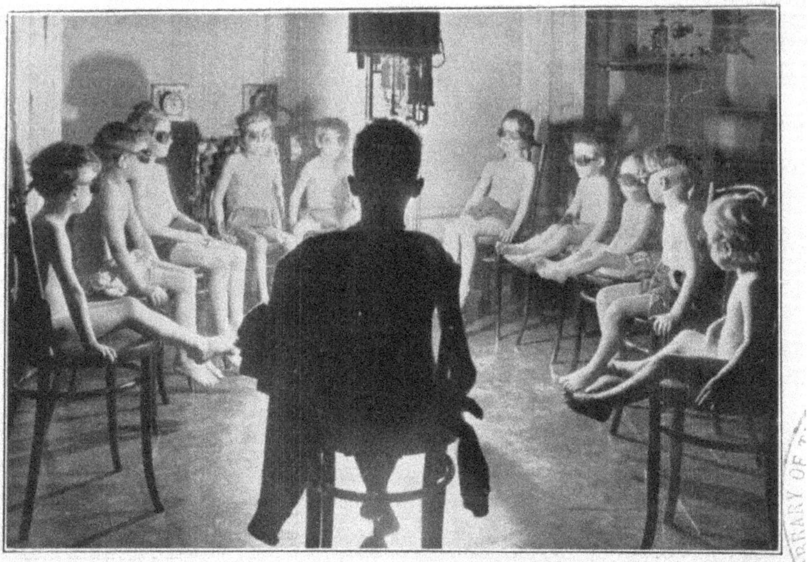

Children receiving sunlight treatment in a London hospital.

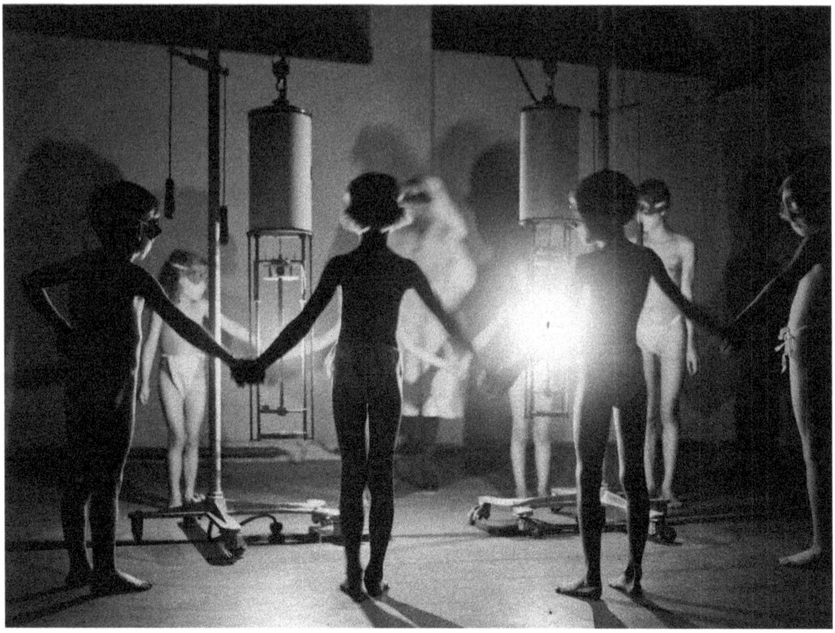

Figure 3.4 'Ray Therapy' [Institute for Ray Therapy, Camden], undated (*c.* 1930s).
Hulton Archive, Fox Photos/Getty Images.

legible print – was, like Figs. 3.3 and 3.4, that of the carbon arc lamp, and only under carefully controlled mediation by the photographer.

In Chapter 2, I opened my discussion with a reproduction of Niels Finsen's photographed forearm, a photograph that represents the researcher's sensitive sunburnt skin as a testing ground to visually analyse the effects of actinic light, especially those rays invisible to the human eye: the ultraviolet rays (Fig. 2.1). In that chapter I made it clear that although Finsen's skin appeared to have acted as a satisfactory register for the solar erythema test – to himself and other practitioners influenced by his work – the photograph (and its reproductions) attempting to represent and disseminate the results failed to convey them legibly. This obscurity of the photograph prompted me to consider the solar erythema itself as an uncooperative, highly transitory, and highly individualised physiological phenomenon that resisted being 'fixed' by practitioners in order to enable clear dosage standardisation. I used the specific phrase 'Finsen's photographed forearm' in reference to Figure 2.1 in two distinct but fundamentally interrelated ways: both to mean Finsen's sunburnt arm and the actual photograph of it. As photosensitive surfaces, both the subject and its material representation act as latent *light registers* and can be understood literally as 'photo-graphs'; that is, as 'written' or produced by light.[8]

Throughout the present chapter I discuss the frequent analogies made by light therapists between photographs and skin, and perceptions of the resemblances between photography and light therapy as 'light technologies': technologies that both depended upon light as a source in order to function. Their similar photochemical operations would make them appear at first to be natural bedfellows. Certainly it seemed this way to practitioners, who looked to photographic processes and larger developments in photochemistry in order to understand how and why light therapy worked on patients. This is evident in the epigraph above, by Drs Eleanor H. Russell and William K. Russell, who made a direct analogy between the actinic light of flash photography and that of phototherapy.

In Section I of this chapter I explore this alliance, but in Section II, I want to tease out the tensions in what came to be an uneasy, incestuous relationship between photography and light therapy, between the visualising and therapeutic powers of light. This was especially the case with phototherapy, a therapy that relied upon artificial light originally intended for electric lighting; in other words, for vision. Tudor-Hart's negative, newly available as a positive printed for public view, presents light therapy with exceptional delicacy and skill, in which the treatment appears as a highly controlled, well-managed, and technologically progressive practice of bodily exposure to actinic light. The control or management of this powerful actinic light was only further emphasised and validated by the fact that the photograph of the therapeutic process was equally in control of that light. Because of what it is and what it represents, Figure 3.1 offers itself as evidence of both phototherapy and photography skilfully controlling the 'injurious' light rays that quickly blinded eyes and burnt skin and film.

But what of the historic photographs that do not wholly contain this blinding, burning therapeutic light, what can they communicate about light therapy? Submerged in archival folders throughout the UK are numerous 'bad' photographs of light therapy, injured with photographic accidents known as 'artefacts': 'black suns', engulfing masses, and legible splays of white light visibly mark numerous overexposed photographs, the results of lens flare and 'solarisation'. The latter, in which extreme overexposure produces reversals of light and dark in the photograph, is a particularly relevant word here since it was a synonym for light therapy itself. In her 2008 book, *The Burning Mirror*, Melissa Miles reconceptualises these 'accidents' as productive and instructive examples of light's volatility in the history of photography – of light not as an agent of truth, revelation, and 'enlightenment' but as a blinding, excessive, and immaterial force. Throughout this chapter I defer to Miles's work to understand the complex relationship between actinic light's therapeutic and visualising powers in the intertwined histories of light therapy, photography, and electric lighting. Like the previous chapters, I continually return to Figure 3.1 as a poignant visual representation and material object driving my argument: that light therapy was encountered and represented photographically as an *obscure* (literally 'dark', unclear, or unknown) practice, in which these light technologies do not so much converge as collide.

I Material convergences

As Tanya Sheehan demonstrated in *Doctored*, the close relationship between light therapy and photography began early on in the nineteenth century. She argued they were both perceived as agents of social and physical health, focusing specifically on blue-light therapy and commercial photography studios in mid-nineteenth-century Philadelphia. Sheehan discussed the experiments of General Augustus Pleasonton, who analysed the effects of coloured lights on the growth of grapes and pigs during the 1860s. He reported that blue light, emitted through panes of blue glass, was far more stimulating to vegetative and animal growth than ordinary, clear glass. In his 1872 patent application, Pleasonton claimed similar beneficial, rejuvenating effects for humans using blue glass. According to Sheehan, these claims initiated a blue glass 'craze' in Philadelphia in the 1870s and 1880s. She noted that contemporaneous photographers perceived their sky-lit studios as physically and psychologically beneficial spaces for their sitters and workers, and they equally incorporated panes of frosted blue glass for their pleasing light effects on the sitters' complexions in photographs. Her chapter discussed the fascinating correspondences and 'material resemblance' between Pleasonton's blue-light therapy (what she termed 'phototherapy') and studio portrait photography using blue glass, between 'two technologies of light'.[9] Indeed, she even argued that beyond mere similarity these two technologies converged, in which this kind of photography 'emerged as a powerful phototherapy' in its rehabilitating social powers.[10]

Like Sheehan, I view the relationship between photography and phototherapy as more than a 'material resemblance' between two light technologies. If, for Sheehan, studio photography using blue light acted as a kind of social 'phototherapy', for me phototherapy acted as a kind of excessive, risky form of photography – a blinding, burning practice of 'light writing'.[11] This relationship came to be less one of material resemblance or even material convergence than a material *collision*. Pleasonton's blue-light therapy was but one of many, international examples of light therapy correlating to photography's practices and its technical processes. As a light technology, it was born not simply from older medical practices but out of technologies bound up with vision. For light therapy, and especially phototherapy, to emerge fully in the 1890s, two technologies needed to be embedded within the sciences (broadly here encompassing physics, chemistry, engineering, and medicine), and both of them were fundamentally tied to the visual: photography and electric lighting. Actinic light took centre stage in the intertwined histories of photography, electric lighting, and therapies utilising the wavelengths of the electromagnetic spectrum. As Kelley Wilder made clear,

> photography's real calling card is its reputation for widening the scope of what could be observed by the eye. Ultraviolet radiation, called variously the chemical spectrum and the actinic spectrum, formed the basis of nineteenth-century photography. When it was found that photography was also sensitive to a whole host of other 'invisible' radiation in the 1890s, the discovery did no more than reinforce Talbot's opinion, written in 1844, that 'the eye of the camera would see plainly where the human eye would find nothing but darkness'.[12]

As I explain in the next chapter, this 'darkness' or optical invisibility led to vanguard techniques of representation, particularly montage, to visualise these invisible, therapeutic, and risky rays.

This is not to suggest that photography, as a light technology, did not possess its own tensions and ambiguities as a major form of representation for the sciences. As numerous historians of photography have asserted, through its claims to objectivity as a so-called unmediated and passive mechanical tool, photography gained tremendous authority as a medium for scientific observation, dissemination, and experimentation despite overt awareness of its faults.[13] The uneven photosensitivity of emulsions to certain light wavelengths over others,[14] and the reliance on 'doctoring' or retouching negatives to correct errors are two significant examples.[15] Photography's limitations as a visualising medium are especially resonant by studying 'bad' photographs of light therapy, but they are certainly not exclusive to this medical treatment or to medical photography in general during the nineteenth or early twentieth centuries. As a medical treatment that relied primarily on photography to document and disseminate its efficacy, light therapy was like any other therapy of its day. It was exceptional, however, because actinic light was the source of the cure *and* the means to its visual representation. In this respect it bears close similarity to X rays, which were used almost immediately upon discovery, in 1895, as both a therapy (radiotherapy) and a diagnostic tool (radiology). The visualising and therapeutic capacities of light collapse onto each other in light therapy literature through the practitioner's scientific knowledge of light's generative, transformative role in photography. The more we think about this odd convergence, the stranger it becomes: imagine, by analogy, if the history of hydrotherapy was primarily encountered through archival images made with watercolours. Pushing the analogy further, imagine if hydrotherapists formulated their theories about the therapeutic efficacy of water based on their understanding of watercolour painting, its techniques and material processes.

In this sense, any photograph we find of or about light therapy could be said to present this convergence: it is a visualisation simultaneously *of* and *with* actinic rays.[16] But, as is evident by looking carefully at Figure 3.1, the photographer faced significant difficulties when attempting to represent light therapy. That practitioners continued to rely on photography despite these difficulties of representation says as much about photography's authority as it does about its limitations as a medium. This collision of light technologies occurred at the juncture where the *therapeutic* utilisation of light exceeded the possibilities of its utilisation to *visualise*. Put another way, the blinding powers of actinic light were reconfigured and expanded for therapeutic purpose at the expense of photographic representation. When these technologies came together – when photography was called upon in the service of phototherapy – their volatile interaction resulted, more commonly than not, in photographic accidents and representations of technological failure of one or both media: we encounter images in which the delicate photosensitivity of the camera's film, badly injured, could not legibly represent the lamp's burning light (photography's failure), while legible photographic representations exist by means of manipulation and fakery, of patients standing around an unlit lamp (phototherapy's failure). Even in rare instances of photographic success, like Figure 3.1, our access to the therapeutic process remains obscured. And so we begin, like the occupants in Tudor-Hart's photograph, in darkness: in the darkroom.

The dark room

Pleasonton's blue-light therapy was not, within the history of medicine, defined as 'phototherapy' (artificial light therapy) but rather referred to as chromotherapy or colour therapy, and for practitioners Pleasonton was perceived as an early pioneer in the therapeutic benefits of visible, coloured light.[17] As outlined in previous chapters, the historical narrative of phototherapy proper is bound up with Finsen in the 1890s.

Finsen's experiments with light began during the early 1890s through an observation of its negative influence on variola, also known as smallpox.[18] He discovered that if the patient was placed in a room totally devoid of all but red light within the first stages of smallpox, known as the stage of vesiculation or blistering of the skin, the disease did not develop into the stage of suppuration (in which pus would discharge from the small blisters). By doing so, the patient could heal with little or no scarring. It therefore was not a cure, per se, but a method of managing the illness and minimising risk, including complications and fatalities, at a time when smallpox vaccination was not yet fully widespread throughout Europe. To carry out the treatment he created a room where all the windows were covered with thick, red cloth or a dense red glass, to filter out all but the red rays. He stated in an 1895 article in the *BMJ* that,

> The exclusion of the chemical rays must be absolute; even a brief exposure to daylight may produce suppuration and its sequelae. In other words, the skin during small-pox is as susceptible to daylight as a photographic plate, and must be kept from the chemical rays in the same way and almost as carefully.[19]

As Finsen made clear, red-light therapy operated according to knowledge gained from photographic practices. The patient's skin was as photosensitive to actinic light as a photographic plate. His treatment room, consequently, emulated a darkroom. He made sure the conditions were right before allowing his patients to enter by hanging a photographic plate in the centre of the room.[20] Any blackening of the emulsion on the plate indicated actinic light was somewhere filtering into the room and therefore it was not safe for patients to enter.[21] Perhaps unsurprisingly, I have been unable to find photographs of the process. Such conditions purposely excluded the possibility of photographs being taken or subsequently developed, the light enabling photographic impressions a risk to the equally photosensitive skin of his smallpox patients. Instead, Finsen included in that 1895 article only a 'before' photograph, of a patient in the stage of vesiculation, and a chart of her temperature fluctuations to mark the progress of the disease. No 'after' photograph was provided, only a reassuring text to explain that, following red-light treatment, the patient recovered. This is an overt and early example of light therapy being encountered as an 'obscure' practice: it was a short-lived therapy, vaccination rendering it redundant; it was carried out in the dark; and, as a result, no visual representations of it appear to exist.

The knowledge gained from the darkroom, however, did not pass into oblivion. As Edwin Ash wrote in *Facts about Artificial Sunlight*, in 1925:

> One can always remember how it is the violet or red series of rays which have most active chemical properties by calling to mind that the photographer works with a red lamp. This gives him just enough light to see by, whilst the red rays do not appreciably influence the sensitive films he exposes to them.[22]

Modelling their treatments on photographic practices provided lessons to light therapy practitioners about the physiological action of light as well as its psychological actions. Finsen noted the difficulty of continually excluding the injurious rays to his darkroom, explaining that nurses as much as patients desired to fling open the curtains for their own mental well-being.[23] Further direct references to photographic darkrooms and developing processes relayed the perceived psychological effects of coloured light rays. There are multiple, international references in light-therapy literature to the photographic factory in Lyon of the famous Lumière brothers, who reported that their workers became very agitated, excited, and disruptive after extended periods in darkrooms illuminated by red light. Thomas Nogier, in his 1904 medical dissertation, *La Lumière et la vie*, described the workers as displaying 'all the symptoms of an abnormal cerebral excitement: they talked, gesticulated, sung and… manifested in their actions a certain bawdiness that harmed the good [working] order of the factory'.[24] Earlier, in 1898, Dr Léon Bouchacourt stated that red lighting was especially excitable to women in this situation, causing 'incessant disputes'. He explained that it was only by substituting 'ruby' red lighting for a 'cathedral' green that calm was restored – as if by 'enchantment' – to the factory, claiming that one of the Lumière brothers had asserted this to him directly.[25] This well-known case was cited for decades by several international light therapists, including British practitioners.[26]

Finsen also experimented with the biological effects of coloured light on the growth of living things such as tadpoles and insects, and he knew of Pleasonton's experiments with blue glass (though professed little confidence in Pleasonton's blue-light therapy).[27] When projecting beams onto these creatures he lapsed into the vocabulary of photography, discussing a focused beam of actinic light as a 'luminous pencil'.[28] Returning to Finsen's photographed forearm (Fig. 2.1), it becomes evident that this experiment, in which he glued various coloured glasses to his arm and then exposed it to actinic light in order to test the glasses' transmitting properties, was but one of many he conducted in the 1890s with coloured light to understand its physiological effects on the animal world. I am fascinated that physicians looked to practices adopted within photography as models for direct application in light therapy. These darkrooms and photographic factories served unwittingly as testing grounds for phototherapy, on par with laboratories like the MRC's Hampstead institute, the NIMR (Chapter 2), providing evidence of light's chemical and physiological effects.

The chemistry of light

Like other physicians and scientists, Finsen knew that the red light of the spectrum was the weakest in terms of concentrated chemical (actinic) action. Red light is furthest on the spectrum from blue, violet, and ultraviolet light, which are highest in chemical as well as bactericidal action. The naturally bactericidal powers of sunlight had been known since the late 1870s, primarily from the experiments of Arthur Downes and Thomas Blunt in 1877 on the destructive action of actinic light on bacteria.[29] However, awareness of its lethal action on bacteria was not the only influence on the earliest experiments with and hypotheses about the 'injurious' rays' therapeutic application. Nor can these origins of light therapy be solely attributed to Finsen. Dr Theobald Palm, a medical missionary trained in Edinburgh and stationed in Japan between 1874 and 1884, cited Downes and Blunt at length in an 1890 article, but he also spoke of photography and developments in photochemistry as explanations to substantiate his belief that rickets could be cured by the systematic use of sunbaths (heliotherapy):

> I would now urge that the physiological and therapeutic actions of sunlight have hitherto met with too scanty recognition, and that though our knowledge of them is at present vague, it is sufficient to warrant the belief that careful study of them would lead to valuable results. The study of the Chemistry of Light as regards inorganic compounds has led to the marvels of photography, and the effect of light in organic chemistry must be still more full of interesting facts.[30]

Palm's direct reference to the 'chemistry of light', and particularly its capitalisation, would strongly suggest a citation to the well-known photographer and photochemist Hermann Wilhelm Vogel's 1875 book, *The Chemistry of Light and Photography*.[31] Vogel (1834–89) contributed greatly to developments in photography, researching dye sensitisation that led to new emulsions, inventing instruments such as an improved photometer and spectroscope, and even teaching Alfred Stieglitz in the early 1880s. Vogel's research on the 'chemistry of light' (photochemistry) was directly cited by light therapists well into the twentieth century.[32]

The sun's ability to blacken silver salts was discovered in 1725 by anatomy professor Johann Heinrich Schulze and confirmed in the 1770s by Swedish apothecary Carl Wilhelm Scheele.[33] The experiments by German chemist Johann Wilhelm Ritter clarified that it was the invisible, ultraviolet rays of the spectrum that had the most chemical effect, using paper coated with silver chloride in a dark room, following the earlier research of botanist Jean Senebier in 1782.[34] Ritter is credited with discovering ultraviolet rays in 1801, one year after Sir William Herschel discovered the infrared rays. Like Wilhelm Röntgen (X rays) and Henri Becquerel (gamma rays) almost 100 years later, these invisible ultraviolet rays were first detected and discovered by photographic action.[35] Photography's ability to detect invisible phenomena, and specifically wavelengths on the electromagnetic spectrum invisible to the human eye, proved an invaluable resource for scientists. Simultaneously, photography's ability to visualise and, through photographic reproduction, to disseminate data on that phenomena doubly served the sciences.[36] This is exemplified by the contemporaneous growth of spectroscopy as a field.

Spectroscopy emerged, according to Klaus Hentschel, as a visual culture that came to dominate the sciences from the late nineteenth century onwards, in part because of the use of photography to aid it visualising and measuring the electromagnetic spectrum.[37] Spectroscopes, alongside various models of photometers (actinometers, actinographs, heliographs, etc.), were equally relied upon by light therapists, who mention it frequently when discussing natural and artificial light intensities.[38] Spectrum photographs sprinkle light therapy texts and, as Hentschel and Wilder

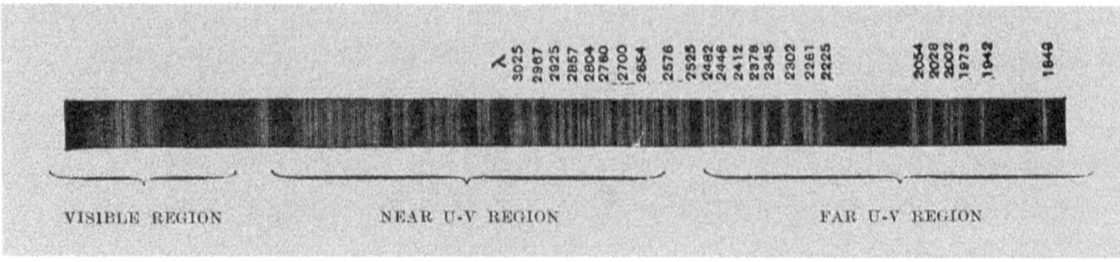

Figure 3.5 'Spectrogram showing part of the visible and ultra-violet regions.'
In Eleanor H. Russell and William K. Russell, *Ultra-violet Radiation and Actinotherapy* (Edinburgh: E. & S. Livingstone, 1925), Figure 4, p. 38. Author's collection.

both noted, highly specialised knowledge was required in order to interpret or 'read' them (Fig. 3.5). Like Finsen's photographed forearm (Fig. 2.1) these photographs were impenetrable to the ordinary viewer. Looking at the images together, they present important similarities. Beyond any visual resemblance of what is pictured as various kinds of vertical bars or lines, we are looking at layers of *light registers.*[39]

Light registers

When American physicist Henry Augustus Rowland published his impressive spectrum photograph, *Photographic Map of the Normal Solar Spectrum*, in the late 1880s, he described it as follows: 'The photograph is the work of the sunlight itself and the user of this map has the solar spectrum itself before him.'[40] A veritable self-portrait of the sun, the spectrum photograph is a representation *of* light rays made *with* light rays, just as Figure 2.1 acts as a light register (photograph) of a light register (sunburnt forearm). In this sense it also presents layers of authorships and subjects: it a photograph of Finsen, by Finsen, but also of, and by, actinic light.

The notion of the sun as the photograph's rightful author is historically traceable back to the very inception of photography. Corey Keller explained:

> The metaphor most widely used to characterize the photographic process was that of nature 'drawing her own picture' – a peculiar rhetorical construct that implies an unmediated translation of the natural world into a self-generated representation, removing any notion of authorship. As such, the photograph could be understood as replicating and standing in for the scientific specimen rather than merely representing it.[41]

Miles added that, 'As the sun was designated the true author, photography's prints could be deemed as trustworthy as fingerprints.'[42] This belief in the photograph as a direct trace or referent of the subject explains its historic (and ongoing) status as a faithful and true document, but this could be said of any photograph. Something different, something more, is happening in the photographs of sunburnt skin scattered throughout light-therapy texts (Figs. 2.1–2.3, 2.13). In their 'material resemblance' as photochemically active surfaces, photograph and skin are separate layers of light registers but here collapse onto each other; not simply index and subject, they are conceptually one and the same.

Devices for light registration make obvious this conflation of photograph and skin. Some measuring devices relied upon a comparison between photographic paper and the skin's erythema production to measure actinic light (see Chapter 2). The Russells explained they used 'printing-out paper', which they exposed for different lengths of time to a light source and then compared the various 'tints' to measure light intensities.[43] The same method is used to produce a photographic test strip in a darkroom when developing a positive from a negative, ensuring the ideal exposure time. As explained in the last chapter, Saidman's 'sensitometric test' was a clockwork mechanism with progressive timed openings, pressed against the patient's abdomen, which measured how rapidly the skin reacted to actinic light (Figs. 2.12–2.13). In doing so, Saidman used the patient's skin itself as a photographic test strip in order find the correct 'dose' of light for the patient. These gradations of erythematous markings on the flesh were measured and, furthermore, photographed – a register of a register, like Finsen's photographed forearm.

In looking at these photographs of sunburnt skin, we encounter separate layers of light registers or, as Sophia Zweifel discussed in relation to the French psychoanalyst Didier Anzieu's writings on the 'skin-ego', layers of 'pellicules'. A pellicule is a thin membrane or 'skin' enveloping parts of plants and animal organisms, such as the skins of an onion, but it also is used to mean photographic film, onto which the photosensitive emulsion is coated.[44] Zweifel, analysing the early visual culture of radiology, asserted that the layers of skin displaced by the process of irradiating the body with X rays are reconstituted onto the photographic film of the radiograph itself (Chapter 4). For light therapists, the receptivity of the skin to light and that of photographic media was more than a metaphorical connection; it was literal.[45]

NIMR researchers Albert Eidinow and Sir Leonard Hill had relied upon spectroscopy to measure light intensity and dosages, but they found the process 'tedious', preferring to measure intensities and dosages by erythema (sunburn) production.[46] Underpinning light therapy as a medical treatment was the fundamental notion that the skin is a natural photometer for detecting and measuring actinic light. Eidinow noted the crucial similarities between skin and photographic plates:

> The normal white skin is sensitive to ultra-violet rays from 2,970 to 2,500 A.U., and this sensitiveness is comparable to the effect of visible rays on the

> photographic light sensitive plate. There is, in all probability, some photobiochemical effect produced, which controls these reactions, which are typically characteristic of light erythema.[47]

But for Eidinow the skin's erythema production triumphed over both spectroscopic and photographic readings of light – measuring either intensities or varieties of wavelengths emitted from a particular source – because it provided evidence of the light's physiological (termed 'biological') effects.[48] This was the only reason that measuring light was useful to the physician, in Eidinow's mind. What good was it, after all, for a physician to measure light if not for therapeutic application? His belief only served to confer more authority and dependence upon the solar erythema as the main light registration 'system' for practitioners (Chapter 2). Put simply, the sunburnt skin *was* the photograph. It superseded photography and rendered photographic registration redundant, at least as a form of measurement. Eidinow, and other British practitioners who guided their practice according to erythema production, clearly still relied upon photography as a form of representation and would push this light technology to its limits in the pursuit of medical progress.

The complicated convergence of aesthetic and therapeutic light occurs in other photographs of light therapy, not only those presenting sunburnt skin. In the 1901 English translation of his book, *Phototherapy*, Finsen included several plates of his patients and described them as evidence of light therapy's good effects on patients (see also Fig. 2.4). His many before and after photographs of lupus vulgaris patients may *obscure* the therapeutic process – it is visually absent, merely implied in the spaces between the two photographs – but once again viewers are presented with images produced of and about actinic light. Like other medical and scientific researchers of his time, Finsen had no issue exploiting the 'slippery' nature of photography: he used photography both to explain photochemical processes, for therapeutic application, and to act as a recording device for his results with actinic light.[49]

The same might be said of any of the light-therapy facilities known to have numerous photographers and darkrooms on site, producing photographs and radiographs: the famous Swiss heliotherapist Dr Auguste Rollier's sanatoria in Leysin; the Royal London Hospital's Light Department; and the British light therapy sanatorium, the Lord Mayor Treloar Hospital for Crippled Children in Hampshire, where hand-held cameras were apparently in abundance (see Chapter 1 on these institutions).[50] Treloar's archives additionally contain several reprints of the same image in various states of light intensities and quality, suggesting the nurses or even the patients practised developing prints in its darkroom using negatives about light therapy.[51] These images depict photography as a representational (aesthetic) tool absorbed into daily practice at the light clinic, for medical purposes and for entertainment.

Electric light

The Finsen lamp is the most well known of historic examples of phototherapy lamps. As an object it marks light therapy's inception as a modern and systematised treatment, first utilised to treat skin diseases (Fig. 2.6). But absent within the secondary literature on the therapy's history, scant as it is, are discussions of the wider context for such an invention. The Finsen light was a modified carbon arc lamp, a form of electric lighting that had been invented at the beginning of the nineteenth century by the British chemist and proto-photographer, Sir Humphry Davy, contemporaneous with his photographic experiments and Ritter's discovery of ultraviolet light.[52] By the mid-nineteenth century the carbon arc was used in welding and to light railway stations, public streets, theatres, and even the low-lit interiors of photographic studios. The carbon arc lamp emitted a brilliant white light in an arch formation when an electrical current was passed between its two rods of carbon, which made it ideal for lighting large public spaces or, when focused with a mirror, for spotlights and searchlights (illuminating distances up to six kilometres).[53]

In his modifications, Finsen's attached focusing devices, channelling the emitting light of the arc into brass telescopic arms that were fitted with quartz lenses.[54] In addition to using pyrogallic acid (a staple in photographic darkrooms[55]) alongside light therapy to treat lupus lesions, Finsen experimented with various lenses, coloured glass, and additional filters, as well as coloured stain solutions applied to the lens in order to absorb heat, again reminiscent of photographic practices.[56] This use of lenses to focus and concentrate sunlight was not without precedent, in optics or medicine. Various references throughout the late eighteenth and the nineteenth centuries exist about physicians who used concentrated sunlight to treat surface lesions.[57] Finsen was perfectly aware of previous experiments to treat lupus vulgaris by focusing lenses, known as 'burning glasses' or 'burning mirrors', as well as contemporaneous cases of physicians using incandescent electric and carbon arc lights therapeutically; he cited them directly in his publications. Focusing natural light through lenses and mirrors to produce intense heat had ancient origins in Archimedes, and during Finsen's time physicians were still attempting to cauterise skin lesions, including tumours, using lenses that concentrated natural and artificial light.[58] Some even designed their lenses using photography equipment, such as filters.[59] Original to Finsen was filtering out the heat rays with blue filters and coatings, concentrating the most chemically active visible rays (blue and violet) and, when using quartz lenses, the ultraviolet rays, in order to destroy tubercle bacilli. As noted above, his point of origin lay in photographic experiments common to the developing field of photochemistry.

The Finsen light was known to be extremely costly to buy and to run, and while Finsen may seem to have been the most famous to employ the carbon arc lamp's output of ultraviolet rays therapeutically – beyond its function to illuminate surroundings – there were other early practitioners who modified his working methods using their own devices. In Britain, Dr J. Alfred Codd, based at the General Hospital at Wolverhampton, explained he had built a home-made ultraviolet lamp to treat a variety of skin conditions, much as physicians would do with X-ray machines.[60] Another of these physicians was Dr Margaret Cleaves, operating out of New York, who described her method of phototherapy using not only lenses like Finsen but also marine searchlights (Fig. 3.6). In her 1904 book, *Light Energy*, an early and massive work of over 800 pages, she explained:

> Marine searchlight [carbon arc] mechanisms of from 20 to 80 ampères, provided with large reflecting mirrors of the Mangin type, projecting the beam upon the patient's body at a distance of from 7 to 15 feet, according to the light intensity, are used to a considerable extent in the United States. [...] The author [herself] has had in use for the past 4 or 5 years such a 25-ampère marine searchlight capable when adjusted on a short focus, of picking up and observing the manoeuvres of a vessel at a distance of one and one-fourth miles.[61]

Figure 3.6 'Marine searchlight, with blue glass screen.'
In Margaret A. Cleaves, *Light Energy* (New York and London: Rebman Company, 1904), Figure 21, opposite p. 478.
Wellcome Library, London.

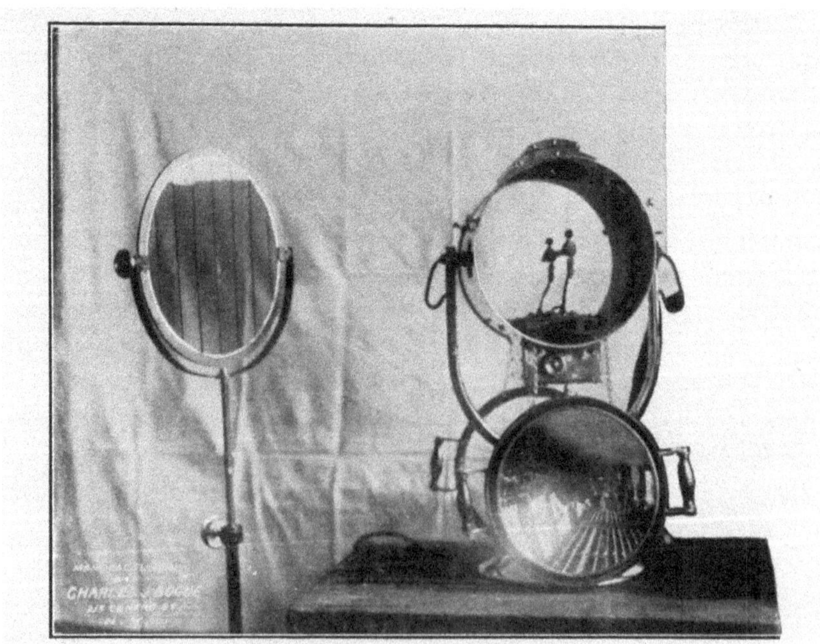

She added that Figure 3.6 showed the lamp with its glass door open, allowing the beneficial ultraviolet rays access to patients' bodies. When open she used the lamp for large surface exposure, for example on patients with pulmonary tuberculosis, aiming it squarely at their chests.[62] When closed, she stated, it could be used as a searchlight. Cleaves further modified her lamp, in collaboration with a manufacturer of marine searchlights, with the creation of an iron funnel that localised the rays onto specific skin lesions, just as Finsen had done with telescopic arms. With her device she treated the skin diseases lupus vulgaris and lupus erythematosus, as Finsen was doing in Denmark, and (ironically) carcinomas.

British practitioners also appropriated searchlights early on for therapeutic use, as evidenced by the catalogues of medical instrument-maker Schall (1905, Fig. 3.7).[63] These examples of modified carbon arc lamps indicate not only that, in its infancy, phototherapy developed out of great and creative experimentation, but also that it was indebted to knowledge of artificial light's abilities first and foremost to visualise and only second to heal.

The modifications by manufacturers and physicians also evince how a light technology intended for use in large, public spaces or at long-range distances was transformed into a new, far more intimate, interior use while still retaining its original function. After all, carbon arc lamps continued to be used for public lighting, theatre lighting, and as searchlight devices into the twentieth century.[64] Even as late as 1923 the Royal Northern Hospital in London reported using discarded carbon arc railway lamps to treat lupus vulgaris patients.[65] Incandescent lighting, made accessible through Thomas Edison's carbon filament light bulb, was also exploited, but for its heat, since it emitted little in the way of actinic light. 'Light cabinets' multiplied and extended the use of the ordinary light bulb by irradiating patients, especially arthritics in need of the analgesic properties of heat, in enclosed boxes of incandescent light. Much later, in 1931, Dr William Beaumont described a modified stage light, also an incandescent filament lamp, that was used for colour therapy (chromotherapy). It had specially designed filters to obtain specific coloured rays for local application.[66] Intriguingly, manufacturers of photographic equipment, such as the Amalgamated Photographic Manufacturers Ltd, also simultaneously produced light-therapy lamps (see Chapter 1).[67] Returning to the United States, the physicist Matthew Luckiesh considered the visualising and therapeutic powers of light to remain intertwined in light technologies' developments. As director of the Light Research Laboratory at General Electric, a company initially started by Thomas Edison, Luckiesh continued to experiment with light for health and for vision.[68]

Both electric lighting and photography operated as visualising media: to see, to picture, to capture, and to know. Aiding and enabling the development of light therapy, these visualising media were appropriated by physicians and researchers

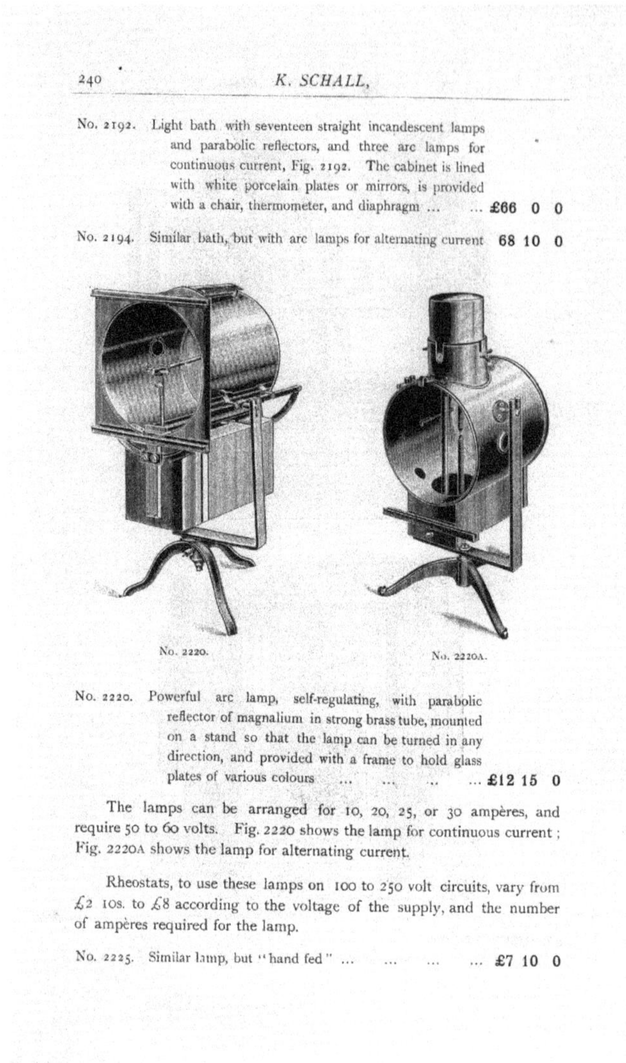

240 *K. SCHALL,*

No. 2192. Light bath with seventeen straight incandescent lamps and parabolic reflectors, and three arc lamps for continuous current, Fig. 2192. The cabinet is lined with white porcelain plates or mirrors, is provided with a chair, thermometer, and diaphragm **£66 0 0**

No. 2194. Similar bath, but with arc lamps for alternating current **68 10 0**

No. 2220. No. 2220A.

No. 2220. Powerful arc lamp, self-regulating, with parabolic reflector of magnalium in strong brass tube, mounted on a stand so that the lamp can be turned in any direction, and provided with a frame to hold glass plates of various colours **£12 15 0**

The lamps can be arranged for 10, 20, 25, or 30 ampères, and require 50 to 60 volts. Fig. 2220 shows the lamp for continuous current; Fig. 2220A shows the lamp for alternating current.

Rheostats, to use these lamps on 100 to 250 volt circuits, vary from £2 10s. to £8 according to the voltage of the supply, and the number of ampères required for the lamp.

No. 2225. Similar lamp, but "hand fed" **£7 10 0**

Figure 3.7 Carbon arc lamps.
In K. Schall, *Electro-medical Instruments and their Management and Illustrated Price List of Electro-Medical Apparatus*, May 1905 (London: Bemrose & Sons Ltd, 1905), p. 240. Thackray Medical Museum, Leeds.

to exploit light's therapeutic potential. So far I have focused on the convergence of light's visualising and therapeutic powers in light therapy's early development, describing its archival images as light registers. I have also described photographs of light therapy as multi-layered 'self-portraits' of actinic light, especially Finsen's photographed forearm (Fig. 2.1). But what happened when this self-portraiture went wrong, when the 'luminous pencils' of light obscured rather than illuminated light therapy? I made it clear in Chapter 2 that Figure 2.1 is, by its fuzzy, illegible outlines and poor 'fixing', a 'bad' photograph, one that, despite its best intentions, communicates solar erythema as an equally illegible phenomenon. I now want to explore these 'bad' representations, in which the photograph-as-light register was pushed to its representational limits, rendering light therapy a blinding, obscure practice. Not simply converging, photography, electric lighting, and light therapy materially collide in these 'bad' representations, producing photographic 'accidents' and 'injuries'.

II Material collision

Let us return to Tudor-Hart's photograph of the phototherapy room at the SLHWC (1934, Fig. 3.1). That it failed to make the cut in the photographic selection for the pamphlet only piques my interest in it all the more. Like Finsen's fuzzy, lost photographed forearm, we could consider Tudor-Hart's photograph a 'failure' (despite its high quality) in that it is seemingly tangential or incidental to the larger context of light therapy in Britain: the work of an émigré photographer that was never shown at the time.[69] But Tudor-Hart's practice and this photograph in particular sit at the nexus of a discourse on the visualising and therapeutic powers of light during the early twentieth century. Metaphors of light and darkness prevail in discussions of her work. Her radical political beliefs in Communism, supported by the Popular Front in Britain, fuelled her interest in bringing to light the 'shadow' of social injustice, especially through her documentary photographs of dark slums and abject poverty in both Austria and England.[70] Lobby groups such as the Sunlight League adopted wholeheartedly this rhetoric of bringing light into the slums to eradicate the 'diseases of darkness', as social campaigner Dr Caleb Saleeby so poetically called them.[71] Tudor-Hart's training as a Montessori teacher in the 1920s, through to her photographs of children for the British Medical Association and ministries of information, health, and education in the 1950s, show a lifelong devotion to child health, welfare, and 'enlightened' education.[72] As such, her commission at the SLHWC exemplifies Tudor-Hart's photographic oeuvre, despite receiving merely passing mention in her biographical literature (Figs. 3.1–3.2).[73]

Located in Clapham Common and founded in 1912, by the time of the booklet's publication in 1935 the SLHWC boasted it had become 'the largest general hospital in the country officered by women for women and children'.[74] The expensively produced booklet was intended to help raise £45,000 funds for a considerable extension, including a second level for a 'light and airy' children's ward as well as two maternity wards, and this cost did not include new equipment.[75] Triumphing modern technology, the booklet stated:

> Science is ever finding more accurate, more ingenious – and more expensive – instruments to detect and frustrate disease or to alleviate pain. It is essential that equipment should be up to date, essential for the sake of patients and also for the training in the Hospital of medical women for the general field.[76]

It had a special radium clinic here too, to treat women with breast cancer, for which it also desperately needed funding. The hospital's aims must have resonated with Tudor-Hart, for in addition to serving middle-class women it noted working-class women were in 'appreciable proportion' and many came from the slums.[77] It also spoke forcefully of the need to provide training and support to facilitate more women practising medicine. The many other photographs by Tudor-Hart and Stern throughout the pamphlet represent these female staff members interacting with patients in consulting rooms and hospital wards, examining radiographs, and working in the pathology laboratory. Figures 3.1 and 3.2, as photographs depicting child patients undergoing phototherapy, must therefore be contextualised within the pamphlet's larger purpose: they, like the other photographs, represent the hospital above all as beneficent and as modern – through its forward-thinking beliefs about women as well as its technologically sophisticated equipment.

Significantly, these are not the only photographs Tudor-Hart produced about bodily exposure to therapeutic light: she took photographs of sunbathers at Vienna's bathing area, the Lobau, in the early 1930s and of sunbathing children for the journal, *Sun Bathing Review*, dating from 1935 to the late 1940s (see Chapter 5). Tudor-Hart and her photographs are therefore not incidental but vital to understanding light therapy's history as an 'obscure' practice. Quite aside from the fact that we know her name and can attribute specific photographs of light therapy to her (a rarity in itself), Tudor-Hart is a case study cloaked in layers of invisibility: she produced photographs of heliotherapy and phototherapy that did not in fact circulate within the standard light-therapy literature but rather in an exceptional promotional pamphlet or in non-medical journals; her presence is erased in the production of her photographs by virtue of her position behind the lens;[78] and while taking on various commissions during the 1930s and 1940s in Britain, including photographing children being exposed to therapeutic light, she acted as a Comintern spy. Her clandestine contribution to light therapy's development exemplifies the ongoing dead ends researchers must face if they are to engage with a thorough examination of its history, and in Chapter 6 I discuss the myriad numbers of light therapy's 'invisible' women, including nurses, patients, patrons, and artists. Discussions of success and failure, light and dark, clarity and obscurity, visibility and invisibility, and 'good' and 'bad' photography thus are prompted by Tudor-Hart's photographs of bodily exposure to light.

Accidents and artefacts

In their books, Wolfgang Schivelbusch, Chris Otter, and Graeme Gooday have explained that arc lighting was the first form of artificial lighting that produced too much light for vision, making it practical for use only in large spaces like railway stations, streets, and factories, places Schivelbusch states had an 'insatiable appetite for light'.[79] Its blinding powers meant it needed to be installed high above crowds when used for public lighting, to the point that it not only illuminated streets but entire towns by 'tower lighting'.[80] This penetrating, all-encompassing light proved too harsh and too expensive for ongoing practical use, eventually replaced by Edison's electric incandescent light bulb. Producing dazzling light so alike sunlight, with such intensity that it could not be looked at directly, arc lighting was not, according to Schivelbusch and Gooday, used in the home.[81]

The history of light therapy, of course, indicates that this was not entirely the case. Small, portable carbon arc lamps were produced well into the 1950s for prophylactic tanning within the privacy of one's home. More interestingly, during the 1920s when small arc lamps began to be marketed for home use they necessarily had to be plugged into the home's primary electrical outlet (Fig. 3.8). As is clear from Figure 3.8, this was the central light source in the main living room. Electricity in the British home was not the norm until well into the 1930s, and for those who could afford it the outlets installed were few and far between (see Chapter 4). To operate this Ajax arc lamp, users had to replace the 'normal' incandescent light source with this blinding, therapeutic light. Unless they took the cure outdoors in natural daylight, they found themselves, once again, within the obscurity of the darkroom. Light therapy, and in particular phototherapy, transformed the visualising powers of carbon arc lighting and exploited its abilities to dazzle and blind, bringing its excessive actinic light (as a veritable mini sun) into the interior and close to patients, instead of illuminating surroundings above them.[82] This blindness or obscurity was a condition of its therapeutic use and made photographic representation difficult, if not impossible.

In Tudor-Hart's photograph (Fig. 3.1), the powerful open flame of the carbon arc lamp was the primary light that simultaneously allowed the patients to heal and to be recorded onto the camera's photosensitive negative. In other, similar photographs of London clinics it was the only light source. No additional lights and no flash were used in Figures 3.3 and 3.4, and thus the legible prints were produced by the same and sole light that simultaneously treated the photographs' subjects. In this way we might consider that the camera was as much a participant – even a patient – in this light seance as the subjects.[83] Skin, eye, and film are photosensitive surfaces that were activated, transformed, and imprinted by the lamp's actinic light.

They were also easily burnt and injured by it. As I pointed out in the opening of the chapter, it was only by effectively using the child patient as a shield or 'screen' in Figures 3.1 and 3.3 that these photographs remain legible instead of overexposed. Overexposed photographs, sometimes subtle (as in the case of an overexposed white hat in Fig. 3.9), sometimes not so subtle (Fig. 3.10), are common representations of heliotherapy and phototherapy in process.[84] Both Figures 3.9 and 3.10 depict Treloar

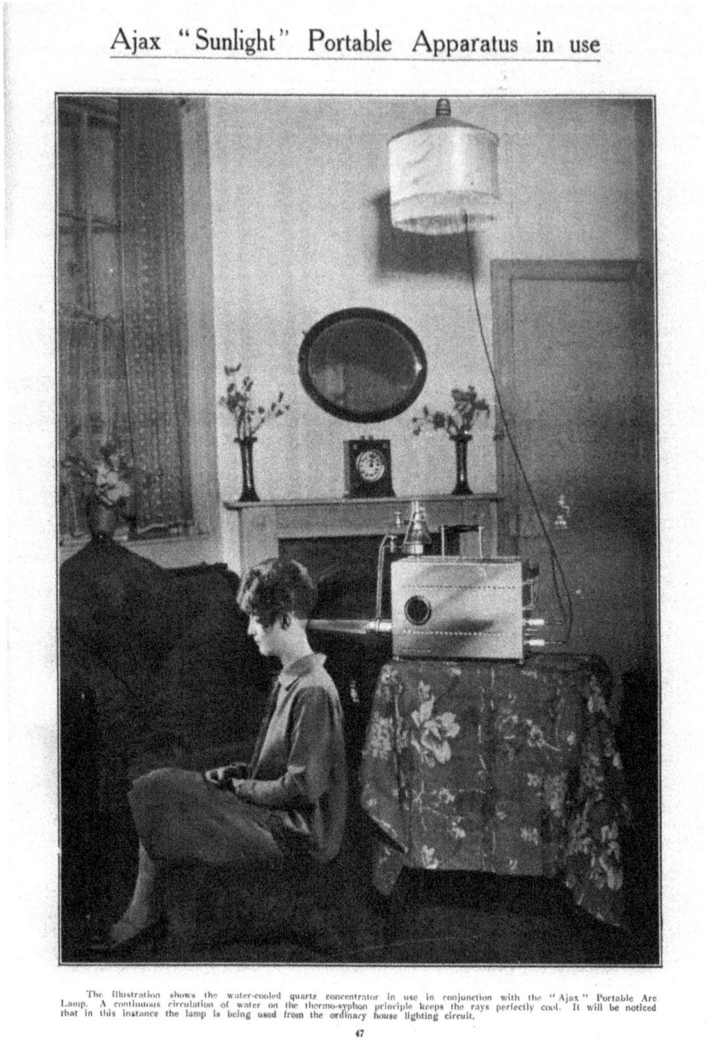

Figure 3.8 'Ajax "Sunlight" portable apparatus in use.' In *'Sunlight' Treatment: A Concise Guide for the Use of Ultra-violet Irradiation in Actino-therapy*, undated (late 1920s), p. 47. Thackray Medical Museum, Leeds.

Hospital, an institution run by Sir Henry Gauvain employing both heliotherapy and phototherapy to treat tuberculous children (see Chapter 1).

Overexposure, visualised by means of sunburn, blistered skin, or a so-called 'unsuccessful' or 'bad' photograph, attests to the light's volatility in therapeutic and photographic processes.[85] Figure 3.10 is a strange depiction of phototherapy, both in

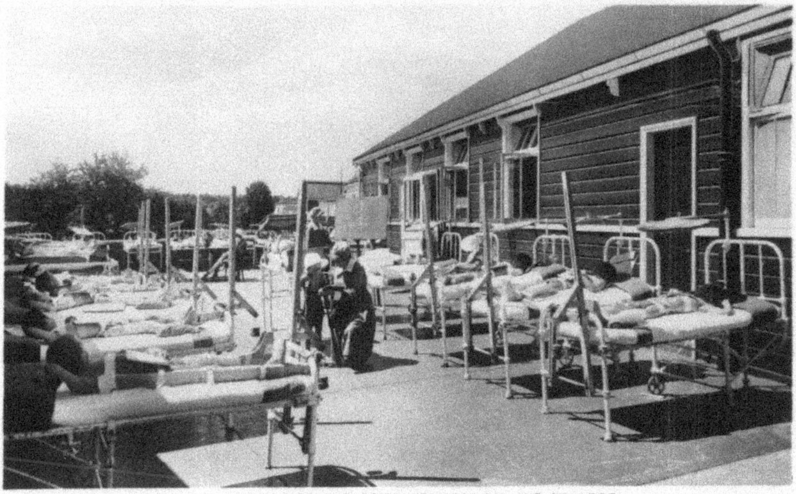

Figure 3.9 'Lord Mayor Treloar Cripples' Hospital and College: solarium at Alton', undated postcard. Author's collection.

the context of what is happening in the image as well as its aesthetic representation. The camera was aimed parallel to the open flame of a tungsten arc lamp. From the photograph it was likely a 'Premier' tungsten arc lamp, aimed directly at the neck of a child patient.[86] Yet, unusually, the arc was unshielded, and, worryingly, the patient wore no goggles and was not attended by a nurse. A skilled operator was particularly needed for this type of lamp, which required almost constant manual adjustments to the tungsten electrodes.[87] That person perhaps was the photographer; the Treloar archives contain several photographs made by the nursing staff.[88] Other comparable photographs were, more logically, taken from behind the lamp's reflector (Fig. 3.11). In Figure 3.11, a child patient suffering from rickets was made to stand for the camera while receiving general treatment with the lamp, supported by an attendant nurse. Both clearly wore the requisite goggles to protect their eyes from the light, and the photographer took the image diagonal to and behind the lamp to avoid overexposure. By contrast, in aiming the camera at the lamp without any protection or 'screens', the photographer of Figure 3.10 produced an injured negative of enveloping black orbs where the actinic light burnt the film, printed as encompassing white globes in the positive. The print is a dramatic example of a photographic 'accident' known as lens flare, in which stray intense light bounces and refracts within the camera, leaving white sprays and streaks, starbursts, rings, circles, or an overall haze across the image. Aside from the striking orbs, streaks are visible in the top right-hand corner

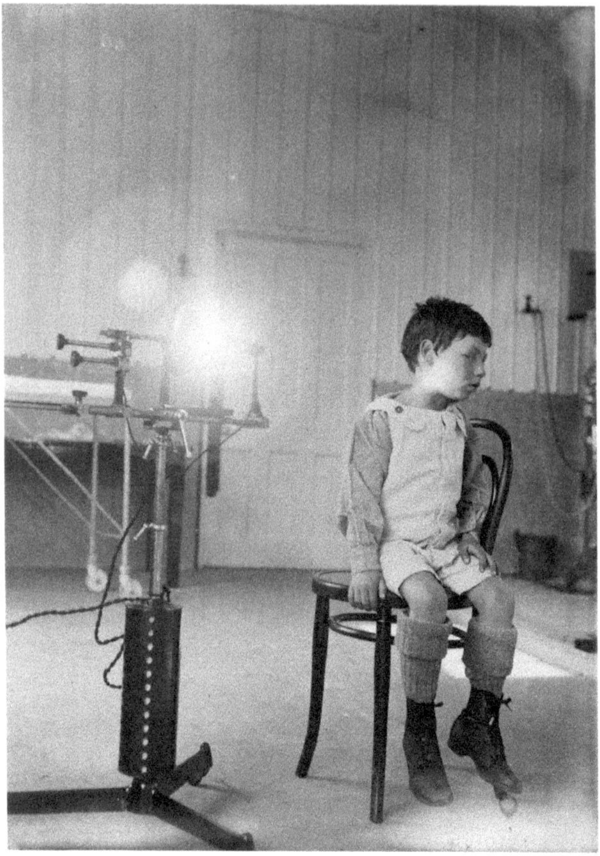

Figure 3.10 A child patient receiving phototherapy by a tungsten arc lamp at Treloar Hospital, undated photograph. Science Museum/Science & Society Picture Library, London.

of the photograph, and a haze is detectable in the lower right-hand corner. These are known as 'artefacts', and, as Wilder pointed out, they can serve as useful pieces of information depending upon who looks at them.[89]

Unintended artefacts are particularly common in photographs of phototherapy (Figs. 3.12–3.13). Figure 3.12 captured the phototherapy room at Guy's Hospital, where multiple suspended open arc lamps were used on masked and goggled children and, in the background, adults. Intense starbursts of actinic light emit from the carbon arcs and radiate translucent orbs, which overlap across the right side of photograph and lead the viewer's eye to the visible spray of light streaking towards its lower corner. Actinic light similarly consumes a mysterious photograph of phototherapy treatment from the *Daily Herald* archives (Fig. 3.13). Goggled unclothed child patients and a nurse, positioned at the outer edge of a dosage circle (see Chapter 2), faced a camera that shared the full blast of open arc treatment. A giant white orb

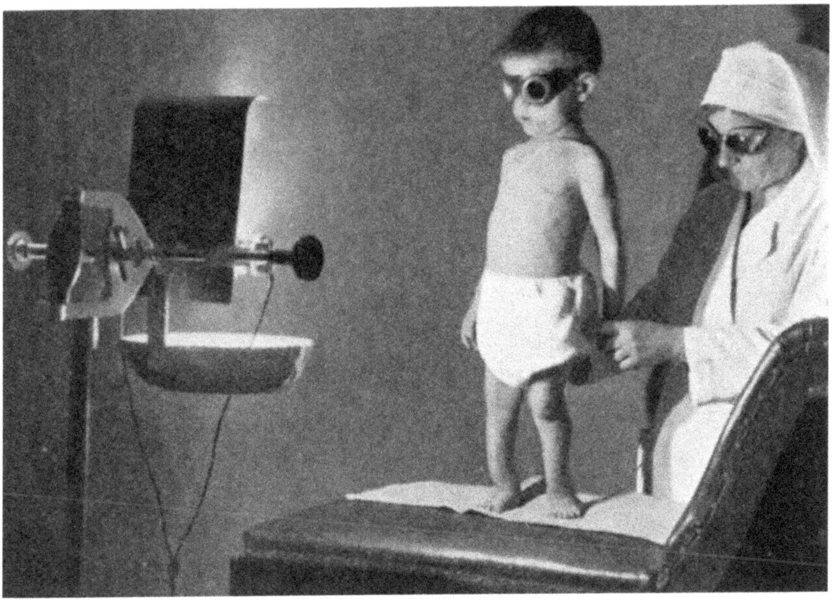

Figure 3.11 'A tungsten arc [lamp] at work at the Hull Corporation Clinic.'
In Katherine Gamgee, *The Artificial Light Treatment of Children in Rickets, Anaemia and Malnutrition* (London: H. K. Lewis and Co., 1927), Figure 20, p. 66. Wellcome Library, London.

radiates in the photograph like the sun itself, while the lower right-hand corner is damaged by the ghostly splaying lines characteristic of lens flare.

Miles perceived damaged prints like these as theoretically productive, revealing light's excesses and photography's dependence upon a mastery over light to function – an issue of control that light therapy also struggled to master (Chapter 2). As marks of excessive or disruptive light visibly present on the photograph, they betray the materiality of the photograph as an object. No longer the transparent stand-in for the thing it represents, the 'injured' photograph announces itself as a material sign, disrupting photography's status as an index of the 'real'.[90] Indeed, the artefacts in Figure 3.10 present significant similarities with Roland Barthes's concept of the *punctum*, which he described as a shocking, piercing wound or mark:

> A Latin word exists to designate this wound, this prick, this mark made by a pointed instrument: the word suits me all the better in that it also refers to the notion of punctuation, and because the photographs I am speaking of are in effect punctuated, sometimes even speckled with these sensitive points;

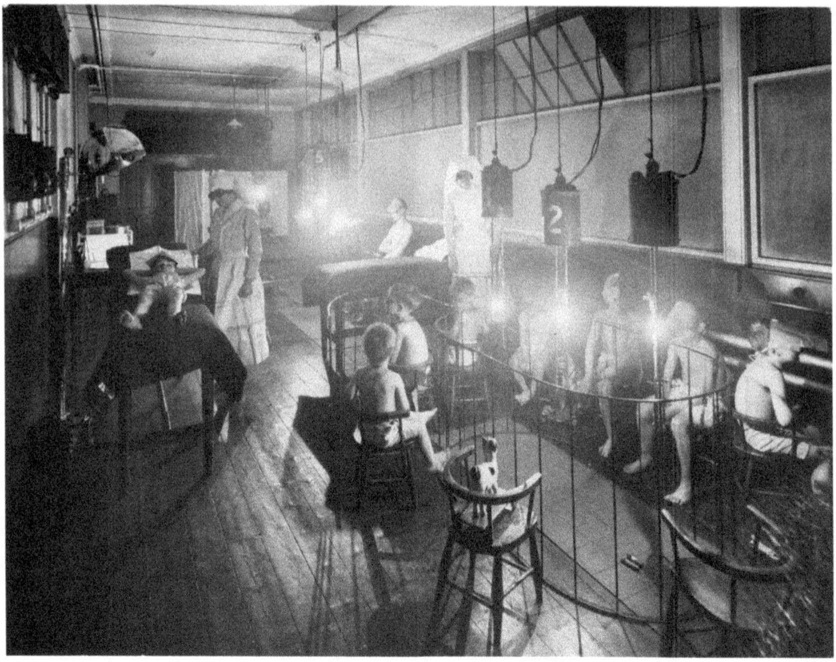

Figure 3.12 [Underwood Commercial Studios Ltd], Light Department, Guy's Hospital, undated photograph.
London Metropolitan Archives, London and courtesy of Guy's and St Thomas' Charity.

> precisely, these marks, these wounds are so many *points*. This ... I shall therefore call *punctum*; for *punctum* is also: sting, speck, cut, little hole – and also a cast of the dice. A photograph's *punctum* is that accident which pricks me (but also bruises me, is poignant to me).[91]

We might add that it is also a burn, an injury to the negative: note the small black circles in the centre of the white orbs in Figures 3.4 and 3.10, 'black suns' burnt by the light's greatest intensity that 'punctuates' like the dot of an exclamation mark. Citing Ansel Adam's *The Black Sun, Tungsten Hills, Owens Valley, California* (1939), Miles explained that black suns, like lens flare, are traditionally considered to be photographic 'accidents' or 'injuries' to the negative due to overexposure.[92] These 'suns' are artefacts made by intense, excessive light, which is so powerful that it reverses negative and positive on the film. As an historic symbol of melancholy and madness, 'the black sun ... does not mark so much an absence of the light of reason and vitality, but a soul-destroying blindness to a light which is expected to nurture, enrich and offer hope'.[93] The black sun photograph was but one example in Miles's arsenal

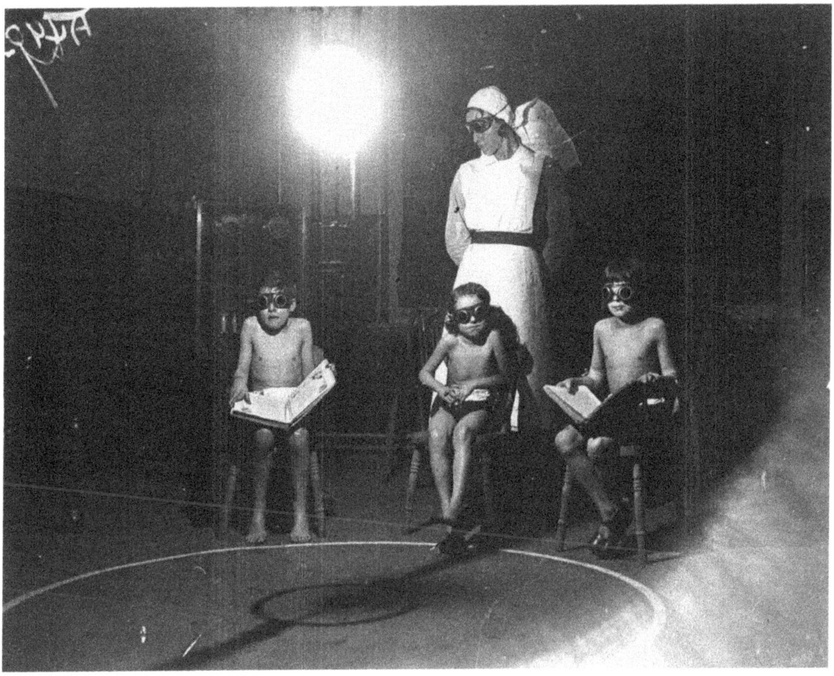

Figure 3.13 'Ultra violet (sun lamp) therapy', undated. Silver gelatin contact print from a glass plate negative. Daily Herald Archive/NMEM/Science & Society Picture Library, London.

to deconstruct or 'exceed the limits' of 'reductive photographic dualisms', the most potent of course being that of light versus dark.

Solarisation

When it comes to analysing photographs of light therapy, the word 'solarisation' is particularly apt. First reported by British photographer William Jackson in 1857, solarisation (sometimes called the Sabatier effect) is described as an accidental reversal of dark and light, of negative and positive.[94] Through overexposure the film loses its photosensitivity, setting into effect the reverse process. It can occur at the point of photographing, as in the case of Figure 3.10, or during the development process, if an extra flash of light is introduced into the darkroom. During the early twentieth century Surrealist artists such as Man Ray and Maurice Tabard adopted solarisation as a vanguard technique in photography, calling attention to the photographic surface as an experimental ground (Chapter 4).[95] Like Nicolai Howalt's photography (Chapter 6), chance and happenstance were welcomed with open arms, the results of these photographic exposures unknown until the finished print was revealed and thus deliberate attempts to make productive accidents.

But solarisation has other meanings. As a verb, to 'solarise' is to affect, modify or, in the specific case of photography, to injure by the influence of the sun's rays. One can solarise vegetation and soil, inhibiting photosynthesis, or solarise glass, altering its transmission of light wavelengths, through prolonged exposure to intense light. With respect to the latter a peculiar irony occurred with the manufacture of glass that permitted ultraviolet rays, such as 'Vita' glass, which was widely installed throughout Britain during the late 1920s and 1930s in hospitals, factories, and schools to allow the buildings' occupants greater access to sunlight. The rays 'Vita' glass permitted quickly altered its properties, through the unavoidable process of solarisation, and eventually made it block their passage, effectively becoming ordinary glass.[96]

Significantly, American physicians referred to solarisation to mean light therapy itself, whether heliotherapy or phototherapy, and sociologist Simon Carter used it to describe light therapy in Britain.[97] R. A. Houstoun, a specialist in optics at the University of Glasgow, intriguingly included a section on solarisation in photography within a chapter on phototherapy, in his 1923 populist book, *Light and Colour*.[98] Photographs like Figures 3.4 and 3.10 are marked by small, distinct instances of solarisation as 'black suns', but glimpses of these strange reversals can be found that altered the entire photographic surface (Fig. 3.14): in this photograph of Rollier's child patients taking a fortifying walk in the Leysin countryside, the beginnings of solarisation take place to the patients' bodies and contours. The fine line between light therapy's success and failure, between desirable sunburns and dangerous injuries, is usefully captured in the word 'solarisation'. At once positive and negative, desired and feared, the solarised photograph does more than metaphorically refer to the accidents of overexposure on the patient's sensitive flesh and eyes. For practitioners, the connection between photosensitive film and body was literal. In the words of Daniel Freund, 'the benefits from therapy *reversed with overexposure*: bodies became more susceptible to disease and less able to heal themselves'.[99] Figures 3.10 and 3.12–3.14 are therefore poignant examples in which light therapy's tensions – as beneficial or dangerous – are materially (physically) and conceptually embedded.

Blinding light

Like red-light therapy, the conditions for open carbon arc treatment necessitated emulating the photographic darkroom, but this time a fully functioning one where photochemical development took place. Some practitioners considered visible light – the red to violet rays, detectable by the human retina but which in excess produced glare or dazzlement – a nuisance that interfered with ultraviolet light's therapeutic action, and consequently they shut out daylight by closing doors and curtains, as is

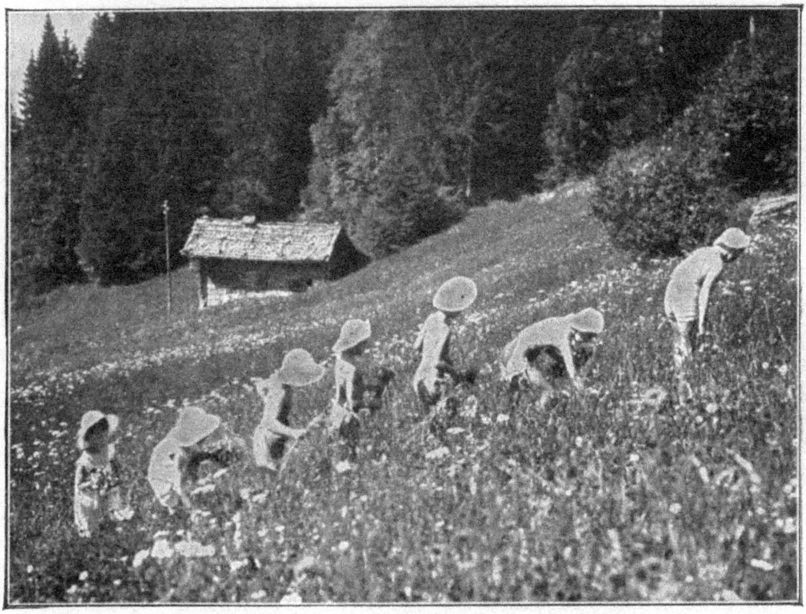

Figure 3.14 'Little convalescents in battle dress. Walk amongst the flowers (Rollier).' In Alexandre Aimes, *La Pratique de l'héliothérapie* (Paris: A. Maloine, 1914), Figure 4, unpaginated plate, opposite p. 104. Martine Gagnebin and author's collection.

evident in Tudor-Hart's photograph (Fig. 3.1), or by practising phototherapy in windowless rooms (Fig. 3.11).[100]

Awareness of ultraviolet light's explosive photochemical action and its blinding effects, analogous to a camera flash, did not deter the Russells from their enthusiasm for light therapy, as is apparent from this chapter's first epigraph. In their section on ultraviolet light's chemical properties, the Russells offered the following quote from the Bible: 'Truly the Light is sweet, and a pleasant thing it is for the eyes to behold the sun.'[101] Sidestepping metaphor here, in practice, the therapeutic use of actinic light necessitated *never* beholding the light of the sun or lamp, at least not directly. Mediated by the strategic use of screens – the judicious use of goggles or facemasks for both patient and operator – light therapy was encountered as an obscure visual practice, one literally performed 'blind'. In the phototherapy room interior, contrasts of light and dark were at their most extreme, the goggled patient and operator encountering the blinding light of the lamp, or total darkness: not only because the lamp often acted as the sole artificial illuminant in a windowless room but furthermore because the tinted goggles darkened one's visual field (or, if masked, partially or wholly restricted it). An article of 1925 in the *Yorkshire Post*, explaining the treatment, advised the public that, 'So fierce is the glare … that very dark glasses must be worn, and, for greater protection, the eyes themselves should be closed when facing the light.'[102] This blindness or obscurity is thus the result both of darkness *and* excessive light.[103] As Michel Foucault put it, 'Dazzlement is night in broad daylight, the darkness that rules at the very heart of what is excessive in light's radiance. Dazzled reason opens its eyes upon the sun, and sees *nothing*, that is, it does not see.'[104]

In the production of Figure 3.1, Tudor-Hart was doubly photographing 'blind'. In the first instance, one could argue that any photograph is the product of a moment of blindness; a photographer cannot know in advance if a shot will be successful until the negative is removed, developed, and subsequently printed into a positive. Geoffrey Batchen, referencing Jacques Derrida, elucidated: 'The photographer points his camera at a scene and removes the lens cap for a certain duration; only later, after development, will he see exactly what the camera has seen. Thus … during the extended moment of photographing he does not see it. He photographs blind, from memory.'[105] Beyond this, however, in these particular circumstances at the SLHWC Tudor-Hart, holding her camera at waist height (instead of in front of her eyes, as a kind of filter), needed to be wearing goggles just like every other person in that room. Looking through the camera's viewfinder with tinted goggles in such extreme contrasts of light and dark, little would have been discernible. Had she refused to wear them, her vision would have been sorely affected nonetheless, suffering from acute conjunctivitis (inflammation of the conjunctiva) from the ultraviolet light soon afterwards. In her 1928 manual, the nurse Myrtle Vaughan-Cowell warned,

> Our eyes like our bodies are extremely sensitive to ultra-violet light, therefore it follows that it is imperative for both patient and operator to be protected by proper goggles. Conjunctivitis is an extremely painful condition which should never occur if care is taken. The patient is generally awakened at night by a sensation of grittiness when movement of the eyelid takes place. This is an inflammatory condition, which in a mild case only lasts a few hours, and should completely clear up within a few days if the necessary rest to the eyes is taken.[106]

Photographs do exist that show children unmasked and ungoggled in front of these open arc lamps (e.g., Fig. 3.10), contrasted by reports in local newspapers of practitioners blinded by ultraviolet lamps.[107] Conjunctivitis due to ultraviolet light was also known as snow blindness, the bane of Arctic and Alpine explorers, and some described it as the optical equivalent of sunburnt skin.[108] It was particularly problematic for actors and directors when creating early films, since arc lights were commonly used for studio lighting.[109]

At its most extreme, phototherapy as a blinding or obscure practice even extended into the treatment of eye diseases, the localising extensions and applicators of mercury vapour lamps aimed directly at the eye.[110] In such instances, blindness could be both produced and rectified, the stimulating flash of actinic light emitted from these lamps a particularly risky tool that, if overdosed, could ironically cause permanent blindness in an effort to restore unimpaired and healthy vision.[111]

While the mechanical functions of a camera and a phototherapy lamp might seem at first to work in oppositional ways – one absorbing actinic light, the other producing it – they both operate by harnessing and manipulating light through focusing devices, and this is because they share similar apparel inside them: lenses and reflectors (mirrors, chrome surfaces, etc.), as mentioned in Section I.[112] But in the 1930s flash photography *did* produce its own light source, and, as the Russells pointed out, its actinic output closely resembled that of a mercury vapour lamp. Miles provided ample evidence throughout photography's history about the dangers of using flash powder, an explosive concoction of chemicals (especially magnesium) ignited to produce a dazzling white light. Invented in the 1860s and in use until the 1930s, flash powder provided temporary artificial illumination for interior or night-time photography. Highly volatile, it could cause physical harm to sitters and photographer, cause fires, and produce shocked and blinded faces under harsh lighting in resultant photographs.[113]

The notion of the flash's actinic light as a weapon finds important parallels with practitioners' belief in the perceived beneficial 'light shock' of therapeutic exposures. The phrase was used by Gauvain (Treloar Hospital), who stated in 1927 that, 'It has long been recognized that morning light is most therapeutically valuable. This, in my opinion, is not due solely or even chiefly to the nature of the light but because the light shock evokes a greater response as immediately following the darkness necessarily antecedent.'[114] While not yet at its highest intensity, the dawning sun was effective for patients in Gauvain's mind precisely because it acted like a stimulating flash emerging out of the darkness. As I explain in Chapter 4, Gauvain's notion of the 'light shock' was metaphorical and unintentionally literal: electric shocks, severe burns, and even death occurred during treatments, risks that came to be part and parcel of therapies using the invisible ultraviolet, X, and gamma rays during the early twentieth century. Gauvain proudly reproduced photographs in his publications about Treloar's revamped Light Department, newly equipped with the latest phototherapy lamps in 1924 (Fig. 3.15). In this postcard, the multiple, suspended open arc lamps emitted so much visible and ultraviolet light that they appear to consume patients. Because of their even higher output of ultraviolet radiation, mercury vapour lamps were also photographically represented as irradiating patients to the point of eradication (Fig. 3.16).[115] Figure 3.16 is a photograph

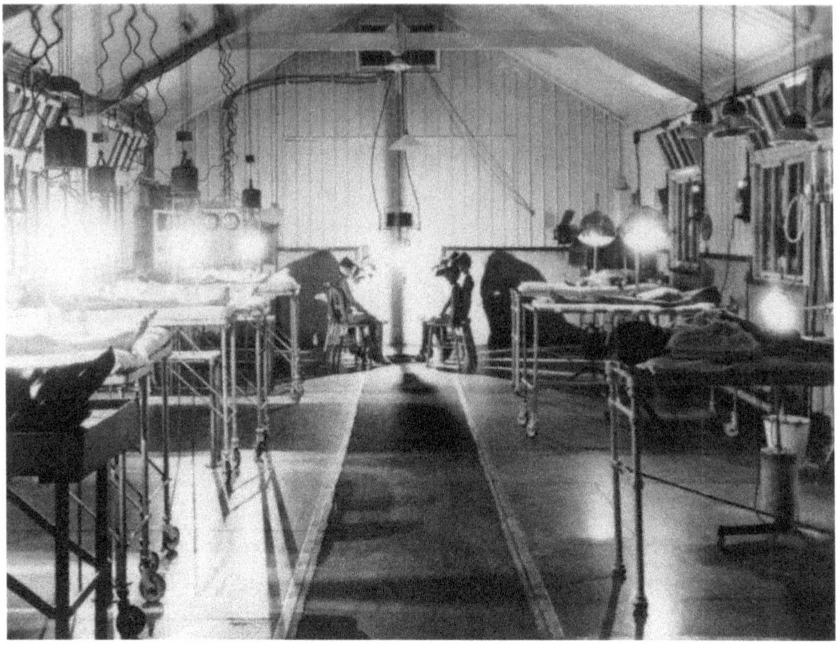

Figure 3.15 'Lord Mayor Treloar Cripples' Hospital and College: the Light Department at Alton', undated (mid-1920s) postcard. Author's collection.

of St Thomas's electro-therapy department, where light therapy was used in conjunction with X-ray therapy and diagnostic imaging, shown on the left-hand side of the photograph.

In such difficult circumstances of photographing while the therapy was in process, some resorted to alternative photographic tactics to reproduce 'reality'. A simple solution was to photograph the open-flamed carbon arc lamp, surrounded by patients but not actually on. In Figure 3.17, a 1930 photograph of the 'Sun Ray Room' at White Oak School Hospital in Swanley (Kent), nurses and patients were fully goggled, masked and in the correct position to receive the actinic rays, but the light source enabling this photograph to exist was the bright sunlight flooding into the room from the large open windows. The arc lamps were conspicuously unlit, no doubt because of difficulties presented to the photographer.[116] Such artifice went without comment in the literature. The primary focus of Chapter 4, these limitations of photographic *processes* – due to the blinding powers of actinic light – enabled other vanguard representations based on photographic *techniques*, that of heavy retouching and montage. It brings me to my final point: what exactly are we 'seeing' in these photographs, and what remains obscured? In Figure 3.17, the viewer is

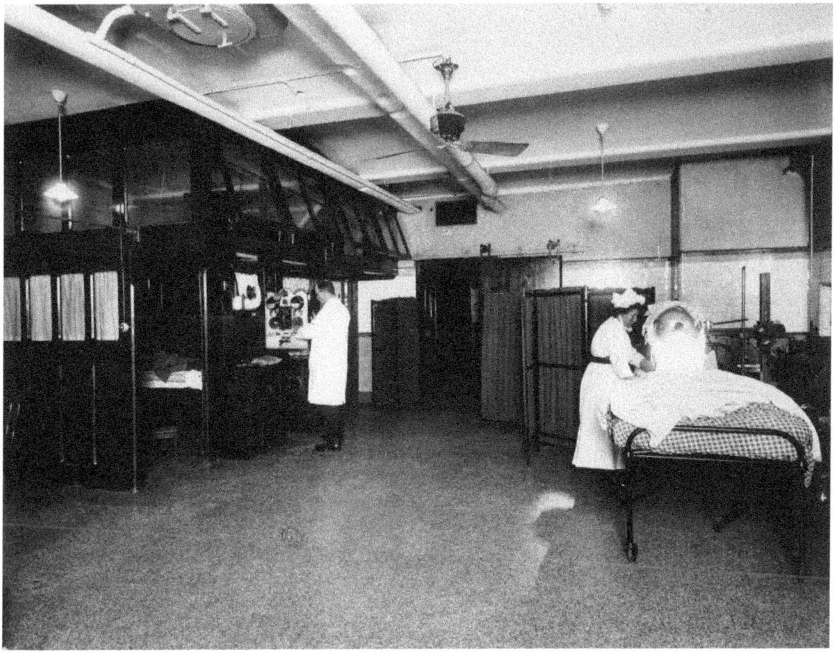

Figure 3.16 'Electro-therapy: X-ray treatment rooms – mercury lamp on right', St Thomas' Hospital, undated photograph. London Metropolitan Archives, London and courtesy of Guy's and St Thomas' Charity.

presented with what is intended as documentary 'evidence' of light therapy in practice, a so-called objective visual record about how the cure was carried out. It was meant to function, in other words, as a visualisation of phototherapeutic technology in operation. Yet it did not and cannot: upon closer inspection it presents a falsified version of phototherapy in order to exist as a legible photographic representation. The one light technology only truly functioned at the expense of the other. One had to remain, to some extent, inoperative and impotent, lest photographic accidents result.

In their complicated, incestuous relationship, photography acted as both a parent to light therapy, guiding and nurturing its development (Section I), and its difficult lover, materially converging and clashing with it (Section II). In those rare instances in which we find 'successful' photographic representations of phototherapy in action, like Tudor-Hart's exceptional image (Fig. 3.1), we must understand that this fruitful resolution was only enabled through the careful mediation of an exceptionally skilled photographer. The light, used both aesthetically and therapeutically, was heavily controlled and so were the patients, offering their bodies as screens to enable legibility.

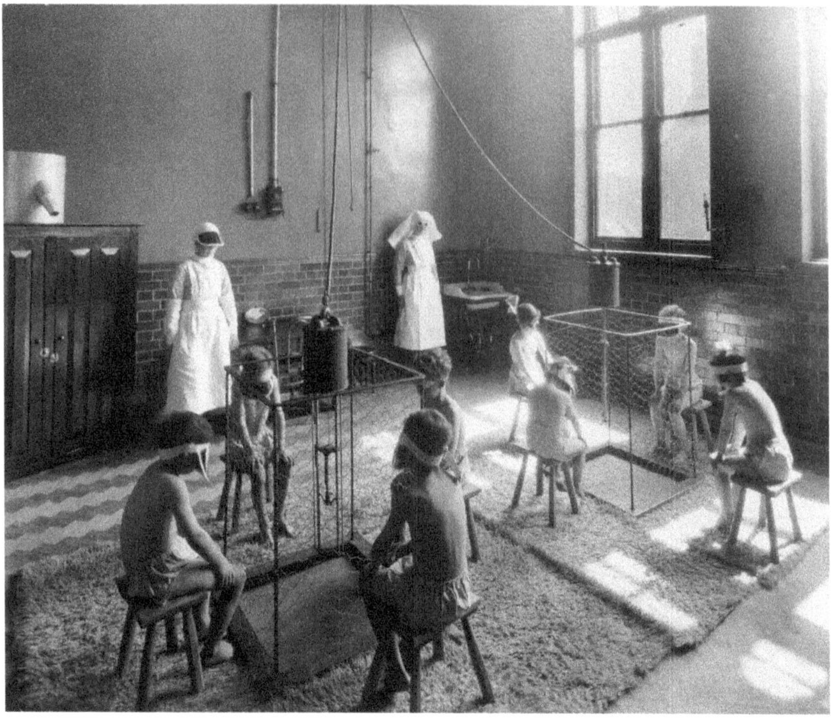

Figure 3.17 'Sun Ray room', White Oak (Swanley), June 1930.
London Metropolitan Archives, London.

Conclusion

When it comes to 'seeing' ultraviolet light, we are always in the dark. 'The two ends of the spectrum gradually fade away into darkness', stated Shelford Bidwell in his popular book *Curiosities of Light and Sight* (1899), and 'we cannot see them; they fall upon our eyes without exciting the faintest sensation of light'.[117] Yet he persisted in making analogous the physiological action of the human eye and the camera, a long-held connection in photography's history.[118] Photography offered to enlighten the eye to these invisible rays, detecting and visualising that which it cannot naturally see, just as telescopes, camera obscuras, magic lanterns, and microscopes provided an 'extra-ocular way of observing the world'.[119]

Again we must ask ourselves, what are we 'seeing' in these photographs of light therapy? What were viewers at the time? Since photographic film registers wavelengths differently to the human eye (including the invisible ultraviolet rays), how can these photographs function as purely 'documentary'? How could viewers recognise the visible wavelengths from the invisible ultraviolet ones in these photographs simply by looking at them?[120] The remarkable beams of light and alternating shadows projecting within Tudor-Hart's photograph contain a combination of visible and ultraviolet light, producing a dramatic and eerie image (Fig. 3.1). But what did the patients, nurses, and photographer actually 'see' during the experience of light therapy in process? On the one hand, we will never be privy to the 'real' experiences optically witnessed by the patients, nurses, and photographers present at the moment of photographing light therapy. What they saw can never be seen by us through the photograph as a mediating object; that will always be obscure to us. Yet on the other hand, we will always be privy to seeing light obscure to the subjects. The photograph registered not only ultraviolet wavelengths but also the excesses of visible and invisible light that blinded subjects, whether by glare, dazzlement, or acute conjunctivitis. These are marked on the photosensitive surface as the 'accidents' or artefacts of lens flare and solarisation (Figs. 3.10, 3.12–3.16).

In attempting to understand light therapy's processes and methods through archival photographs as 'documents' or as evidence, this conundrum may lead one to wonder why I should invest in these objects at all as points of access to the past. Like Miles, I believe that it is precisely these photographic 'accidents' that present the opportunity to critically engage with light therapy's history in a new way. Indeed, that they are problematic documents makes them productive to my analysis. Submerged and hidden in numerous archival boxes, the handful of photographs I discuss in this chapter, exemplified by the photography of Tudor-Hart (Figs. 3.1–3.2), remain obscured from view. Rarely are they looked at in the first place, and as damaged prints they are just the sort of documents others historians interested in light therapy or particular institutions like Treloar's have passed over without comment.[121] But photography's historic role in the development and dissemination of light therapy provides significant insights about how we access and understand medical history.

In many cases, employing black-and-white photography to visualise the effects of light therapy seems to have been extraordinarily difficult or ineffective, as I discussed at length both here and in Chapter 2 in relation to Finsen's photographed forearm (Fig. 2.1). These difficulties of representation communicate much about light therapy's own tensions as a nascent series of treatments struggling to gain legitimacy. In light treatments such as red-light therapy, photography proved impossible as a means of representation. Yet, even in this instance, in photography's absence, we learn how practitioners conceptualised the dangers and advantages of particular wavelengths of light by emulating photographic practices. Lastly, through 'bad' photographs we become aware of photography's limits of representation and how these limitations revolved around picturing the excessive actinic light considered so therapeutically valuable. They also act as notable contrasts to the photographs which succeed where they apparently 'fail': Figures 3.1–3.3 depict excessive, therapeutic light in control, produced by cameras shielded from the open arc lamp by patients, and we come to appreciate the high level of skill, strategies of composition, and sheer determination of certain photographers to produce legible negatives in such blinding circumstances.

Physicians found evidence for the efficacy of the actinic rays, whether natural or artificially produced, *in* photography itself as a light-sensitive medium. This was asserted over and over again by British physicians interested in light's therapeutic potential.[122] The logic went that if these rays acted on photographic surfaces, they must act in a like manner on the patient's skin; that is, photochemically. Batchen described photosynthesis as a form of photography, writing, 'there has never not been a photography. What is photosynthesis, after all, but an organic world of light writing?'[123] We might well ask, in a similar vein, what is light therapy but a deliberate invention and intervention with skin as an excessive, therapeutic form of 'light writing'? The skin was so effective acting as a photograph (photogram) that for practitioners like Eidinow it superseded photographic devices for measuring light intensities, such as photometers and spectroscopes. Developing from, merging with, and eventually superseding photography, light therapy was a stimulating and excessive form of photography itself.

As a 'light shock' for the patient, bodily exposure to actinic light was a therapeutic practice that exploited the excessive light of electric arc lighting and exceeded the limits of photography as visualising media. Yet, as we have seen, this did not signal the end of their interaction, however volatile. Photography remained in the service of phototherapy, despite commonly producing illegible representations ('accidents'). That practitioners continued to rely on photography in spite of these difficulties says as much about photography's authority as a medium of representation as it does about light therapy's unstable reputation. As with the case of 'fixing' sunburn, much was at stake in producing visible results that could effectively legitimise light therapy during its nascent development. Legible representations, fit for dissemination, were only enabled by a high degree of control and mediation: unusual skill, fakery, and manipulation such as heavy retouching or montage – the subject of my next chapter. But legible or illegible, these representations unsettle precisely because they communicate light therapy's obscurity, as revealing manifestations of its light that, ultimately, leave us in the dark.

Notes

1 Eleanor H. Russell and William K. Russell, *Ultra-violet Radiation and Actinotherapy* (Edinburgh: E. & S. Livingstone, 1925), pp. 84–5.

2 Melissa Miles, *The Burning Mirror: Photography in an Ambivalent Light* (North Melbourne: Australian Scholarly Publishing, 2008), p. 43. My thanks to Miles for bringing Edith Tudor-Hart's work to my attention.

3 *The South London Hospital for Women and Children* (Birmingham: Kynoch Press, 1935), p. 25. The prints are now housed at the London Metropolitan Archives.

4 Duncan Forbes, 'Edith Tudor-Hart: In the Shadow of Tyranny', in Duncan Forbes (ed.), *Edith Tudor-Hart: In the Shadow of Tyranny* (Osfildern: Hatje Cantz Verlag, 2013), pp. 11–18, at p. 17. He added that this camera allowed 'speed of execution in a way that encouraged dialogue with the person photographed'.

5 Duncan Forbes, 'Politics, Photography and Exile in the Life of Edith Tudor-Hart (1908–1973)', in Shulamith Behr and Marian Malet (eds), *Arts in Exile in Britain, 1933–1945: Politics and Cultural Identity* (Amsterdam and New York: Rodopi, 2005), pp. 45–87, at p. 60.

6 Figure 3.12, for example, was taken by Underwood Commercial Studios Ltd. See also *Ultra Violet (Sun Lamp) Therapy*, undated silver gelatin contact print from a glass plate negative, Science and Society Picture Library, 10630203, Daily Herald archive (A4903).

7 Owen Logan, who printed this photograph for the exhibition, explained that Figure 3.1 'needed some "dodging" to retain detail in the shadows', meaning parts were exposed for different lengths of time to create even lighting. This is, according to Logan, a standard process in the darkroom. Email correspondence, 8 August 2013.

8 Many photography historians have noted the conceptual similarities between photographs (especially photograms) and skin, see Tanya Sheehan, *Doctored: The Medicine of Photography in Nineteenth-Century America* (University Park, Pa.: Pennsylvania State University Press, 2011), pp. 95–6; Kelley Wilder, *Photography and Science* (London: Reaktion, 2009), p. 11; Geoffrey Batchen, *Burning with Desire: The Conception of Photography* (Cambridge, Mass.: MIT Press, 1999), p. 171. See also the work of contemporary artist, elin O'Hara slavick, and the essay by James Elkins in *After Hiroshima* (Hillsborough: Daylight Community Arts Foundation, 2013).

9 Sheehan, *Doctored*, pp. 83–4. See also Richard Dyer, *White* (London and New York: Routledge, 1997), p. 14.

10 Sheehan, *Doctored*, pp. 84–5.

11 It should be stated that there is now a therapy known as 'Photo Therapy' or 'therapeutic photography' – not to be confused with phototherapy – which, like art therapy, uses photography as a rehabilitative practice for patients. See http://phototherapy.org.uk/. Even in its choice of title we see this material collision taking place, in which a therapeutic photography and artificial light therapy merge as modern-day synonyms. Like Sheehan, Sander Gilman discussed the perceived psychologically therapeutic benefits of photography, writing on Diamond's psychiatric photography in the 1850s. Sander L. Gilman (ed.), *The Face of Madness: Hugh W. Diamond and the Origin of Psychiatric Photography* (New York: Brunner/Mazel, Inc., 1976).

12 Wilder, *Photography and Science*, p. 19, citing William Henry Fox Talbot, *The Pencil of Nature* (1844–46).

13 See, for example, the work of Wilder, Miles, Batchen, as well as Klaus Hentschel, *Mapping the Spectrum: Techniques of Visual Representation in Research and Teaching* (Oxford: Oxford University Press, 2002), pp. 199–200; Lorraine Daston and Peter Galison, *Objectivity* (New York: Zone Books, 2010); Josh Ellenbogen, *Reasoned and Unreasoned Images: The Photography of Bertillon, Galton, and Marey* (University Park, Pa.: Pennsylvania State University Press, 2012); and Jennifer Tucker, *Nature Exposed: Photography as Eyewitness in Victorian Science* (Baltimore, Md.: Johns Hopkins University Press, 2005). Vogel stated that because photography, unlike our eyes, detects and visualises ultraviolet rays, 'it is natural that photography should represent many objects in a false light'. Hermann Vogel, *The Chemistry of Light and Photography* (New York: D. Appleton & Company, 1875), p. 64. Early attempts by physicians to measure the light intensities of lamps noted the difficulties of using photography

for precisely this reason, see Hugh Walsham, 'On the Ultra-violet Light from a Rapid Oscillation High-Tension Arc, for the Treatment of Skin Diseases', *Lancet*, 1 February 1902, pp. 285–8.

14 Hentschel, *Mapping the Spectrum*, p. 176. See also Wilder, *Photography and Science*; and Kelley Wilder, 'Visualizing Radiation: The Photographs of Henri Becquerel', in Lorraine Daston and Elizabeth Lunbeck (eds), *Histories of Scientific Observation* (Chicago, Ill.: University of Chicago Press, 2011), pp. 349–68.

15 See Sheehan, *Doctored*; and Hentschel, *Mapping the Spectrum*, p. 221.

16 See Wilder, *Photography and Science*, p. 43; and Miles, *Burning Mirror*, p. 42. This is not to be confused with the development of ultraviolet photography.

17 On chromotherapy, see, for example, R. Douglas Howat, *Elements of Chromotherapy: The Administration of Ultra-violet, Infra-Red and Luminous Rays through Colour Filters* (London: Actinic Press, 1938).

18 Niels R. Finsen, *Phototherapy*, trans. J. H. Sequeira (London: Edward Arnold, 1901), p. 1.

19 Niels R. Finsen, 'The Red Light Treatment of Small-Pox', *BMJ*, 7 December 1895, pp. 1412–14, at p. 1414. See also Finsen, *Phototherapy*, p. 27; and Niels R. Finsen, 'Remarks on the Red-Light Treatment of Small-Pox', *BMJ*, 6 June 1903, pp. 1297–8, at p. 1297. This quote is also cited by Hobday, though he does not discuss the connection between photography and phototherapy: Richard Hobday, *The Healing Sun: Sunlight and Health in the 21st Century* (Forres: Findhorn Press, 1999), p. 93.

20 Charles Warrenne Allen, *Radiotherapy and Phototherapy* (New York and Philadelphia, Pa.: Lea Brothers & Co., 1904), pp. 450–1.

21 The darkroom, for Finsen, may have been conceptualised as a place of safety for smallpox patients – a treatment room or site of health – but darkrooms were also historically understood as places of risk, danger, and disease and were associated with magic and alchemy. See Sheehan, *Doctored*, pp. 106–31.

22 Edwin L. Ash, *Facts about Artificial Sunlight* (London: Mills & Boon, 1925), p. 48. See also Mihran Krikor Kassabian, *Röntgen Rays and Electro-Therapeutics* (London and Philadelphia, Pa.: J. B. Lippincott Company, 1907), p. 511.

23 Finsen, *Phototherapy*, p. 27; and also, 'The Red Light Treatment of Small-Pox', p. 1414.

24 Thomas Nogier, *La Lumière et la vie*, medical dissertation (Lyon: Imprimerie Waltener, 1904), p. 332.

25 Léon Bouchacourt, *De l'Exploration des organes internes à l'aide de la lumière éclairante et non éclairante* (Paris: G. Steinheil, 1898), p. 34. On the Lumière brothers' involvement in providing photographic products for medical and scientific research, see Lisa Cartwright, *Screening the Body: Tracing Medicine's Visual Culture* (Minneapolis, Minn.: University of Minnesota Press, 1995).

26 See Oskar Bernhard, *Light Treatment in Surgery* (London: Edward Arnold, 1926), pp. 107–8; Allen, *Radiotherapy and Phototherapy*, p. 451; and William Beaumont, *Fundamental Principles of Ray Therapy* (London: H. K. Lewis & Co. Ltd, 1931), pp. 86–7.

27 See Finsen, *Phototherapy*, pp. 37–55. In particular, Finsen found Pleasonton's experiments faulty and his view that blue light could act as a universal panacea to be 'coloured', p. 54.

28 Finsen, *Phototherapy*, p. 40. This is a reference to Talbot's *Pencil of Nature* (1844–6).

29 Arthur Downes and Thomas P. Blunt, 'Researches on the Effect of Light upon Bacteria and Other Organisms', *Proceedings of the Royal Society of Medicine*, 26 (1877), 488–500.

30 Theobald A. Palm, 'The Geographical Distribution and Aetiology of Rickets', *Practitioner*, 45:4 (1890), 270–9, and 45:5, 321–42, at pp. 338–40, 336. See also Simon Carter, *Rise and*

Shine: Sunlight, Technology and Health (New York and Oxford: Berg, 2007), p. 41; Richard Hobday, *The Light Revolution: Health, Architecture and the Sun* (Forres: Findhorn Press, 2006), pp. 52–3; and Jadesola Ekpe, 'The Chemistry of Light: The Life and Work of Theobald Adrian Palm (1848–1928)', *Journal of Medical Biography*, 17 (August 2009), 155–60.

31 Vogel, *Chemistry of Light*. See also Wilder, *Photography and Science*; and Corey Keller, 'Sight Unseen: Picturing the Invisible', in Corey Keller (ed.), *Brought to Light: Photography and the Invisible, 1840–1900* (New Haven, Conn.: Yale University Press with SFMOMA, 2008), pp. 19–35, at p. 20.

32 Bernhard, *Light Treatment*, pp. 22, 110. As Barthes declared, 'It is often said that it was the painters who invented Photography (by bequeathing it their framing, the Albertian perspective, and the optic of the *camera obscura*). I say: no, it was the chemists.' Roland Barthes, *Camera Lucida: Reflections on Photography* (London: Vintage Books, 2000), p. 80.

33 Miles, *Burning Mirror*, p. 134.

34 Miles, *Burning Mirror*, p. 42; and Hentschel, *Mapping the Spectrum*, p. 178.

35 See Albert Eidinow, 'Observations on Some of the Principles of Artificial Sun Treatment', *British Journal of Tuberculosis*, 19:3 (1925), 113–26, at p. 117. See also Russell and Russell, *Ultra-violet Radiation*, p. 24, on Ritter and the discovery of the ultraviolet rays; and Vogel, *Chemistry of Light*, p. 64. On Edmund Becquerel's contribution to registering the invisible rays of the spectrum with photography in 1842, see Kelley Wilder, 'Photography Absorbed', *Bildwelten des Wissens: Kunsthistorisches Jahrbuch für Bildkritik*, 4:2 (2006), pp. 43–53.

36 As Wilder makes clear, 'photography is not only a method for *illustrating* science, it is also a method for *doing* science'. Wilder, *Photography and Science*, p. 103.

37 Hentschel, *Mapping the Spectrum*, pp. 6, 274. Wilder provides a different, nuanced analysis of photography's role and place in spectroscopy in 'Photography Absorbed'.

38 See, for example, Leonard Hill, *Sunshine and Open Air: Their Influence on Health, with Special Reference to the Alpine Climate* (London: Edward Arnold, 1925), pp. 63–70; Russell and Russell, *Ultra-violet Radiation*, pp. 90–1; Beaumont, *Fundamental Principles*, p. 20; Albert Eidinow, 'Some Observations on the Dosage of Ultra-violet Rays in Artificial Sun Treatment', *Lancet*, 15 August 1925, pp. 317–23, at p. 318; Bernhard, *Light Treatment*, pp. 22–3.

39 Cartwright, *Screening the Body*, pp. 29–30; Sophia Zweifel, 'Pellicular Penetrations: The Skins of the Early X-Ray Image' (MA dissertation, University College London, 2012), p. 38; Wilder, *Photography and Science*, p. 11. This of course is only further complicated by the fact that in this book we encounter many more layers of reproductions, far removed from the original negative: the positive print, reproduced in the book, scanned as a digital jpeg, reproduced in a printed book or, in the case of the e-book, viewed through the screen. See Patrick Maynard, *The Engine of Visualization: Thinking through Photography* (Ithaca, NY: Cornell University Press, 1997), p. 18; and Dyer, *White*, p. 85.

40 Henry Augustus Rowland, *Photographic Map of the Normal Solar Spectrum* (Baltimore, Md., 1889), p. 80, cited in Wilder, 'Photography Absorbed', p. 48.

41 Keller, *Brought to Light*, p. 24.

42 Miles, *Burning Mirror*, p. 34.

43 See Russell and Russell, *Ultra-violet Radiation*, p. 148.

44 Didier Anzieu, 'The Film of the Dream', in Sara Flanders (ed.), *The Dream Discourse Today* (London and New York: Routledge, 1993), p. 137, cited in Zweifel, 'Pellicular Penetrations', pp. 25–6, 30–1. See also Barthes, *Camera Lucida*, pp. 80–1; and Steven Connor, 'Integuments: The Scar, the Sheen, the Screen', *New Formations*, 39 (winter 1999), 32–54. Auguste Rollier used the word 'pellicule' in relation to skin during heliotherapy

treatment in *Le Pansement solaire: héliothérapie de certaines affections chirurgicales et des blessures de guerre* (Lausanne and Paris: Librairie Payot & Cie., 1916), p. 27. See also Victor Roditi, *Contribution à l'étude du traitement des brûlures par l'héliothérapie*, medical dissertation (Montpellier: Imprimerie Firmin et Montane, 1914), p. 19.

45 See Allen, *Radiotherapy and Phototherapy*, p. 403. Some of the earliest attempts to 'fix' light-generated impressions were printed on skin (white leather) by Davy and Wedgwood, see Batchen, *Burning with Desire*, p. 28.

46 Eidinow, 'Observations on Some of the Principles', p. 123.

47 Albert Eidinow, 'The Action of Ultra-violet Rays on the Skin', *British Journal of Tuberculosis*, 22:3 (1928), 136–9, at p. 137.

48 Eidinow, 'Observations on Some of the Principles', p. 123. See also *Actinotherapy Technique* (Slough: Sollux, 1933), p. 13; and *Actinotherapy Technique* (1943), p. 205.

49 See Wilder, 'Visualizing Radiation', pp. 349, 364. Finsen likely used a large format camera for this purpose; a photograph of a patient portrait being made with this camera model at the Institute exists in the Medical Museion. My thanks to Nicolai Howalt for bringing this to my attention.

50 Respectively, on Leysin, see Tania Woloshyn, 'Patients Rebuilt: Dr Auguste Rollier's Heliotherapeutic Portraits, *c.* 1903–1944', *Medical Humanities*, 39:1 (2013), 38–46; on the London Hospital, see Anne Kinloch Jamieson, 'An Intolerable Affliction: A History of Lupus Vulgaris in Late Nineteenth- and Early Twentieth-Century Britain' (Ph.D. dissertation, University of Leeds, 2010), p. 51; and on Treloar's, see William Treloar, 'The Cure of Tuberculous Children', *Graphic*, 21 December 1918, p. 739. Both professional and amateur photographers were on site at Treloar's. Many of its archival photographic prints are stamped with an agency's name on the reverse. Images of nurses with cameras in hand include Treloar Archives, Hampshire County Records Office, 47M94/F2/5/4/18, [Keystone View Company, London], *Founders Day*, undated, and 47M94/F2/5/2/19, [Alfieri Picture Service, Fleet Street, London], *Founders Day*, 1930. Small handheld cameras for the public were available, notably through Kodak, from the 1880s, see Hentschel, *Mapping the Spectrum*, p. 187. Kodak's famous slogan, 'You push the button, we do the rest', finds important similarities with advertising rhetoric by manufacturers of home-use phototherapy lamps, which professed to provide sunlight on demand with the 'flick of a switch'.

51 See undated and untitled reprints of heliotherapy patients in the Treloar Archives, 47M94/F2/3/6/12 and 13.

52 On Davy as a 'proto-photographer', see Batchen, *Burning with Desire*.

53 Wolfgang Schivelbusch, *Disenchanted Night: The Industrialization of Light in the Nineteenth Century*, trans. A. Davies (Berkeley, Calif.: University of California Press, 1995), p. 55. See also Chris Otter, *The Victorian Eye: A Political History of Light and Vision in Britain, 1800–1910* (Chicago, Ill.: University of Chicago Press, 2008), pp. 186–7; Charles Bazerman, *The Languages of Edison's Light* (Cambridge, Mass.: MIT Press, 1999); and Hollis Clayson, *Electric Paris: The Visual Cultures of the City of Light in the Era of Thomas Edison* (Chicago, Ill.: University of Chicago Press, forthcoming).

54 Valdemar Bie, 'On Finsen's Phototherapy', *BMJ*, 30 September 1899, pp. 825–30, at p. 826. These tubes or telescopic extensions, like mirrors and lenses, were commonly found in scientific instruments such as spectroscopes and solar microscopes, in order to focus or extend vision. They were also affixed to cameras to photograph astronomical or microscopic phenomena, aided by artificial light sources. See Vogel, *Chemistry of Light and Photography*, pp. 91–2, 195, 206–8.

55 Finsen, *Phototherapy*, p. 77. Miles noted, 'The inventory of hazardous chemicals commonly stocked in these darkrooms includes mercury, potassium cyanide, ether, alcohol, iodine, bromine, potassium iodide, silver nitrate and pyrogallic acid, and it was not uncommon for photographers to become seriously ill or die from the fumes of these chemicals or direct exposure.' Miles, *Burning Mirror*, p. 61. See also Jamieson, 'An Intolerable Affliction', p. 34; and Sheehan, *Doctored*, pp. 106–31.

56 Niels R. Finsen, *Om Anvendelse i Medicinen af Koncentrerede Kemiske Lysstraaler* (Copenhagen: Gyldendalske Boghandels Forlag, 1896), pp. 5–52, cited in Kirsten Iversen Møller, Brian Kongshoj, Peter Alshede Philipsen, Vibeke Ostergaard Thomsen, and Hans Christian Wulf, 'How Finsen's Light Cured Lupus Vulgaris', *Photodermatol Photoimmunol Photomed*, 21:3 (2005), 118–24, at pp. 119–20.

57 Finsen cited the work of Thayer, Otterbein, Mehl, Ziegelroth, and Lahmann with burning mirrors and lenses, and 'electric light baths' displayed in Chicago, in Finsen, *Phototherapy*, pp. 54, 64. See also Margaret Cleaves, *Light Energy: Its Physics, Physiological Action and Therapeutic Applications* (London and New York: Rebman, 1904), p. 437.

58 See Miles, *Burning Mirror*, p. 200; and Gregory Lynall, '"Bundling Up the Sun-Beams": Burning Mirrors in Eighteenth-Century Knowledge and Culture', *Journal for Eighteenth-Century Studies*, 36:4 (2013), 477–90. John Harvey Kellogg stated he had used lenses and concave mirrors to concentrate sunlight first in 1883; see 'Heliotherapy, Phototherapy, and Thermotherapy', in Solomon Solis Cohen (ed.), *A System of Physiologic Therapeutics* (London: Rebman, 1902), pp. 210–60, at p. 222. In relation to tumours, Cleaves referenced epitheliomas being treated with sunlight concentrated through lenses in *Light Energy*, p. 437. An epithelioma is a benign or malignant tumour of the epithelium, sometimes loosely or incorrectly used as a synonym for carcinoma.

59 A Dr Kime, reporting from his sanatorium in Iowa, spoke of using a 'modification of the ray filter employed in photography' to focus natural sunlight onto a lupus patient. See J. W. Kime, 'Light in the Treatment of Lupus and Other Chronic Skin Affections', *Journal of the American Medical Association*, 11 April 1903, pp. 966–8, at p. 966.

60 J. Alfred Codd, 'Some Results of Treatment by X Rays, High-Frequency Currents, and Ultra-violet Rays', *BMJ*, 23 July 1904, pp. 176–80.

61 Cleaves, *Light Energy*, p. 477.

62 Cleaves, *Light Energy*, p. 477.

63 See Finsen, *Phototherapy*, p. 67. Cleaves was aware of the lamps on offer through Schall in Britain; see *Light Energy*, p. 481.

64 Schivelbusch similarly explained how lighting technologies informed each other, of gas lighting to arc lighting, and arc lighting to the electric light bulb. He wrote, 'Lighting technology appears to have progressed in logical steps from the hearth flame via the torch, the candle and the Argand lamp to gaslight, without faltering or looking back. But technical progress is more than a resolute stride forward; it also involves the developmental stages that have been left behind. Often, these do not simply disappear, but live on, in modified – that is, modernised – form.' Schivelbusch, *Disenchanted Night*, p. 49. He may not have meant the medical uses of electric lighting, but arc lights clearly found a new market in the 1890s in the wake of Edison's incandescent bulbs' tremendous popularity and commercial exploitation. See also Bazerman, *Edison's Light*, p. 337.

65 'Light Treatment in Hospitals', *The Times*, 'Sunlight and Health' special supplement, 22 May 1928, pp. xxxi–xxxii, at p. xxxii. This is also cited in Jamieson, 'An Intolerable Affliction', pp. 121–2.

66 See Beaumont, *Fundamental Principles*, p. 66. By this time stage lighting had already been using reflectors to concentrate artificial light for centuries: Schivelbusch, *Disenchanted Night*, p. 197.

67 An advertisement for 'Marion Therapeutical Multi-carbon Arc Lamps' can be found in the advertisement section in Myrtle Vaughan-Cowell, *Artificial Sunlight: Its Use and Application* (London: H. Edgar Smithers, 1928), unpaginated.

68 Matthew Luckiesh, *Artificial Sunlight: Combining Radiation for Health with Light for Vision* (New York: D. van Nostrand, 1930). On Edison and General Electric, see Bazerman, *Edison's Light*, p. 259.

69 Despite intense searching, Howalt and the staff of the Medical Museion cannot locate Finseon's original. Frustratingly, a narrative of 'failure' dominates the secondary literature on Tudor-Hart: she struggled financially throughout her life, and her activities as a spy haunted her throughout her later years, leading her to destroy much of her photographs; information about her remained inaccessible to photographic historians until the 1980s, closed off in classified archives; her marriage failed, her son had to be institutionalised due to mental disability, and she lost her studio during the Blitz; above all, her Communist beliefs came to nought and much of her photography was forced to pander to mainstream advertising to get by. See Forbes, 'Politics, Photography and Exile', pp. 65–6. See also the essays in the catalogue, *Edith Tudor-Hart*, especially Forbes, 'Edith Tudor-Hart in London', pp. 65–74, at p. 70; and Roberta McGrath, 'Passport No. 656336', pp. 119–25, at p. 125.

70 Forbes, 'Edith Tudor-Hart in London', p. 65. On photography's role in these metaphors, Miles wrote, 'Photography's metaphorical alliance with light ensured that the medium could serve as a valuable weapon against the obscurity of darkness.' Miles, *Burning Mirror*, p. 58. She cited the documentary photographs of dark slums by Jacob Riis and Lewis Hine in the United States.

71 The light's additional abilities to disinfect/cleanse only further cemented these metaphors; see Otter, *The Victorian Eye*; and Carter cites Salvation Army founder William Booth's 1890 book, *In Darkest England*, in *Rise and Shine*, p. 84.

72 Incidentally, she married a British physician, Alexander Tudor-Hart, enabling her to immigrate to England in 1933. For details on Tudor-Hart in relation to her Montessori teacher training, her political beliefs and connections, her activities in espionage, her links with the Bauhaus and the Worker Photography Movement, her interest in child health and welfare, and more, see Wolfgang Suschitzky, *Edith Tudor Hart: The Eye of Conscience* (London: Dirk Nishen, 1987); Forbes, 'Politics, Photography and Exile'; and the essays by Forbes, Anton Holzer, and Roberta McGrath in *Edith Tudor-Hart*.

73 Figures 3.1 and 3.2 have not been discussed in the Tudor-Hart literature, though the former featured, without commentary, in *Edith Tudor-Hart* at the National Galleries of Scotland, where the exhibition opened in 2013 and where her negative archive is now housed.

74 *The South London Hospital for Women and Children*, p. 1. McGrath notes that the SLHWC was referred to as an 'Adamless Eden' (McGrath, 'Passport No. 656336', p. 123). See also Mary Ann Elston, '"Run by Women (Mainly) for Women": Medical Women's Hospitals in Britain, 1866–1948', in Lawrence Conrad and Anne Hardy (eds), *Women and Modern Medicine* (Amsterdam and New York: Rodopi, 2001), pp. 73–107.

75 On the back cover it stated it was 'expensively produced' and should be passed on rather than discarded.

76 *The South London Hospital for Women and Children*, p. 3.

77 *The South London Hospital for Women and Children*, p. 5.

78 We might say this of most photographs, except in instances when discernible shadows, reflections, or visible appendages record the maker's presence. My thanks to Natasha Ruiz-Gómez for pointing this out.

79 See Schivelbusch, *Disenchanted Night*, pp. 54, 120; Graeme Gooday, *Domesticating Electricity: Technology, Uncertainty and Gender, 1880–1914* (London: Pickering & Chatto, 2008), pp. 24, 155–7; and Otter, *The Victorian Eye*, p. 8.

80 See Schivelbusch, *Disenchanted Night*, pp. 120–34, for American and French examples, including the fascinating unrealised project of Sébillot and Bourdais, 'Colonne-Soleil', a sun tower proposed to light up all of central Paris for the competition for a monument to commemorate the 1889 Exposition, ultimately and famously won by Gustave Eiffel.

81 As Gooday explained, 'The *aesthetic* problems of electric lighting ... were not merely transitory inconveniences, they were serious enough to become a real challenge to those seeking to domesticate electricity.' Gooday, *Domesticating Electricity*, p. 153.

82 Schivelbusch stated, 'The introduction of arc lighting for the first time made good the metaphorical description of street lanterns as artificial suns. The arc-light *was*, in fact, a small sun and the light it cast had a spectrum similar to that of daylight'. Schivelbusch, *Disenchanted Night*, p. 118. Lamps were commonly named after the sun, Hanovia's 'Alpine Sun Lamp' and 'Homesun' mercury vapour lamps but two notable examples. Hill helped manufacture a carbon arc lamp called the 'Sun-Rae', by Watson & Sons; see Vaughan-Cowell, *Artificial Sunlight*, pp. 36, 38.

83 Photography was no stranger to medical metaphors, exemplified by the word 'doctoring' to speak of manipulating images: Sheehan, *Doctored*.

84 Overexposure was not only common when attempting to capture phototherapy in process, it occurred in photographing heliotherapy too: 'Owing to the large proportion of ultra-violet rays in the sunlight of the high mountainous districts, one must give shorter exposures in photography, and one also finds that the fading and loss of colour proceed unpleasantly fast.' Bernhard, *Light Treatment*, pp. 20–1.

85 We might consider such photographic 'accidents' or 'injuries', made through excessive light, analogous to the upper degrees of solar erythema – of blisters and bad burns on the skin, presently defined by Cancer Research UK as signs of acute 'bodily damage' (see Chapters 2, 4, and 6).

86 Russell and Russell, *Ultra-violet Radiation*, p. 59.

87 See Katherine Gamgee, *The Artificial Light Treatment of Children* (London: H. K. Lewis & Co., 1927), pp. 66–7.

88 See Treloar Archives, Hampshire County Records Office, 108A09/1, Miss Barbara M Davis, *The Light Department of Lord Mayor Treloar Cripples' Hospital*, undated (*c.* 1929), album of photographs.

89 '*Artifact*: A visible sign of the process by which an image is made. Artifacts can be a result of the camera or lens technology, the exposure, the emulsion or the development of the film. What is an undesirable artifact for some is a useful piece of information for others.' Wilder, *Photography and Science*, p. 129.

90 Miles, *Burning Mirror*, p. 203. See also Batchen, *Burning with Desire*, p. 149.

91 Barthes, *Camera Lucida*, pp. 26–7.

92 Miles, *Burning Mirror*, p. 161. For another example of a 'black sun' produced in phototherapy, see Treloar Archives, 47M94/F2/1/7/25, Alfieri Picture Service (London), 'The Lord Mayor [right, with Henry Gauvain, left] seen during his inspection of the Artificial Light Section', Founders Day at Lord Mayor Treloar Cripples' Hospital, 8 June 1934.

93 Miles, *Burning Mirror*, p. 167.

94 Miles, *Burning Mirror*, pp. 234–5. The terms 'positive' and 'negative' are attributed to Talbot: Batchen, *Burning with Desire*, p. 34. Solarisation caused particular havoc in spectrum photographs, confusing the reading of the image's dark and light stripes; see Hentschel, *Mapping the Spectrum*, pp. 211, 275.

95 See Wilder, *Photography and Science*, pp. 122–3; and Miles, *Burning Mirror*, p. 235. Miles also discussed the work of several contemporary photographers who deliberately play with volatile light, by aiming their cameras directly at the sun (Danielle Thompson), shining light with mirrors into the camera (Tokihiro Sato), or lighting their exhibitions with carbon arc lamps (Doug and Mike Starn).

96 On 'Vita' glass, see John Stanislav Sadar, 'Unpacking the Latent Bodies of Interwar Ultraviolet Health Glass' (Ph.D. dissertation, University of Pennsylvania, 2010); John Stanislav Sadar, *Through the Healing Glass: Shaping the Modern Body through Glass Architecture, 1925–35* (London and New York: Routledge, 2016); and John Stanislav Sadar, '"Vita" Glass and the Discourse of Modern Culture', in Grace Lees-Maffei (ed.), *Writing Design: Words and Objects* (London and New York: Berg, 2012), pp. 103–17. See also W. W. Coblentz and R. Stair, 'Data on Ultra-violet Solar Radiation and the Solarization of Window Materials', *Bureau of Standards Journal of Research*, 3, ref. PR113, 629–89. Coblentz and Stair's tests proved that 'Vita' glass could lose its transparency to ultraviolet rays through solarisation within days of constant exposure to natural or artificial light during test conditions.

97 The word 'solarisation' is used in American references to heliotherapy: see 'Sunshine and Clothing', *Journal of the American Medical Association*, 10 August 1929, pp. 461–2, at p. 461, and Allen, *Radiotherapy and Phototherapy*, p. 427. Carter used the word 'solarisation' to describe insolation in Simon Carter, 'The Medicalization of Sunlight in the Early Twentieth Century', *Journal of Historical Sociology*, 25:1 (2012), 83–105, at p. 85.

98 R. A. Houstoun, *Light and Colour* (London: Longmans, Green & Co., 1923), pp. 154–5.

99 Daniel Freund, *American Sunshine: Diseases of Darkness and the Quest for Natural Light* (Chicago, Ill.: University of Chicago Press, 2012), pp. 90–1.

100 Leonard Hill, 'Discussion on Influence of Sunlight and Artificial Light on Health', *BMJ*, 12 September 1925, pp. 470–7, at p. 472. As Hill noted, evidence was lacking to prove this, and it is curious some physicians believed this since a carbon arc lamp produced infrared, visible, and ultraviolet light, much like the sun. The confusion over the action of different rays of light is discussed in Chapter 4.

101 Ecclesiastes 11:7, King James Bible, cited in Russell and Russell, *Ultra-violet Radiation*, p. 84. Interestingly, Hobday declared, 'one person's glare is another's phototherapy'. He stated this while discussing architects impeding bright light into buildings to avoid glare or overheating for occupants, to which Hobday objected. Hobday, *The Light Revolution*, p. 27.

102 'Violet Ray Treatment', *Yorkshire Post*, 14 March 1925, p. 10.

103 My thanks to Keren Hammerschlag for her perceptive comments on blindness being the product of both too much and too little light.

104 Michel Foucault, *Madness and Civilization: A History of Insanity in the Age of Reason* (New York: Vintage, 1973), p. 108, cited in Jonathan Crary, *Techniques of the Observer: On Vision and Modernity in the Nineteenth Century* (Cambridge, Mass.: MIT Press, 1999), p. 139. Miles pointed out that the word 'glare' has similar ambiguous, 'transgressive and slippery' meanings in photography, meaning both to stare intently (verb) and 'dazzling or oppressive light' (noun), both 'an agent of fixity and dispersion'. Miles, *Burning Mirror*, p. 225.

105 Jacques Derrida, *Mémoires d'aveugle: L'autoportrait et autres ruines* (Paris: Réunion des Musées Nationaux, 1990), cited in Batchen, *Burning with Desire*, p. 119.

106 Vaughan-Cowell, *Artificial Sunlight*, p. 23. See also *Actinotherapy Technique* (1933), p. 14.

107 See, for instance, 'Blinded by Violet Rays', *Western Gazette*, 2 October 1925, p. 14. The dramatic and mesmerising flame of the lamp may have even drawn patients to stare intently at it during treatment. On technology's 'magnetic pull' on operators and patients, see Margarete Sandelowski, *Devices and Desires: Gender, Technology, and American Nursing* (Chapel Hill, NC: University of North Carolina Press, 2000), p. 30. Nicolai Howalt described his photographic project *Light Break* as exploring the compulsion to look at something one should not, in keeping with his earlier projects on car crashes and boxing facial injuries (see Chapter 6).

108 See John Harvey Kellogg, *Light Therapeutics* (Battle Creek, Mich.: Modern Medicine, 1927), pp. 42–3.

109 See J. C. Elvy, 'Kinematograph Illumination: The Use and Abuse of Light in Studios for Kinema Film Production', *Lancet*, 19 February 1921, p. 413.

110 See *Actinotherapy Technique* (1933), pp. 117–20, in which both general and local treatments were employed for conditions such as chronic blepharitis, chronic (bacterial) conjunctivitis, trachoma, and corneal ulcers. See also W. Stewart Duke-Elder, 'The Therapeutic Action of Ultra-violet Light upon the Eye', *BMJ*, 29 May 1926, pp. 891–5. Duke-Elder names Hill and Eidinow as colleagues of his at the NIMR, with funding from the MRC. He noted that in some local applications, including diseases of the conjunctiva, photophthalmia (the acute conjunctivitis caused by actinic light, also known as snowblindness) was produced purposefully, just as an erythema is provoked on the skin, to stimulate healing. In too high dosages, however, he recognised photophthalmia could become permanent. Rollier included hand-coloured before and after photographs of a patient treated by heliotherapy for tuberculosis of the conjunctiva (upper eyelids) in *La Cure de soleil* (Lausanne and Paris: Baillière & Fils and Constant Tarin, 1914), pp. 172–5. He also cited a physician, Lundsgaard, at the Finsen Institute, who reported using phototherapy on ocular manifestations of lupus erythematosus already by 1906. Gauvain reported, with accompanying photographs, treating the under-surface of a child's eyelid with local treatment at Treloar's in Sir Henry Gauvain, 'Organisation and Work of a Light Department in a Hospital for Surgical Tuberculosis', *Lancet*, 4 July 1925, pp. 10–16, at pp. 14–15.

111 Crary mentioned several scientists whose research into retinal afterimages, involving deliberately staring at the sun, resulted in severely damaged eyesight and even permanent blindness, and concluded, 'What this work often involved was the experience of staring directly into the sun, of sunlight searing itself onto the body.' Crary, *Techniques of the Observer*, p. 141. See also his discussion of J. M. W. Turner's representations of sunlight, pp. 138–41.

112 Miles argued that the camera in fact can be understood to operate as a 'burning mirror' itself by analysing photographs of black suns, lens flare, and solarisation. The camera could thus confusingly be likened to the lamp, the patient, and the treatment room (its origins in the camera obscura literally translating to 'dark room').

113 See Miles, *Burning Mirror*, pp. 147–53. See also Vogel, *The Chemistry of Light*, pp. 18–19.

114 Sir Henry Gauvain, 'Discussion on Light Treatment in Surgical Tuberculosis', Proceedings of the Royal Society of Medicine, 20:6 (1927), 805–15, at p. 809. This notion of the value of the 'light shock' is also discussed in Hobday, *The Healing Sun*, pp. 109, 154–5. Bernhard described light's stimulating action on the body, via the retina to the central nervous system, in *Light Treatment*, p. 54.

115 Miles similarly described excess light that 'burns away visual detail' in photography in *Dreams and Imagination: Light in the Modern City* (Wheelers Hill: Monash Gallery of Art, 2014), p. 46.
116 See also Treloar Archives, album F2/3/15, 'The Light Department', Treloar Cripples' Hospital, undated photograph.
117 Shelford Bidwell, *Curiosities of Light and Sight* (London: Swan Sonnenschein & Co., 1899), pp. 13–14.
118 Bidwell, *Curiosities of Light and Sight*, p. 23. See also Keller, 'Sight Unseen', p. 29; Crary, *Techniques of the Observer*, p. 129; and Batchen, *Burning with Desire*, pp. 82–3.
119 Wilder, *Photography and Science*, p. 9. See Chapter 5 on the role of visual culture in communicating suntan as a form of racial transgression.
120 See Wilder, *Photography and Science*, pp. 65–6; and Miles, *Burning Mirror*, p. 41.
121 Not only by being a damaged or 'bad' photograph but, as part of an archival collection, by 'sinking in among its companions, relinquishing its individual character in order to further a much larger narrative history'. Wilder, *Photography and Science*, p. 100.
122 See Eidinow, 'Observations on Some of the Principles', p. 116; W. E. Dixon, 'Discussion on the Therapeutic Value of Light', *BMJ*, 19 September 1925, pp. 499–504, at p. 499; Beaumont, *Fundamental Principles*, p. 85; Russell and Russell, *Ultra-violet Radiation*, pp. 85–6, 90; and Troup, *Therapeutic Uses of Infra-Red Rays*, p. vi.
123 Batchen, *Burning with Desire*, p. 183.

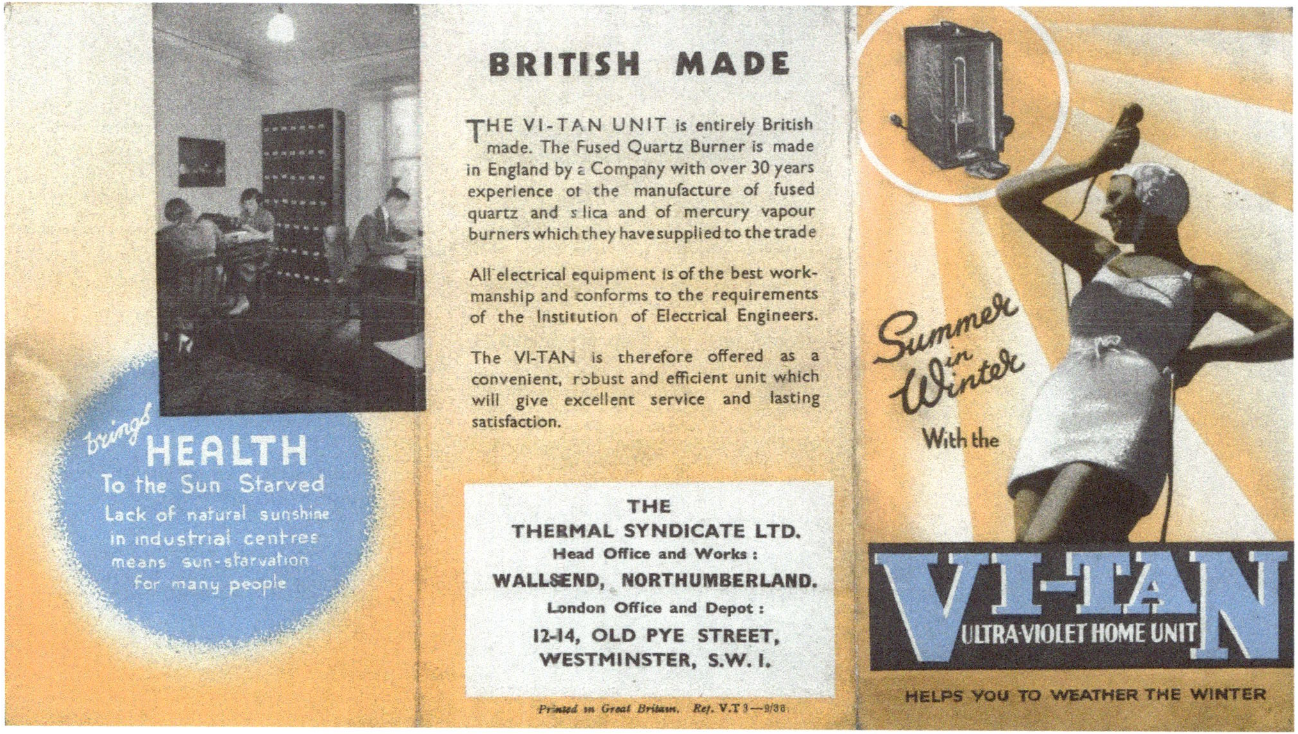
brings HEALTH
To the Sun Starved
Lack of natural sunshine in industrial centres means sun-starvation for many people
BRITISH MADE
THE VI-TAN UNIT is entirely British made. The Fused Quartz Burner is made in England by a Company with over 30 years experience of the manufacture of fused quartz and silica and of mercury vapour burners which they have supplied to the trade
All electrical equipment is of the best workmanship and conforms to the requirements of the Institution of Electrical Engineers.
The VI-TAN is therefore offered as a convenient, robust and efficient unit which will give excellent service and lasting satisfaction.
THE
THERMAL SYNDICATE LTD.
Head Office and Works :
WALLSEND, NORTHUMBERLAND.
London Office and Depot :
12-14, OLD PYE STREET,
WESTMINSTER, S.W. I.
Printed in Great Britain. Ref. V.T 3—9/36
Summer in Winter
With the
VI-TAN
ULTRA-VIOLET HOME UNIT
HELPS YOU TO WEATHER THE WINTER

Plate 1 *Summer in Winter with the Vi-Tan Ultra-violet Home Unit*, *c.* 1936, colour pamphlet, by the Thermal Syndicate.

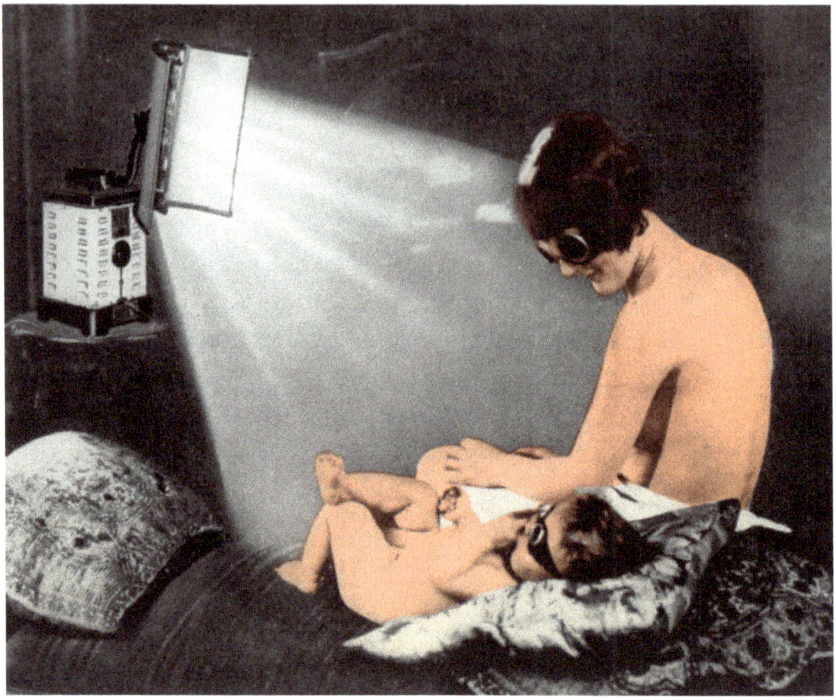

Plate 2 Hanovia, *Get Back in the Sun with a 'Homesun'*, pamphlet, 1940, p. 7. Thackray Medical Museum, Leeds.

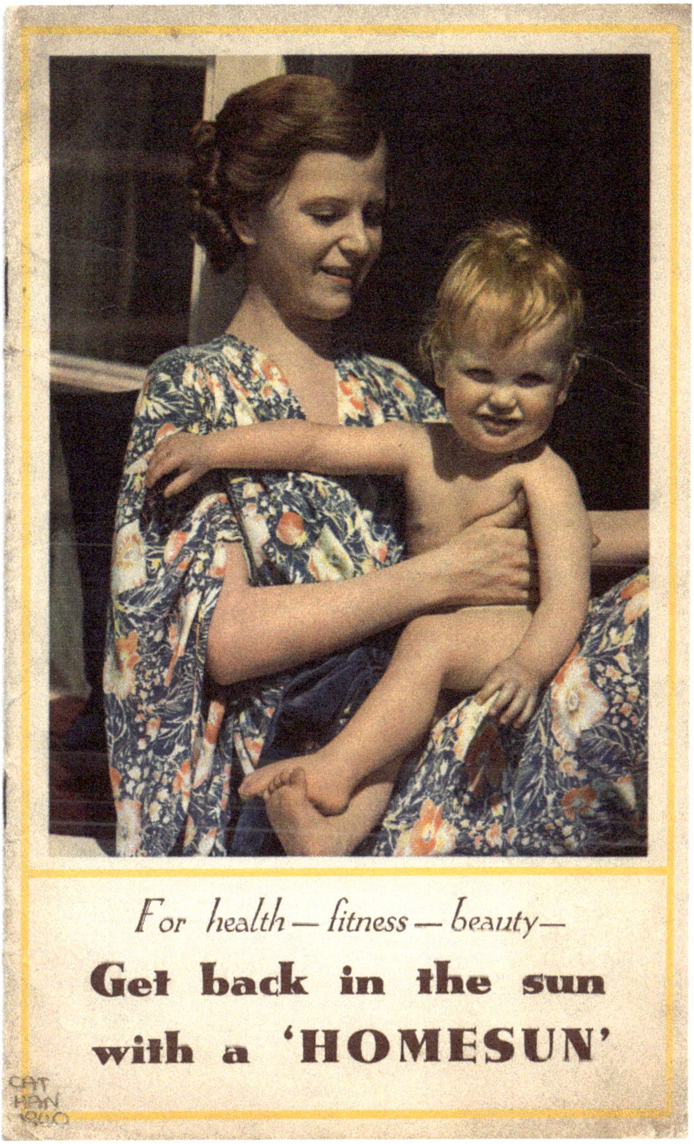

Plate 3 Hanovia, *Get Back in the Sun with a 'Homesun'*, pamphlet, 1940, cover.
Thackray Medical Museum, Leeds.

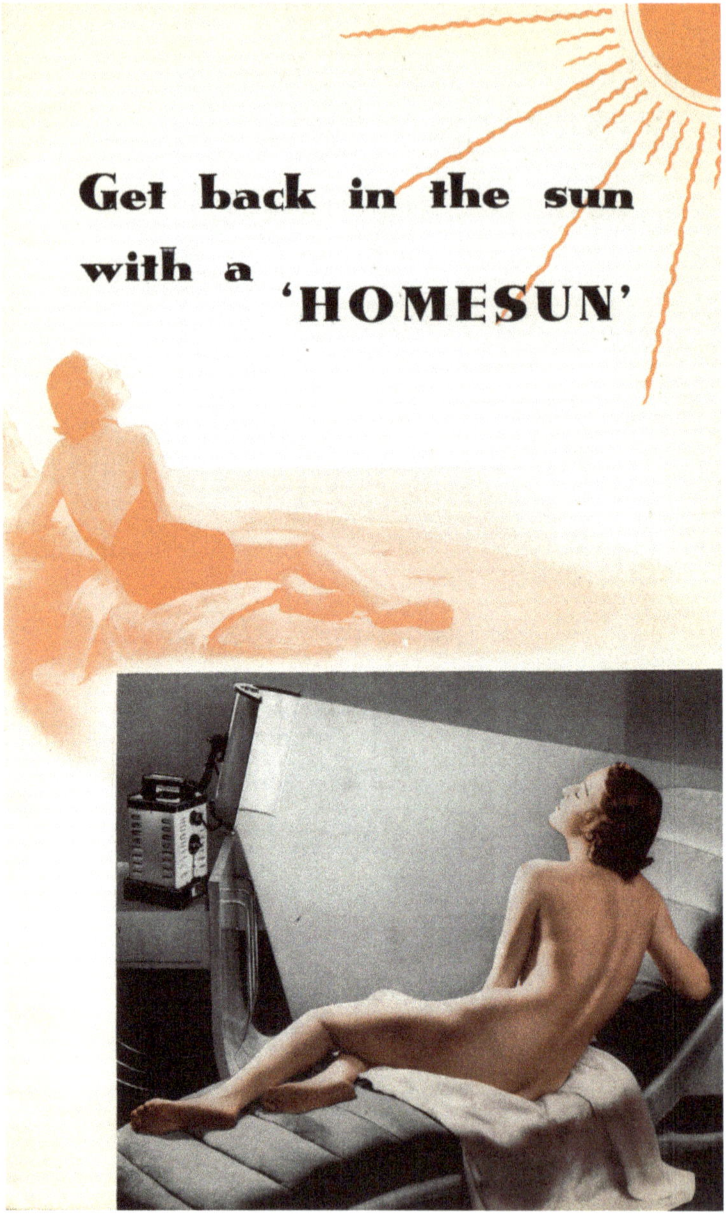

Plate 4 Hanovia, *Get Back in the Sun with a 'Homesun'*, pamphlet, 1940, p. 1. Thackray Medical Museum, Leeds.

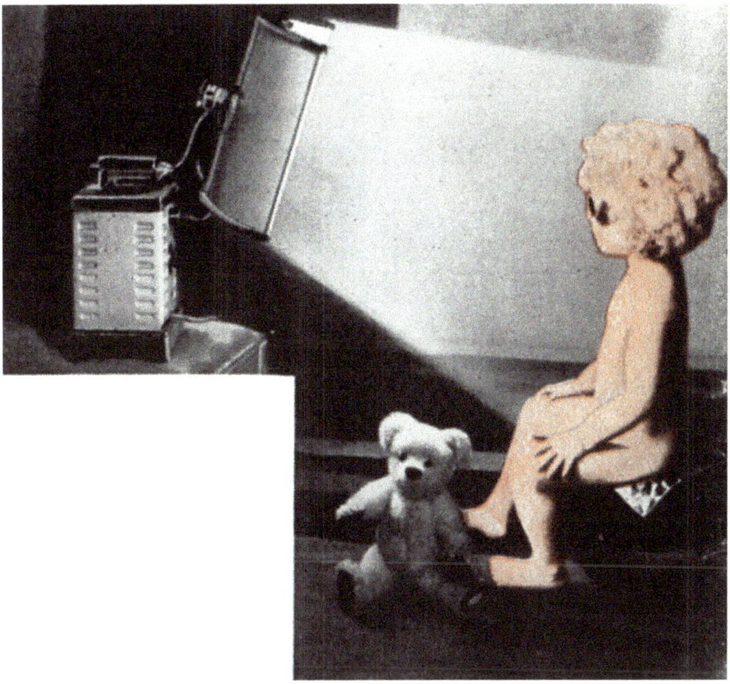

Plate 5 Hanovia, *Get Back in the Sun with a 'Homesun'*, pamphlet, 1940, p. 14. Thackray Medical Museum, Leeds.

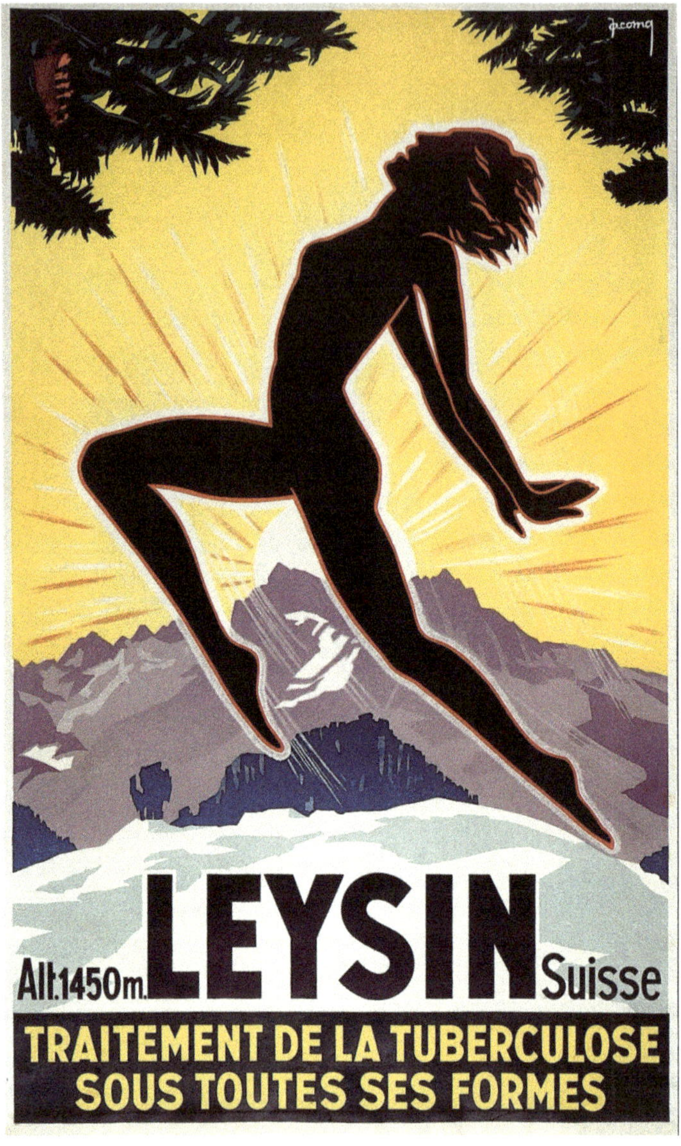

Plate 6 Jacomo Müller, *Alt. 1450m, Leysin, Switzerland: Treatment for Tuberculosis in All Its Forms*, c. 1930, colour lithograph, 99.5 × 61.8 cm.
Wellcome Library, London.

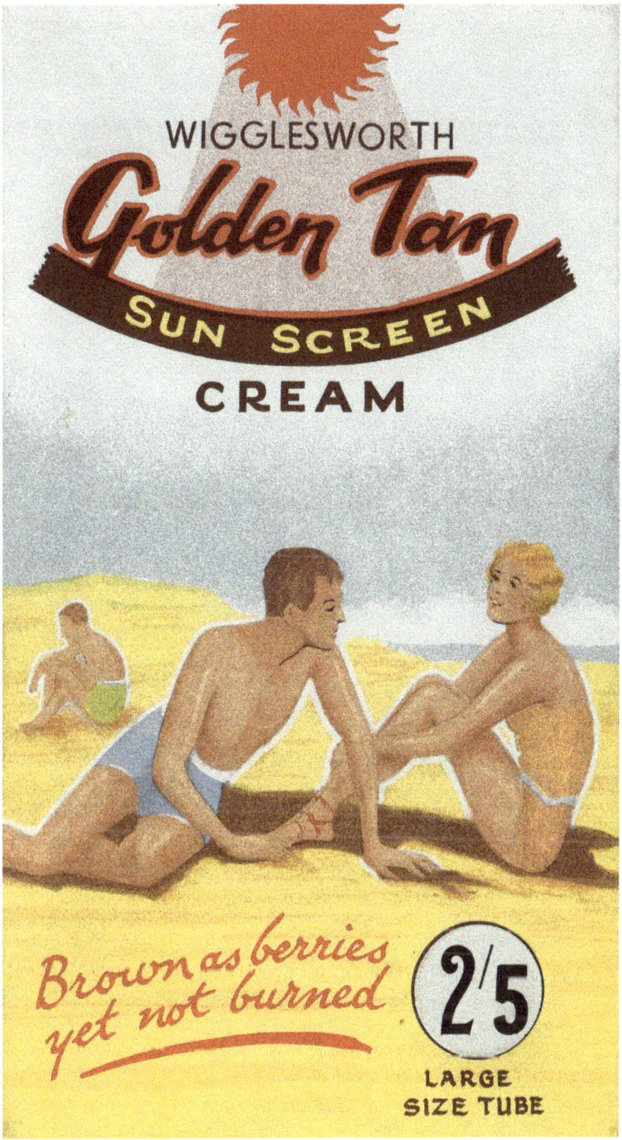

Plate 7 Advertisement for Wigglesworth, 'Golden Tan sun screen cream', *c.* 1930s.
Wellcome Library, London CC BY-NC 4.0.

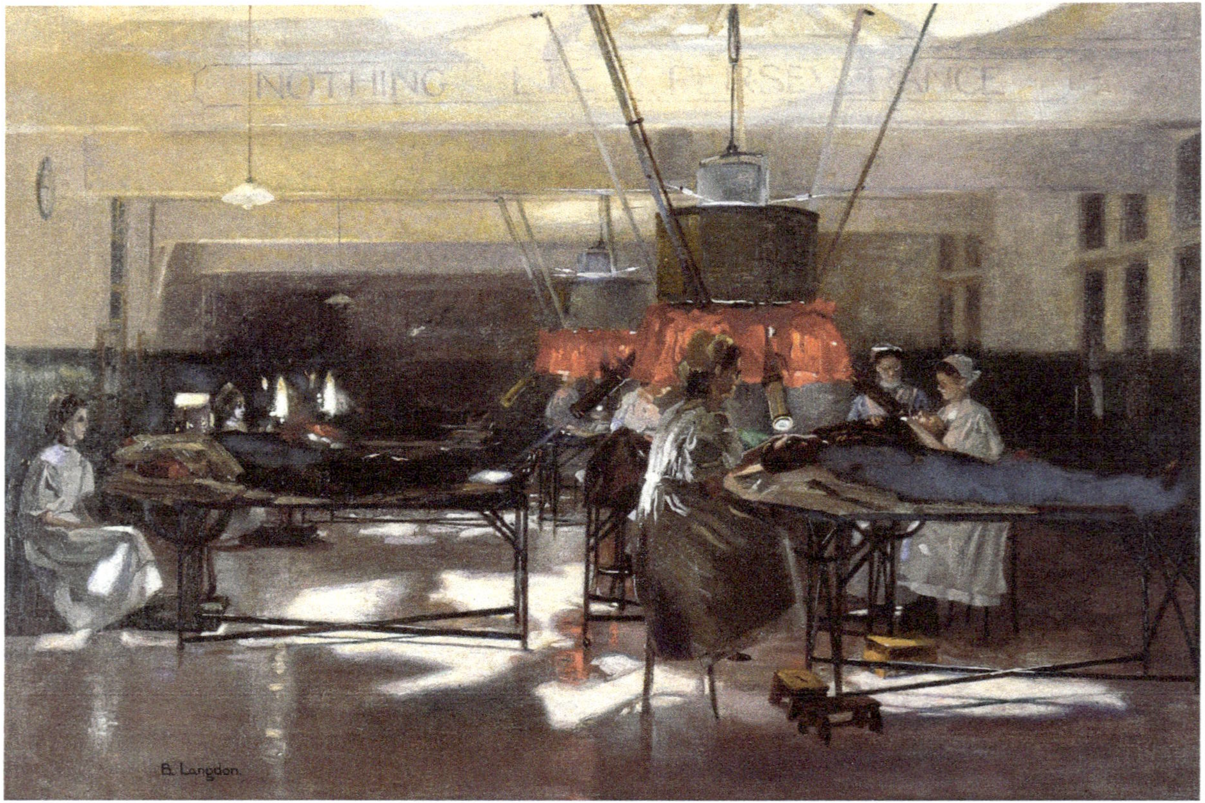

Plate 8 Beatrice Langdon, *The Finsen Light Treatment at the London Hospital*, *c*. 1938, oil painting. Wellcome Library, London.

4

Vanguard rays

> It must be acknowledged that ... our knowledge of the physiological action of light and its effects, whether good or bad, is very limited. In undertaking now the study of one of the properties of the chemical rays, viz., their *injurious* influence upon the animal organism, I do so, not because I regard this property as the only influence of the chemical rays, but *because it constitutes the very foundation of our subject*.[1]
>
> (Niels Finsen, 1894)

> Solar energy, received through the ether and transmuted on arrival into various forms, is responsible for all our activities. What the effect of radiation on human bodies may be, we are only beginning to find out. Pigmentation produced in the skin shows that the effect is by no means negligible; and now clinical work on the effect of radiation, both natural and artificial – especially radiation of frequency too high to affect, except prejudicially, the retina of the eye – is leading to results of obviously great interest even to a layman.[2]
>
> (Oliver Lodge, 1925)

ART Deco sunbeams splay out dynamically behind a deeply tanned, smiling woman (Plate 1). In contrast to their flat graphic pattern, her beautiful and scantily clad body is highlighted by the natural shadows playing across her rounded form. She is positioned in such a way that we look up at her from below, desiring her, desiring to be her: beautiful, vivacious, tanned, happy, fashionable, and healthy.[3] Plate 1 is the cover of a *c.* 1936 pamphlet advertising a home-use lamp, the 'Vi-tan' mercury vapour lamp, designed by the British manufacturer, the Thermal Syndicate.[4] It is a vanguard montage fusing photographs and graphic illustration in both black-and-white and high-keyed, saturated colour. The advertisement delights our eyes with its complementary colours of orange and blue and its modern mix of serif and sans-serif typefaces.[5] But our attention is inevitably drawn back to the model, larger than life and as glamorous and graceful as a dancer on the stage. Placed before the theatrical background of orange and white rays, she twists her body playfully towards (and presumably under) the large orb that is the sun. Yet it is not the sun per se that she worships, but modern technology. A heavily retouched black-and-white photograph of the 'Vi-tan' lamp was cut out and stuck within this orb, adding another disjunctive layer of mismatched scales and spatial dislocation. It is the lamp itself that usurps the sun's primacy as bringer of health and happiness, a sophisticated device to 'help weather the winter' by providing artificial summer sunshine.

With its attractive polished oak casing, chromium reflector, and state-of-the-art fused quartz mercury vapour bulb, the 'Vi-tan' lamp was an object at once homely *and* technologically sophisticated (Fig. 4.1). Supplied with the lamp were brown-tinted, leather goggles (Fig. 4.2), a requisite piece of apparel for exposure to a bulb that the manufacturer declared emitted a whopping (and, frankly, highly unlikely) 99 per cent of invisible ultraviolet light. According to contemporaneous textbooks, standard mercury vapour lamps emitted approximately 28 per cent.[6] If genuine, the Vi-tan's immense output had the capacity to severely burn and blind its users.

Yet looking at the object, we do not get a sense that it is a dangerous device. Any potential dangers of ultraviolet light or electricity appear safely contained in its rich, polished wooden casing.[7] Its promotional advertising, as evident in Plate 1, only further emphasised its polish, its sophistication, as an object not simply of vitalising health but glamorous beauty.

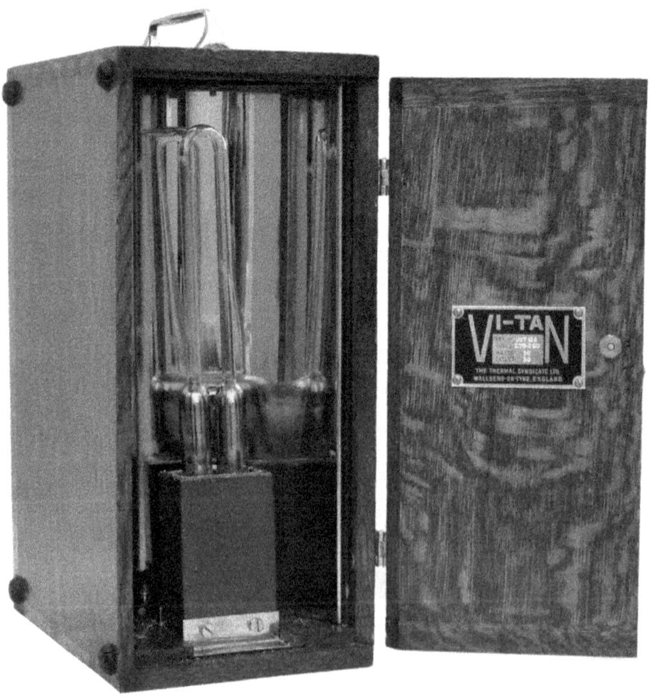

Figure 4.1 The Thermal Syndicate 'Vi-tan' mercury vapour lamp, mid-1930s.
Oak, chromium plating, and quartz glass.
Author's collection.

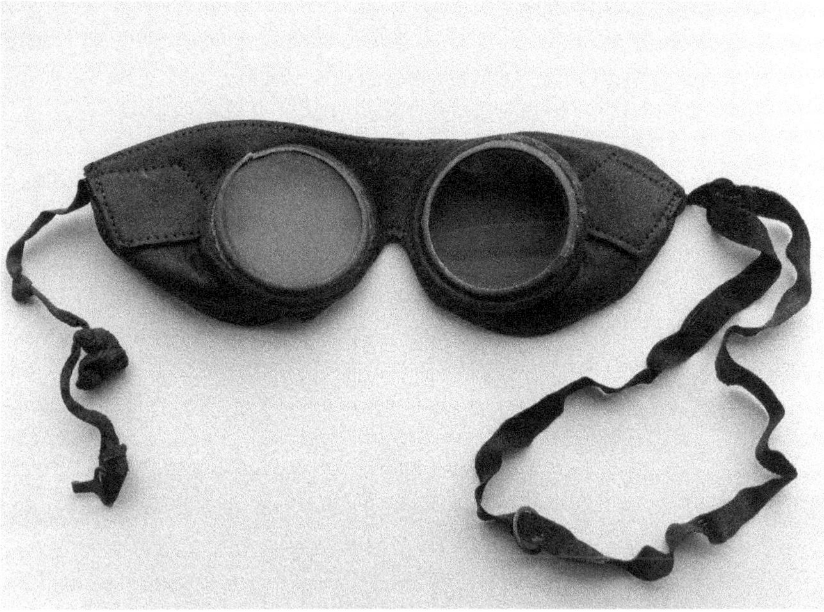

Figure 4.2 The Thermal Syndicate 'Vi-tan' goggles, mid-1930s. Brown-tinted glass, leather, and elastic. Author's collection.

Reputable medical men and quacks alike promoted home-use lamps for public use as the ideal preventive means to health in the absence of natural sunlight. Other medical practitioners, however, urged caution towards these devices, both in the interests of public safety and light therapy's reputation. While continuing to discuss light therapy's appeal and legitimisation, this chapter shifts focus from the previous chapters, moving from the hospital and clinic to the home. It explores the ambivalent reception of home-use lamps when they emerged on the market during the 1920s and 1930s, as objects simultaneously of benefit and risk. Just as they could animate life and bring vitality, so could they cause suffering and even death: life-threatening burns, electrocution, and miscarriage were all reported in popular and medical literature. The history of home-use lamps bears important relation to that of 'domesticating' electricity; both were a haphazard business. As Graeme Gooday showed, domestic lighting occupied a precarious position in public and private life, somewhere between electro-therapeutic apparatus, which professed to restore life, and the electric chair, which ended it. Tales of electricity 'out of control', causing injury and death, versus those of it marvellously 'tamed' within fashionable upper-class homes, present two very different public perspectives of this natural force in late nineteenth- and early twentieth-century Britain.[8]

Like electricity, artificially produced ultraviolet radiation required 'domestication'. To be consumed en masse it needed to be harnessed, controlled, and 'tamed' within the home. With their emanating penetrative radiation and electrical wiring, home-use lamps were potentially volatile devices that could burn and shock users. To be effectively advertised, these new devices required a new aesthetic, one that could represent their invisible, vitalising energies and convey their bodily effects in an arresting, compelling way. This new look did not materialise from the ether, to cite famous physicist and spiritualist Sir Oliver Lodge (1851–1940; see epigraph). It emerged as an adaptation of vanguard techniques of montage – a composite of multiple layers – and must be contextualised alongside contemporaneous advertisements and perceptions of other kinds of therapeutic radiation, notably X rays and radium. This chapter focuses on visual and therapeutic multiple exposures, on the allied and complicated histories of radiation therapies and their public consumption. As the 'Vi-tan' pamphlet cover demonstrates, vanguard visual tactics were in place to advertise these risky, invisible rays, tactics that productively conflated and confounded their powers for a hungry set of consumers.

The epigraphs by Finsen and Lodge evince that ultraviolet radiation's 'injurious', transformative, and mysterious powers continued to seduce and perplex the medical, scientific, and public imagination for decades.[9] Lodge, once president of the Society for Psychical Research, described ultraviolet light as a mysterious and powerful form of radiation, of interest both to the scientist and the layman. Yet, thirty years on, he provided little more clarity about its bodily effects than did Finsen. Like the ambivalence the medical community expressed towards the relative merits or risks of producing solar erythema ('sunburn'), the confusion over 'fixing' dosages (Chapter 2), and the uneasy role of photography in light therapy's development (Chapter 3), the emergence and representation of home-use lamps are fraught with inconsistencies, confusion, and tension – at once beneficial medical devices and dangerous popular toys. In keeping with the general aim of this book, I want to explore these instead of smoothing out their rough edges.

In the previous chapters, black-and-white photography featured heavily as a light technology and a medium of representation. Much of the discussion focused on photography's ambivalent relationship with light therapy and, most of all, on its *limitations* to register, disseminate, and legitimise the therapy as modern medicine. I ended Chapter 3 by mentioning how often light therapy's photographs were retouched, or faked outright, to avoid the hazards and difficulties of capturing the therapy in process. Manual intervention, whether by retouching, assembling composites, or mixing illustration with photograph, is absolutely ubiquitous in its imagery, though obviously not unique to it.[10] We encounter this intervention so frequently – in illustrated newspapers, advertisements, popular treatises, medical handbooks, and institutional archives – that it epitomises light therapy's visual culture.[11] This intervention is exemplified by an image in a promotional booklet for the Peebles Hydropathic Hotel (Hawick), which offered light therapy to its clientele (Fig. 4.3). Note the 'corrections' of overdrawn contours that have been irradiated and eradicated by the light's excesses, the non-naturalistic visualisation of invisible light by bold blocks of negative space and graphic lines, and the vanguard layering of illustration and photograph. So overworked is the operator that she emerges as machine-like as the equipment surrounding her. Her clumsily overdrawn features, clothing, and goggles move the representation into the realm of fantasy or science fiction. In spite of – indeed *because* of – its extent and clumsiness, the over-working betrays a particular anxiety, if not outright desperation, to represent light therapy as a legitimate and modern form of medicine. Such interventions are typical, rivalled only by the damaged, overexposed prints they attempt to address (see Chapter 3). Like Figure 4.3, the 'Vi-tan' pamphlet cover (Plate 1) is also a montage and employs the same kinds of intervention, including layering, mixed media, graphic lines, bold blocks of negative space, and the resultant flattening of space. Yet, like Edith Tudor-Hart's negative of phototherapy at the SLHWC (Fig. 3.1), the image is atypical precisely because it is so sophisticated.

Figure 4.3 'Mercury vapour lamp', photomontage. In *The Peebles Hotel Hydropathic: For Health and Pleasure*, undated booklet (*c.* 1920–30s), p. 40. Scottish Borders Council Archives, Hawick.

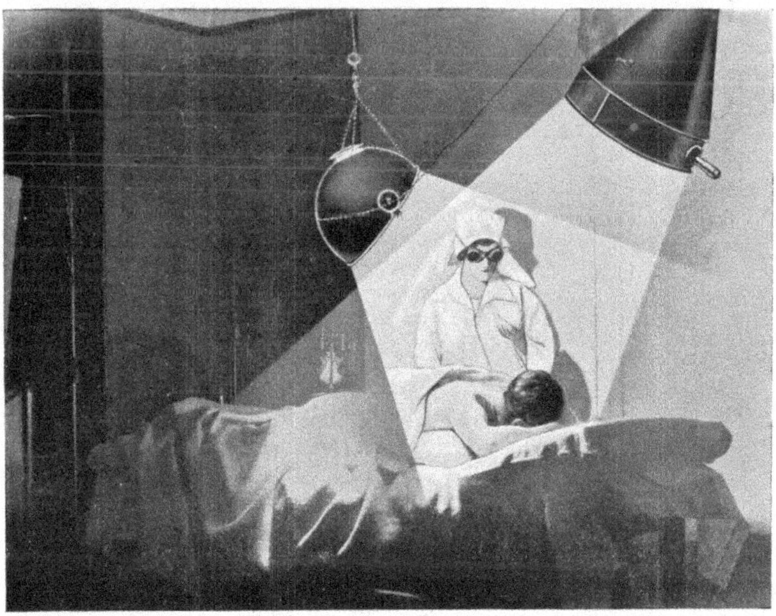

MERCURY VAPOUR LAMP

With the 'Vi-tan' and its vanguard advertisement in mind, in this chapter I examine the aesthetic strategies used to domesticate and sell risky rays (Section I), and why, unlike the incandescent light bulb, the home-use lamp never became a tame *affaire* (Section II).

I Allies

The relationship between ultraviolet, X, and gamma radiation went beyond their cosy position together on the electromagnetic spectrum. Focusing on the contemporaneous, American public reception of X rays and radium, Matthew Lavine argued that, 'The new rays were, in short, the icons of a new and modern science in all its chaotic, fantastic, and ambiguously beneficial glory.'[12] Ultraviolet radiation's place in histories of X rays and radium is consistently dismissed by scholars, Lavine included, and yet it was explicitly understood at the time as a form of radiation therapy and was avidly used alongside them.[13] Finsen himself experimented with X rays and radium alongside ultraviolet rays at his institute shortly before his death and was cited by his successor, Axel Reyn, as advancing the entire field of radiotherapy.[14] This is an integral part of light therapy's history that has only begun to be acknowledged, one connecting the tanning lamp to the atom bomb.[15]

While the existence of ultraviolet rays was known to scientists since 1801, their therapeutic application during the 1890s made them freshly popular and relevant to physicians, physicists, and the public. In the mid-1890s, as Finsen was adapting carbon arc lamps into therapeutic devices, Wilhelm Röntgen announced his discovery of X rays and Henri Becquerel, Pierre and Marie Curie their research on radioactivity and radium (emitting alpha, beta, and gamma rays). It was an unparalleled moment in physics research, and by 1903 these researchers were honoured with the first batch of Nobel Prizes: Röntgen won the first Prize in Physics in 1901; Becquerel and the Curies shared the Prize in Physics in 1903, the same year that Finsen won the Prize in Medicine.[16] The mania for these rays, among physicians, scientists, photographers, and the public, created an 'actinic fever' that was only further fuelled by the prizes.[17] This fever went beyond their entertainment value, as objects of visual spectacle. Citizens sought physical interactions with these rays and their mysterious energies.

Röntgen's and Becquerel's discoveries were enabled by the medium of photography. Both were described as revelatory accidents during experiments with a Crookes tube, in Röntgen's case, and a crystal containing uranium, in Becquerel's case, when invisible wavelengths were unexpectedly registered onto photosensitive surfaces (Figs. 4.4–4.5). Kelley Wilder explained that X-ray photography (radiography) produced a mutually reinforcing relationship between photography and science. Radiation's discovery via photography lent considerable scientific authority to the medium at a time when photography's supposedly objective and infallible character

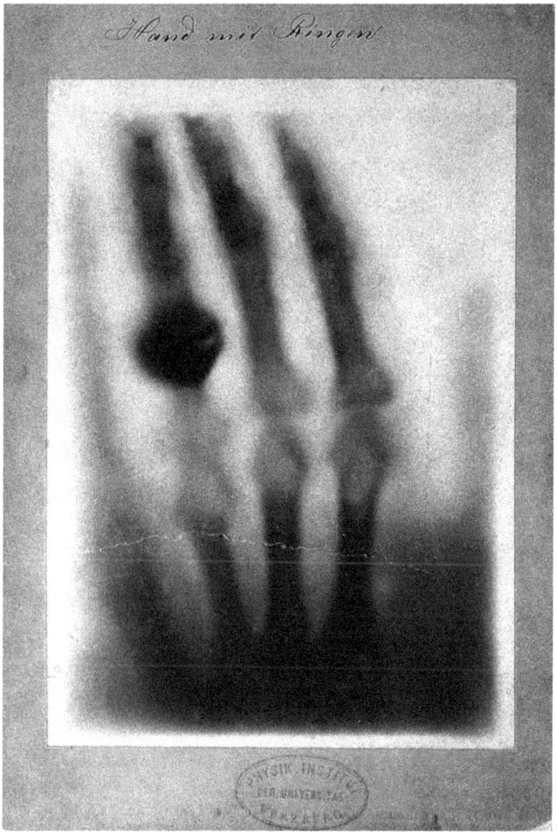

Figure 4.4 Wilhelm Röntgen, X-ray graph of his wife's hand, 1895. Wellcome Library, London CC BY-NC 4.0.

was being seriously questioned amidst growing awareness of its malleability, especially in relation to debates over retouching and the tricks common in capturing 'spirits'. In turn, by giving visual form to these heretofore unknown, invisible rays, photography helped to establish new scientific fields on radioactivity and, later, atomic physics.[18]

Röntgen confirmed the existence and uniqueness of X rays by their difference to ultraviolet rays. Becquerel's experiments were likewise conducted with ultraviolet and Röntgen's rays in mind. His rays were understood in relation to, and distinguished from, the properties of these other rays.[19] Finsen also employed photography in his experiments with ultraviolet light, as both a method of recording and a guide in its technology and processes (Chapters 2 and 3). Early on, Finsen's use of ultraviolet light to treat lupus vulgaris found purpose and understanding through comparison with X rays. Many doctors considered their bodily effects to be analogous.[20] Dr Hugh Walsham, assistant medical officer of St Bartholomew's electrical department, stated in 1902 that,

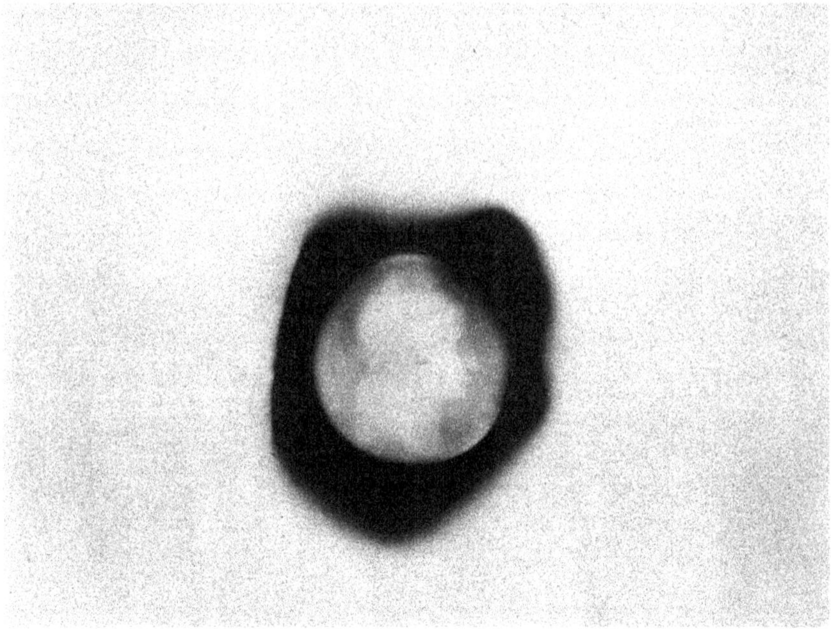

Figure 4.5 Henri Becquerel, 'Original radiography of a medallion, made with uranium, 1903.' In Henri Becquerel, *Recherches sur une propriété nouvelle de la matière* (Paris: Firmin Didot, 1903), Plate 1, No. 2. Wellcome Library, London CC BY-NC 4.0.

> Many observers appear to regard the treatment by x rays and by light as something quite different. When we consider, however, in how many ways ultraviolet light and x rays are alike the distinction between the two almost vanishes. Both act chemically, both produce fluorescence in bodies, both discharge the gold-leaf electroscope. The action on the skin is, however, somewhat different, although they are both capable of producing dermatitis and pigmentation.[21]

The characteristic sign of ultraviolet light's action on the skin, in the form of a solar erythema, could be similarly produced by X and gamma rays. For physicians, the differences lay in the severity of burns and in the latency periods. However, they argued that the way in which each patient reacted to all these rays came down to personal idiosyncrasy. Until the 1930s, the dosages for ultraviolet rays, X rays, and radium were all gauged by their burning action on the individual patient's skin.[22]

Used, like ultraviolet light, both to cauterise lesions by their burning action and to stimulate with shorter doses, X rays found widespread application in clinical medicine. In this they were joined by radium's rays, and all of these were used to treat lupus vulgaris and a host of other skin conditions.[23] These rays were also used to treat forms of cancer and tuberculosis, particularly during their earliest, highly experimental years of application.[24] And while they were understood, almost immediately, to be destructive in their actions, they were also described as stimulating. It depended on the intensity, duration, and method of application. Radium was known to destroy internal cancerous tumours yet was also used to increase fertility: radium fertiliser, for example, was one of its many public applications.[25] They gained even more medical prominence during the First World War, when radium, X rays, and ultraviolet rays found widespread application in treating wounds and scars, and detecting and healing fractures.[26]

Anne Jamieson discovered that the X-ray machine's entry into British hospitals coincided with, or in some cases was attributed to, the entry of the Finsen light for therapeutic over diagnostic applications.[27] She described their early shared history as evidence of a 'growing symbiotic relationship' between X rays (X-ray machines) and ultraviolet rays (notably the Finsen lamp). In this chapter I want to pay equal attention to instances in which this relationship, complicated by the addition of radium, was fraught with tension. Clashing perceptions of their effects made them at once allies and enemies, and this complex union continued well into the 1930s.

From an aesthetic viewpoint, however, the similarities of representation are undeniable. Radiation, whether rays of infrared, visible, ultraviolet, X, or gamma rays, has a long visual history. During the 1800s, photography contributed to and solidified certain visual tropes for representing light wavelengths. By the 1890s, when photography was employed to register and disseminate the discoveries of Röntgen, Becquerel, and the Curies, it crucially made tangible, in Wilder's words, 'previously unseen parts of the spectrum as *fixed, visible entities*'.[28] As we learned in Chapter 2, this 'fixing' occurred as a photochemical process on the emulsion (the fixing of the photograph) that was then used to measure, analyse, and standardise light exposures (the fixing of dosages). But as Wilder noted, by fixing these invisible rays onto the photographic surface, they were also given material form. This is particularly relevant considering practitioners described the very experience of receiving light treatment as an invisible process, warning that 'little or nothing will be felt during the actual treatment', much like receiving X rays or radium.[29]

Representing the rays

In the last chapter I focused on images that were imprinted by excessive actinic light and consequently damaged by marks of overexposure, and argued that these 'artefacts' were particularly poignant examples of the difficulties of undertaking and controlling light treatment. One method of recording the therapy in process was to set up the patients, operators, and equipment as though in the act of treatment but leave the lamps off to avoid overexposing the film (Fig. 3.17). In advertisements this tactic occurred frequently, with the image later undergoing heavy retouching and manipulation to appear as though the lamp was on and functioning. To do so was both practical and creative.

In Figure 4.6, a 1937 advertisement by Hanovia for a popular clinical mercury vapour lamp, the Alpine Sun Lamp, the lower left-hand image fused photograph with hand-drawn and graphic illustration. It appeared in the medical journal, the *British Journal of Physical Medicine*, whose editorial board included some of light therapy's most famous and celebrated international practitioners: Sir Henry Gauvain (Treloar Hospital), Sir Leonard Hill (NIMR), Dr Kurt Huldschinsky (Berlin), Dr Auguste Rollier (Leysin), and Dr Jean Saidman (Aix-les-Bains), among many others. The advertisement was geared therefore to a knowledgeable professional audience and specifically addressed treating wounds and burns with a combination of ultraviolet and infrared light.[30] A photograph of a male patient, lying face down on a hospital bed – his eyes thus conveniently shielded from the emanating actinic light – was cut out and placed onto a black background. A second cut-out of a dual-headed version of the lamp, combining the mercury vapour lamp at the top and an infrared lamp lower down, overlapped the first cut-out and was retouched by hand to emphasise its clean edges and reflective metal surfaces. Note, for example, the added shading to the infrared lamp's focusing head, which appears as swipes of a grey watercolour wash. But most noticeable are the added blocks of white negative space that project, ruler-edged, from the two lamps, signifying overlapping beams of invisible ultraviolet and infrared light. They were subtly shaded as well with graduated grey tones, especially around the patient, to mark out the second beam from the infrared lamp and distinguish their different emanations. It is an image that intriguingly maximises certain photographic *techniques* – retouching, piecing together multiple photographs, and integrating illustration with photograph – in order to correct the limitations of the photographic *process* due to actinic light's volatility.

Many other similar representations exist during this period, for both home-use and clinical lamps (Fig. 4.7).[31] The decision to visualise these invisible emanations in this particular way, as blocks of white negative space, was an extension of their more common representation as graphic lines, shafts, and crepuscular rays (known also as 'God rays', 'Jacob's Ladder', and sunbursts). With their sharply delineated contours and consistently dominant compositional placement, the white blocks materialise something that, by its very nature, is invisible and immaterial.[32] As Shelford Bidwell pointed out to his audience during his popular lectures on light and colour,

> 'Radiation' ... – meaning ether wave-energy – includes what is often improperly called light. Light, people say, takes about eight minutes in travelling from the sun to the earth. But while it is on its journey it is not light in

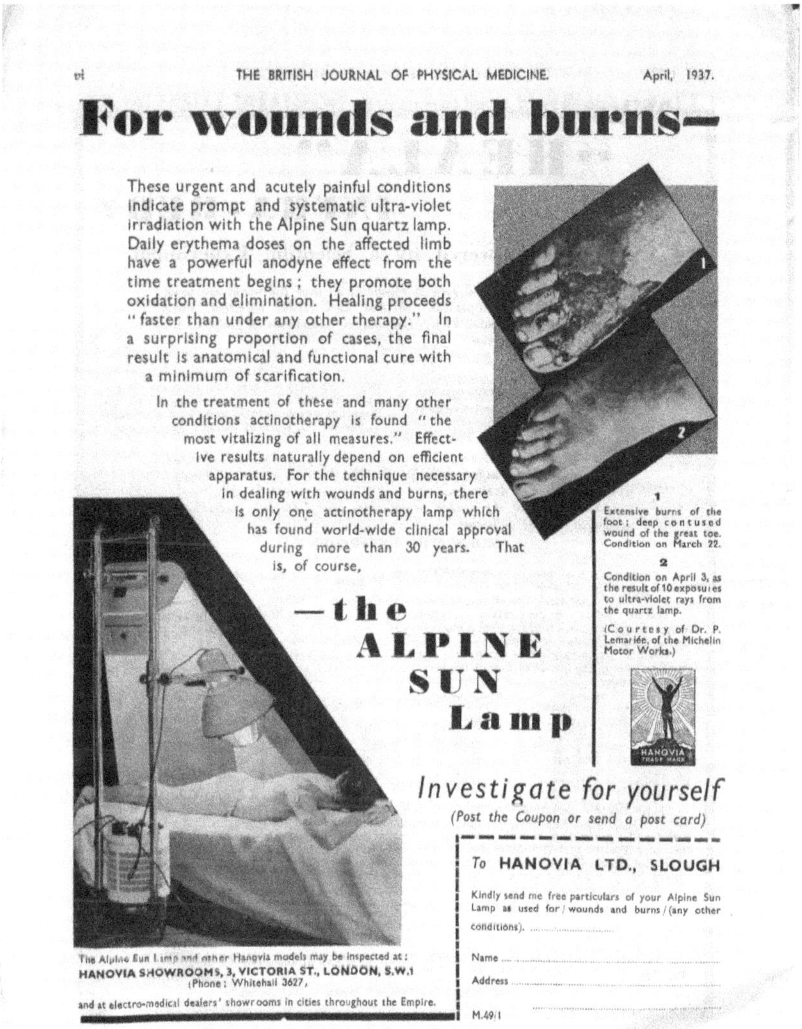

Figure 4.6 Advertisement for the Hanovia 'Alpine Sun Lamp'. In *British Journal of Physical Medicine*, April 1937, p. vi. MSS.292/847.92/4TUC papers, Modern Records Centre, University of Warwick.

> the true sense of the word; neither does anything of the nature of light ever start from the sun. Light has no more existence in nature outside a living body than the flavour of onions has; both are merely sensations.[33]

Given solid, material form, light has substance in these images. It appears tangible and real. Analysing the chronophotography of Étienne-Jules Marey, Josh Ellenbogen

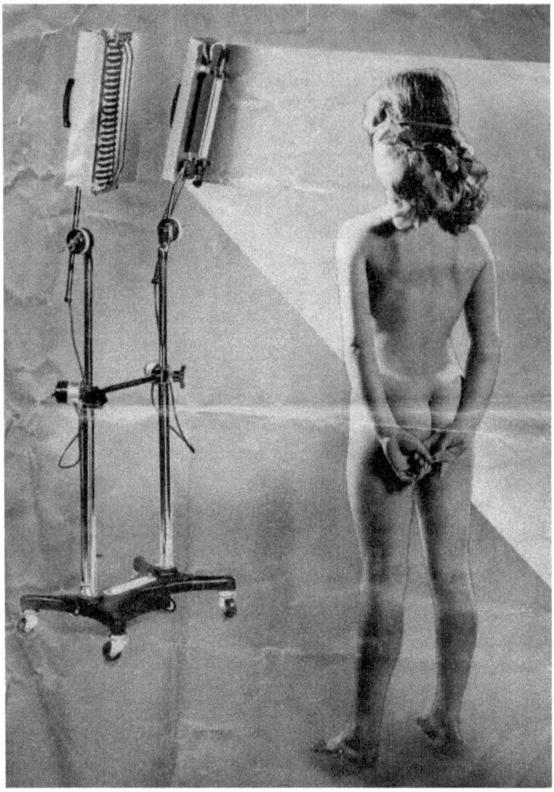

Figure 4.7 Pamphlet cover for the Perihel 'Twin-Ray' (infrared and ultraviolet) lamp, *c.* late 1940s–1950s. Author's collection.

perceptively asked, 'what makes for a useful convention when one visualizes the non-visible?'[34] For ultraviolet rays the obvious reference point was 'visible' light, the red to violet rays that can be seen by the human retina.

Crepuscular rays, emanating boldly from the sun through cloud cover, were the most common representation, and they had an ancient lineage to symbolise the sun, God, and spiritual energies. Light therapists were certainly aware of such representations. In the opening, historical review of heliotherapy in the massive two-volume, internationally authored *Traité d'hélio- et d'actinologie* (1937), the Swiss heliotherapist Oskar Bernhard included a reproduction of the ancient Egyptian relief of Akhenaten, Nefertiti, and their children under the sun's emanating, life-giving rays (Fig. 4.8).[35] Spiritual rays and halos of divine light encircling the bodies of saints, martyrs, and the Holy Trinity transformed this ancient tradition into standard Christian iconography.[36] The 'Alpine Sun lamp' advertisement (Fig. 4.6), like the 'Vi-tan' pamphlet cover (Plate 1), visualises the invisible ultraviolet rays by modernising an ancient iconography. Its hard-edged crepuscular rays appear like theatre spotlights on the stage. The aesthetic choice is doubly ironic: visible rays, on which the depictions are based, were considered relatively useless

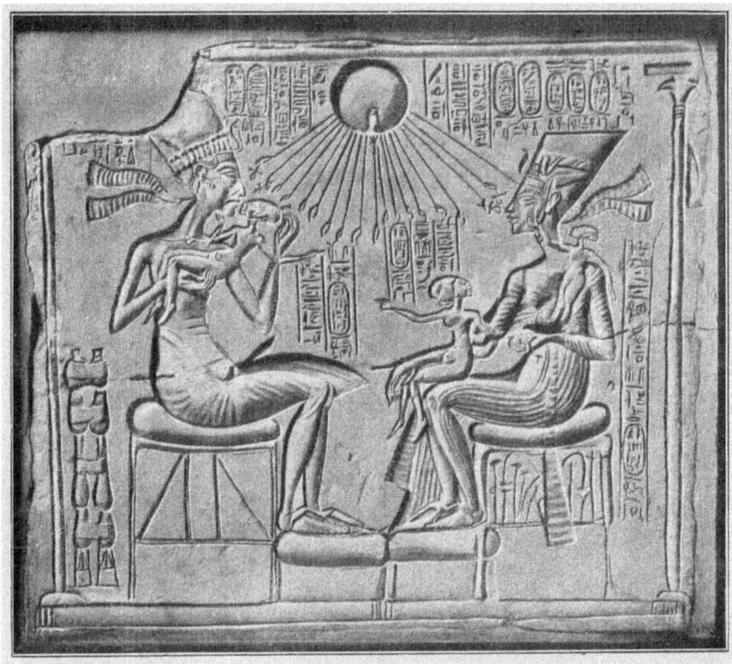

Figure 4.8 Ancient Egyptian relief of Akhenaten, Nefertiti and their children under the life-giving sun, Tell el-Amarna, relief carving, *c.* 1375 BCE.
In Oskar Bernhard, 'L'Évolution historique du traitement solaire', in Charles Brody (ed.), *Traité d'hélio- et d'actinologie* (Paris: Maloine, 1938), vol. I, Figure 1, p. 7. Author's collection.

from a therapeutic interest; and stage spotlights could be incandescent lamps but could also be carbon arc lamps.[37] As we learned in the last chapter, this was neither the first nor the last time that light for vision would prove incompatible with light for healing.

Emanating shafts, beams, and 'pencils' of light depicted as white or black graphic lines were also standard representations for electricity's powers. In number they were exceeded only by lightning bolts, as Carolyn Thomas de la Peña showed.[38] Importantly, both beams and bolts were also used to illustrate the powers of X rays and radium, in Britain and abroad (Fig. 4.9). Analysing an American advertisement for the 'Revigator' radium jar, a product impregnating water with 'healthful' radioactivity, she described the confusing addition of lightning bolts to the streaming irradiated water emerging from the jar, and that, 'The bolts, however [inaccurate], are indicative of the importance of a scientific image to these jars' success. Radium's invisibility necessitated creativity: manufacturers borrowed electricity's cultural cachet, assuming that readers would make the connection.'[39] Indeed, surely they

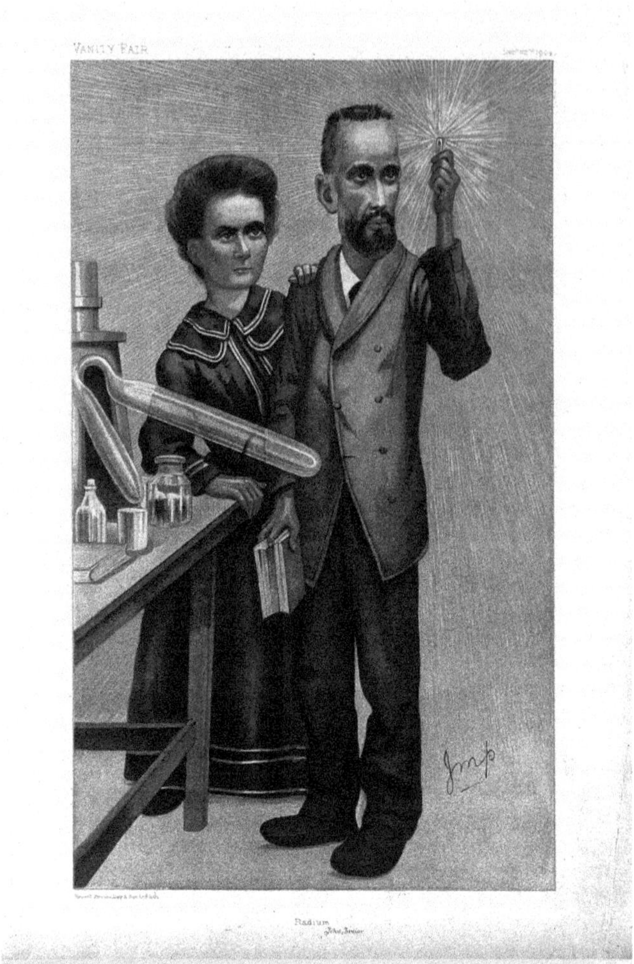

Figure 4.9 After J. M. Price, 'Marie and Pierre Curie, he holding aloft a glowing specimen of radium', 1904. Colour lithograph. Wellcome Library, London CC BY-NC 4.0.

forged this connection between the powers of electricity and radium for their target audience through such visual representations. Like the sun, radium's most powerful appeal to the public was its radiant luminosity. In fact its apparent self-generating, luminescent glow, as well as its limitless energy, made its analogy with the sun seem natural. This continued well into the 1940s with the invention of the atom bomb.[40]

Synthetic nature

Portable, compact, and with a door that cleverly conceals its function, the 'Vi-tan' was designed for the modern, elegant, affluent British home. Its price tag of £12, in 1936, equates to about £760 in 2016.[41] Its cost, as well as the necessity of accessible electrical sockets of the right amperage within the home – during a period when domestic electricity was still out of reach for many – indicates that the 'Vi-tan' was not a staple electrical appliance within the average British household.[42] Yet the Thermal Syndicate's advertising material clearly intended it to appeal to a broad and varied audience. Indeed, in his book *Objects of Desire*, Adrian Forty argued that during the 1930s new domestic electrical appliances actually drove, rather than followed, Britain's market of electricity consumption, leading to the widespread wiring of homes.[43] Advertisements for the 'Vi-tan' were placed in local newspapers and even in naturist journals, notably the *Sun Bathing Review* (Fig. 4.10).[44] Equally glamorous with her contemporary curls and decorative boudoir, the model in Figure 4.10 is stripped to the waist and contentedly faces the 'Vi-tan' while its emanating shafts of light reach out towards her.

The foldable, illustrated colour pamphlet of *c.* 1936 promoted the 'Vi-tan' as an essential device of preventive medicine for all workers in industrial areas and those in indoor, sedentary occupations, including a photograph of clerks in an office (Plate 1). This strategic appeal to the working masses by the manufacturer was certainly not

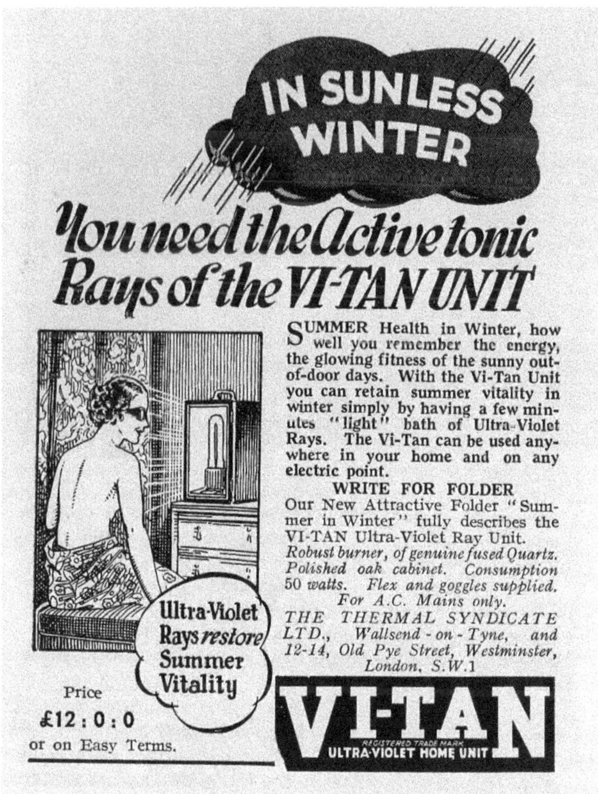

Figure 4.10 Advertisement for the 'Vi-tan' mercury vapour lamp. In *Sun Bathing Review*, 4:17 (1937), 180. Hawk Editorial, publisher of *H&E Naturist* magazine, www.henaturist.net.

unique to the 'Vi-tan'. The most well-known manufacturer, Hanovia, similarly marketed its 'Homesun' mercury vapour lamp (Fig. 4.11) to the ordinary British worker, stuck indoors in the daily grind or commuting under near-constant cloud cover, and consequently suffering from 'sun starvation' (see Chapter 5). Its equivalent price of £18 in 1940 would be over £1,000 in 2016.[45] It was almost twice the size of the 'Vi-tan', and yet its promotional literature also stressed its design aesthetic as ideal for the home. Its user pamphlet declared, 'The sleek, clean design, enhanced by the beautiful finish in cream ivory, with mahogany Bakelite fittings, is an adornment in any surroundings.'[46] Modernity in this case was expressed through hygienic light colours, minimalist contours, and new synthetic materials.[47]

Unlike Hanovia's 'Homesun', the Thermal Syndicate's 'Vi-tan' is curiously composed of both natural and modern materials, an oak shell containing the shiny, chromium-plated reflector and the company's celebrated fused silica (quartz) glass bulb. Simon Carter argued that 'the sunlamp was at the same time both "of nature" and "of science"', while Daniel Freund similarly asserted that home-use lamps were 'modern versions of nature, blurring boundaries between synthetic and real [sunlight]'.[48] The same has been said of other purportedly 'natural' products that rely heavily upon modern technologies

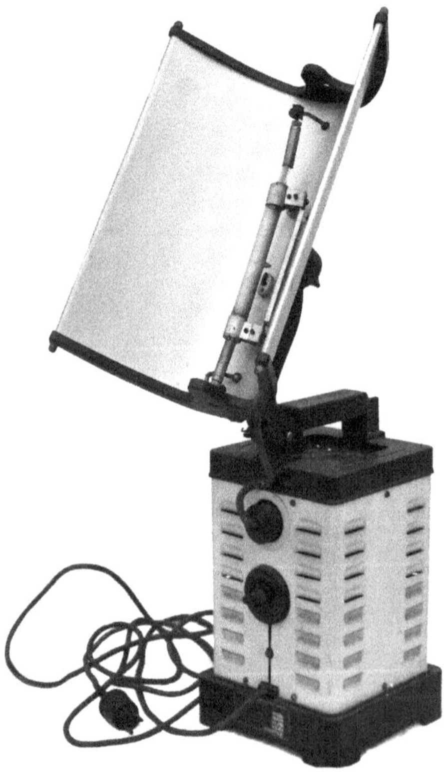

Figure 4.11 Hanovia 'Homesun' mercury vapour lamp, *c.* 1940. Metal, Bakelite, chrome, and quartz glass. Author's collection.

and human intervention, not least cow's milk.[49] Together, the 'Vi-tan' lamp's fusion of components makes materially manifest these arguments, conforming to Freund's notion of the 'hypernatural' – of science exceeding and perfecting nature.[50] Certainly this was the view of the Thermal Syndicate, who confidently declared their lamp's superiority to natural sunlight in its advertising pamphlet by stating that its bulb was 'more effective even than … the sun', since sunlight was impeded by the atmosphere.[51] It was also available on demand, a particular bonus for a nation notorious for its poor weather (see Chapter 1). As Dr William Beaumont put it in 1931, 'artificial sunlight treatment is really an attempt to wrest from science what nature designed us to have'.[52]

If in its design and its function the 'Vi-tan' is an object of synthetic nature, its visual representation through advertising further collapses distinctions between the natural and the artificial, between reality and artifice, between the visible and the invisible. In the cover montage (Plate 1), colour mixes with black-and-white, and photographs with graphic and hand-drawn illustration. Proportions are skewed, flattened shapes overlap as obvious cut-outs, and any sense of naturalistic space is limited to the shadows on the figure's form.[53] The small lamp takes its place within the sun while its serpentine electrical cord, disconnected from its source, is wrapped around the model's body like a fashionable feather boa. Unplugged and detached, the lamp is useless, impotent, while its cord is turned into feminine adornment, and yet the sun's dynamic, crepuscular rays shine on. If the lamp was meant to emit 99 per cent ultraviolet light – wavelengths commonly known to be invisible to the human retina – its vitalising rays nonetheless dominate the composition, given prominent visual form with near-fluorescent complimentary colours as bold blocks separated by graphic lines. These are Art Deco sunbeams, a design commonly found in contemporaneous popular and vanguard graphic representations on travel posters, textiles, doors, jewellery, and tableware.[54] The pamphlet indicated that little visible light was actually emitted by the lamp, and yet they are presented here in a dramatic representation that confounds visible and invisible rays as well as natural and artificial sources.

Phototherapy lamps emitted highly varied light wavelengths, in particular infrared, visible, and ultraviolet, and in diverse proportions as evidenced by the proclaimed output of the 'Vi-tan'. This varied light could be produced by mercury vapour bulbs as well as by rods of carbon or tungsten, in the case of carbon arc or tungsten arc lamps. They also came in a surprising variety of shapes and sizes. In the 1920s large, standing models could be sold for home and clinical use, evidenced by the Ajax advertisement in Chapter 1 (Fig. 1.4), but towards the end of the decade and early 1930s smaller, compact units began to be marketed for home use. These were used by members of the public as well as house-bound patients, who were visited by nurses with these devices. Taken together, the sheer variety of models, manufacturers, lamp types, outputs, required voltages, prices, and competing views from the medical profession about unregulated, unsupervised home use is, quite simply, astounding. This erratic cacophony of information encountered in the popular and medical texts is only further confounded through visual representations, exemplified by the 'Vi-tan' pamphlet cover (Plate 1).

As stated in Chapter 1, noted physicist Sidney Russ spoke of natural sunlight as a beneficent and benign nourisher of children, yet he remained sceptical of artificial substitutes:

> Sources of ultra-violet radiation can now be obtained very easily, perhaps too easily, from those who represent that they have 'artificial sunlight' for sale. It is a bad term, for the radiation from none of these lamps resembles sunlight very closely, and they all contain some ultra-violet rays which normally never reach us [from the sun]. So it cannot be recognized too clearly that anyone using such lamps is using a source of rays with which man is yet quite unfamiliar, and how the body is going to react to repeated doses of these rays is not yet really known.[55]

By replicating nature with scientific technology, lamp manufacturers harnessed a powerful source that, for some, bordered on magic. Although there were home-use lamps advertised throughout the volumes of the Sunlight League's journal (Fig. 4.16), *Sunlight*'s editor Caleb Saleeby wrote in a 1929 issue that,

> The boom in artificial sunlight was inevitable, not only because ultra-violet radiation, rightly used, has real value – as in making Vitamin D in the skin – and because our urban shortage of natural ultra-violet, real sunlight, will persist until we abolish our urban smoke; but also because of our stupid preference for anything novel, unnatural, semi-magical.[56]

His choice of the word 'stupid' is curious; etymologically meaning 'stunned', 'amazed' or 'confounded', the word is surprisingly appropriate considering the man himself proudly owned a Hanovia 'Homesun' lamp.[57] Perhaps this was the lamp's 'magical' pull. After all, 'Any sufficiently advanced technology is indistinguishable from magic', to quote Arthur C. Clarke.[58]

Or was it the magic of advertising? In its spatial distortions, mismatched scales of objects, and layering of photograph and graphic illustration, the 'Vi-tan' pamphlet cover is decidedly non-naturalistic. We have no sense that this is a real person, in a real space under a real sun. We cannot imagine stepping into the picture and joining her there, however much we may wish it. Instead, the image is illusionistic of a different promised reality, one that, however fantastical, did not seem out of reach to the modern British citizen. As Charles Bazerman explained, 'Purveyors of new technologies must … entice risk-taking customers to buy into the dream so as to make the dream real.'[59] They did so through advertising, a 'magic system' that performs 'feats of transformation and bewitchment', as Raymond Williams and Sut Jhally both argued.[60] Ernest Turner noted that the depression only compelled advertisers in the 1930s to produce more aggressive, fear-driven campaigns at a time of desperate competition.[61] Though there were instances of rogue manufacturers who deliberately and duplicitously hoodwinked the public with false product information, the majority of lamp manufacturers certainly did not have nefarious intentions. Hanovia, for example, was a highly respected company that supplied lamps to the medical profession, to schools, factories and light clinics, and to the public. But, as is clear from Russ's statement above, even the names of some of these lamps – notably Hanovia's 'Homesun' (Fig. 4.11) and the 'Alpine Sun Lamp' (Fig. 4.6) – were enough to create obfuscation, from which manufacturers profited. That these lamps were sold both to the public (the 'Homesun') and to practitioners (the 'Alpine Sun Lamp') indicates consumers were not unanimously naive or gullible.[62] In 1929, Dr Maurice Weinbren stated, 'Manufacturers were not slow to see the profitable advantages of mass production of apparatus, some of which is useless from the therapeutic point of view and definitely dangerous from its electrical design. The result is that one is now offered "treatment" by many a barber and apparatus by many an ironmonger.'[63] Russ's and Weinbren's concern may have been with public access and misuse, but instability existed among professional use and beliefs too. The lamps and their advertisements did more than reflect or follow already clear-cut, embedded medical perceptions of light's effects on the body: they actively shaped, mobilised, and confounded them, and they did so to a wide audience.

II Antagonists

In *Naked to the Bone*, Bettyann Holtzmann Kevles described the technology of radiography as eradicating the skin's surface and rendering it 'transparent' – a common reference to the penetrative power of the X ray, with the radiograph presenting the organs and tissues as a 'mist of overlapping layers'.[64] Sophia Zweifel, citing the writings of French psychoanalyst Didier Anzieu, theorised that the radiograph can be understood as a composite of layered 'pellicules', meaning both photographic film and membranes, or 'skins' (see Chapter 3).[65] Lisa Cartwright, discussing microscopy, similarly singled out the microscopic specimen as a 'series of light-penetrated sheets' analogous to Clement Greenberg's description of the flat, skin-like surfaces of Cubist paintings.[66] The reference to avant-garde painting is particularly apt, especially the dynamic layered surfaces in the paintings of Marcel Duchamp, František Kupka, and Francis Picabia. These artists were enamoured with radiography's visual aesthetic, especially its 'cuttings' (layered sections of the body), and popular conceptions of

Theosophy and the Fourth Dimension, as discussed at length by Linda Dalrymple Henderson.[67] Henderson explained that these artists, informed by popular science, sought to visualise the imperceptible, an invisible reality beyond surface appearances that challenged the 'inadequacy of human sense perception'.[68] In their oil paintings they prominently represented the body as a series of 'dematerialised' translucent layers, such as in Kupka's *Planes by Colours* (1911–12, Musée National d'Art Moderne) and Duchamp's *Portrait (Dulcinea)* (1911, Philadelphia Museum of Art).

Like Kupka's and Duchamp's vanguard paintings, photomontage emerged during the late 1910s and 1920s as a sophisticated and modern representation for sophisticated, modern medical and scientific concepts, exemplified by the art, design, and photography of the Hungarian László Moholy-Nagy and the Russian El Lissitzky (Figs. 4.12–4.13). In the catalogue for the exhibition, *Montage and Modern Life: 1919–1942* (Boston, Vancouver and Brussels, 1992–93), Matthew Teitelbaum described montage as offering a 'kaleidoscopic expanded vision', not merely representing the real but an idea of the real as 'something not yet seen'.[69] Above all, montage was attributed to a 'specifically modernist practice of seeing and experiencing', as Maud Lavin made clear.[70] Lavin's examples of montaged advertisements for products such as shampoo similarly feature 'artistic', hand-drawn illustration layered with photographs and crisp cut-outs of modern products.[71]

Figure 4.12 László Moholy-Nagy, *Design Project*, 1935. Photomontage, pencil, Perspex, and silver foil. Private collection. © Hattula Moholy-Nagy/DACS 2016 and Bridgeman Images.

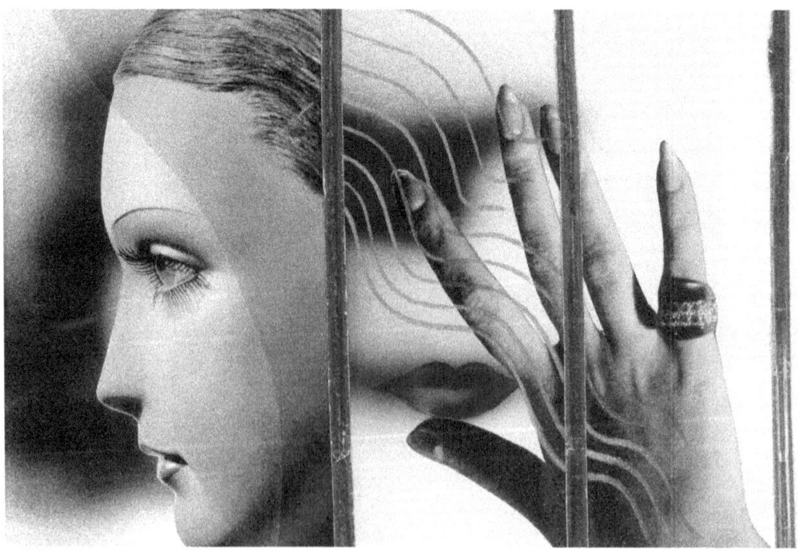

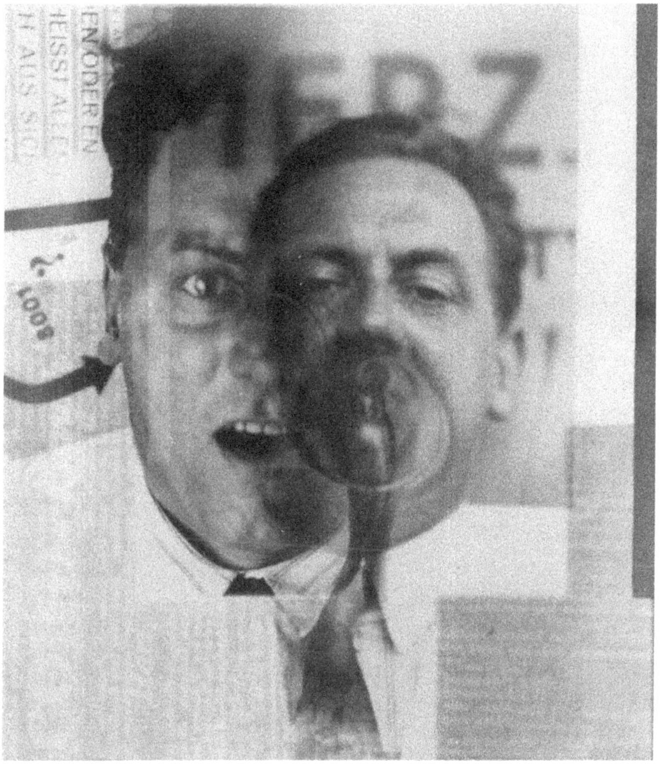

Figure 4.13 El Lissitzky (Lazar Markovich Lissitzky), *Kurt Schwitters*, 1924–25. Silver gelatin print photograph (photomontage). Private collection. © Christie's Images/Bridgeman Images.

Dawn Ades pointed out that art historians and the artists themselves have disagreed, and continue to disagree, on a uniform definition for '(photo)montage', and its definition varies from dictionary to dictionary.[72] Ades also firmly connected it with modernity and modern technology, writing of montage as a product of 'the technological world, the world of mass communication and photo-mechanical reproduction'.[73] Though vanguard montages vary enormously in style, they were commonly produced by the overlaying ('assembling' or constructing) of opaque or translucent layers (Figs. 4.12–4.13). It is fitting that many of them resemble the 'mist of overlapping layers' and light-penetrated 'skins' of X-ray graphs (Fig. 4.4), then, since radiography was a firm influence on montage's development as a new form of representation.[74]

Perhaps unsurprisingly, montage was relied upon heavily to represent invisible radiation in popular advertising; their aesthetics were mutually reinforcing if not interdependent. From the 1920s onwards, montage was widely used in advertising, often produced by commissioned avant-garde artists, and it promoted products with its unique aesthetic in 'strange', 'marvellous', and '*magic*' ways.[75] In advertisements selling invisible energies, montage thus found its ideal place. Revisiting the advertisements for the 'Vi-tan' and the 'Alpine Sun Lamp' (Plate 1, Fig. 4.6), their modernist assembling of multiple, overlapping layers of mixed media, spatial distortions, and dynamic compositions align them with the production of vanguard artists such as Moholy-Nagy and El Lissitzky. Tudor-Hart offers an intriguing connection to these varied images and their makers. Although photomontage held only a minor interest in Tudor-Hart's oeuvre, her training at the Bauhaus, likely under the tutelage of Moholy-Nagy, and her continuing affiliation with him and his wife, Lucia, while in Britain in the mid-1930s exemplify the ongoing ties between developments in light therapy and photography.[76] Curiously, Moholy-Nagy's work was also disseminated in Britain through a journal called *Ray*, 'the only English periodical of the avant-garde'.[77]

The vanguard light aesthetics of Moholy-Nagy, applied to diverse interests in photography, montage, sculpture, and film, were central to what he termed 'the New Vision'.[78] While teaching at the Bauhaus, under the guidance of Walter Gropius and an 'intoxication with all things technological', Moholy-Nagy introduced into the metal workshop modern industrial materials such as chrome, aluminium, nickel, and glass – materials essential to the construction of light-therapy lamps.[79] Eleanor Hight wrote that, 'For many artists of the 1920s, the machine provided the basis for a new universal art', both negatively and positively represented.[80] Both Gropius and Moholy-Nagy considered the machine a tool for social progress, improving the lives of citizens by means of mass production.[81] Moholy-Nagy collaborated with Allgemeine Elektrizitäts-Gesellschaft (AEG), one of Germany's largest industrial companies and, in partnership with Heraeus, founder the Quarzlampen-Gesellschaft mbH in 1906. Together, and until 1973, they designed the Art Deco 'Original Hanau' mercury vapour lamp, one of the most well-known lamps on the market, as well as the 'Sollux' (an infrared lamp that additionally incorporated colour filters for chromotherapy). AEG's design consultant, Peter Behrens (1868–1940), began there in 1907 by designing arc lamps. Later, while still consulting for AEG, he ran a private architectural practice that at one time employed Gropius, Le Corbusier, and Mies van der Rohe.[82] Moholy-Nagy constructed his own vanguard light devices, including his most important project: *The Light-Space Modulator* (1930), a 'kinetic sculpture' built on AEG's premises.[83]

During this same period, the Moholy-Nagys were simultaneously indulging in naturism as part of their interest in physical culture, just as Tudor-Hart began taking a serious interest in sunbathing as a photographic subject (see the next chapter on her photographs in *Sun Bathing Review*).[84] Christopher Wilk made an intriguing connection between the interwar obsession with bodily health and its vanguard art:

> The idea of perfecting and altering the body perhaps found its visual equivalent in the form of the photomontage and the image manipulated in the

> darkroom. Man Ray, László Moholy-Nagy and Herbert Bayer, among others, created photographic prints in which bodies were depicted with parts missing or added, where transparency was much emphasized or where there was a reversal of traditional poles of light and dark that heightened awareness of the subject [solarisation]. These depictions of the human form, and the unusual viewpoints from which they were presented in New Photography, represented strategies for avoiding traditional modes of depiction, suggesting a new view of the body.[85]

We might also include that it was a new view of the technologies designed to produce and perfect the body – of synthetic nature. The 'Vi-tan' pamphlet cover (Plate 1) remakes the body, perfects it, through its 'magical' product (the lamp) as well through its 'magical' aesthetics (montage).

Penetrating rays

For Moholy-Nagy, Hight declared, 'Light became the most important element of his work, whether in painting, sculpture, or photography, from this point [1922] to the end of his career.'[86] Like Kupka and Duchamp, he was influenced by popularised scientific theories of light, such as Max Planck's quantum theory and Albert Einstein's relativity theory, as well as spiritualist understandings of light as regenerative, accessed at the Bauhaus through the writings of Wassily Kandinsky and Expressionist art.[87] Aside from his sculptures he became famous for his photographs of light, especially his photograms (cameraless photographs). Moholy-Nagy's experiments with photograms began in collaboration with his wife in 1922. Like Man Ray and Christian Schad, they experimented with the photosensitive register, placing diverse objects of varying opacities onto the paper and passing various fluids and materials between paper and light source, reminiscent of Finsen's and Hill's photographed experiments with skin and actinic light (Figs. 2.1, 2.3).[88] Although in his photograms Moholy-Nagy gave actinic light a material form and treated it as a medium, he described light as 'dematerialising' and photography as 'the penetration of the body with light'.[89] These complex, even perplexing, notions of actinic light's penetrability and its relative materiality – its transparency, translucency, or opacity – find not only significant visual expression in the diversity of his artwork but also important analogies with competing understandings among light therapists over light's penetrability through the skin and into the body.

Kevles stated that X rays revolutionised medicine by rendering the body transparent. This fantasy of transparency, by using penetrative electromagnetic wavelengths to reveal the body's depths, has fuelled medical imaging ever since.[90] The desire to access the body's interior, reveal its secrets, render it 'transparent' to the eye, and flood it with light, however, predates the discovery of X rays and their diagnostic imaging potential. The practice of transillumination, of penetrating the body's orifices with light by means of mirrors and lenses, and the inventions of endoscopy, laryngoscopy, and cystoscopy are significant nineteenth-century precedents for radiography.[91] For Chris Otter, 'The visceral folds and surfaces of bodily organs were revealed to the surgical eye' by means of the cystoscope.[92]

Just as X rays and radium both visualised the body's interior, by producing photographic imprints, and physically altered it while doing so, these earlier means of penetration were simultaneously metaphorical and literal: a penetrative vision by means of physically entering inside the body and illuminating it with light from within.[93] During the 1896 frenzy over X rays, a correspondent in the *Lancet* pointed out that the celebrated physician and sanitarian, Sir Benjamin Richardson, had demonstrated as early as 1868 that the body could be illuminated by passing light into and around it with various artificial sources, including electric light, gaslight, limelight, and magnesium light. Richardson displayed his method by illuminating the bones of a child's hand as well as the interiors of fish and other animals, and as a result considered the body 'translucent'.[94]

Moholy-Nagy's declaration that photography itself 'penetrated' the body with light (rather than operated by capturing the light *reflecting off* the body's surface) finds an early ally in an 1875 statement by photographer and photochemist Hermann Wilhelm Vogel:

> Photography has been begun to be applied on a large scale to the province of medical science, not only in taking interesting anatomical preparations and morbid phenomena of short duration, but in giving exact anatomical views of the different organs. The apparently impenetrable interior of living organs has been disclosed by eye-mirrors, ear-mirrors, and throat-mirrors, so that their interior is fully disclosed to the eye of the observer. *In like manner*, the image visible to the eye has been successfully retained by photography.[95]

For Vogel, photography's relationship with transillumination was twofold: by penetrating the body's interior, photography operated like transillumination, providing 'exact anatomical views' of organs; and by recording and disseminating transillumination's interior views, it further aided medical science.

By the 1890s, when Röntgen unleashed the penetrative vision of X rays onto the world, physicians and scientists had been for some time, and would continue to be, deeply involved with illuminating the body's interior with light. Finsen was among them, experimenting with the depths of the body's penetrability by blue, violet, and ultraviolet light, and well beyond the skin surface.[96] As previously discussed,

Finsen developed the theories and techniques of phototherapy through self-experimentation. Like the blackening of silver salts on a photographic plate, Finsen witnessed his skin's reddening and subsequent pigmenting as a register to test how transparent substances were to ultraviolet light. On his arm he glued a quartz disc and different coloured glass plates and additionally painted his initials (N. F.) with India ink (Fig. 2.5). He subsequently became interested in testing how deep actinic light could penetrate into the body, again by means of photographic experiments. Using his wife's outer ear (pinna), behind which he had placed photographic paper, Finsen focused a beam of sunlight and noted that no reaction took place even after five minutes of exposure. But when he sandwiched the ear between two plates of glass, compressing it to drain blood from the area, the paper behind it became black within twenty seconds. From this he reasoned that light could penetrate through an organism's skin and tissues if rendered bloodless (anaemic), heightening the rays' effects on tuberculous skin lesions by reaching their bacterial source.[97] Finsen had various devices and instruments to facilitate light's penetration into lesions, including round lenses and skin compressors (Fig. 2.7).

Other physicians and researchers in France, Germany, and America conducted similar experiments during the 1890s, attempting to capture photographic imprints behind or beyond the body.[98] Indeed, it is likely Finsen was influenced by Dr T. V. Godneff (Kazan), who in 1882 reported that he had blackened silver chloride sealed in glass tubes after physically inserting them under the skin of animals and exposing them to sunlight.[99] These experiments convinced Finsen that the skin was penetrable by actinic light but the blood opaque to it, and consequently he considered it a hindrance to the cure. Others were determined to prove that sunlight and artificial light could act just like X rays and penetrate through and beyond the body, blood and all.

The French Dr Joseph Malgat (Nice) claimed that he had blackened photographic paper held behind a whole nude torso, arguing that sunlight penetrated through the entire body, reaching deeply seated lesions within it. Apparently Malgat demonstrated this in 1901, with the implication that sunlight was curative not only for skin lesions but also pulmonary tuberculosis, of lesions within the lungs.[100] In a 1911 publication, he illustrated how he exposed his consumptive patients, seating them in an interior but facing an open window with sunlight directed onto the lungs (Fig. 4.14). Yet, as is obvious by the shadow projected behind the patient in Figure 4.14, sunlight did not penetrate through the chest or torso. Word and image here seem at odds, offering contrasting perceptions of sunlight's penetrability into the human body.

Shortly afterwards in Britain, Dr James Sequeira of the London Hospital began experimenting with skin penetrability to test a new lamp on the market. The Simpson lamp, named after its inventor, was an arc lamp using rods of tungsten (Wolframite), rather than carbon. We encountered the tungsten arc lamp in the last chapter

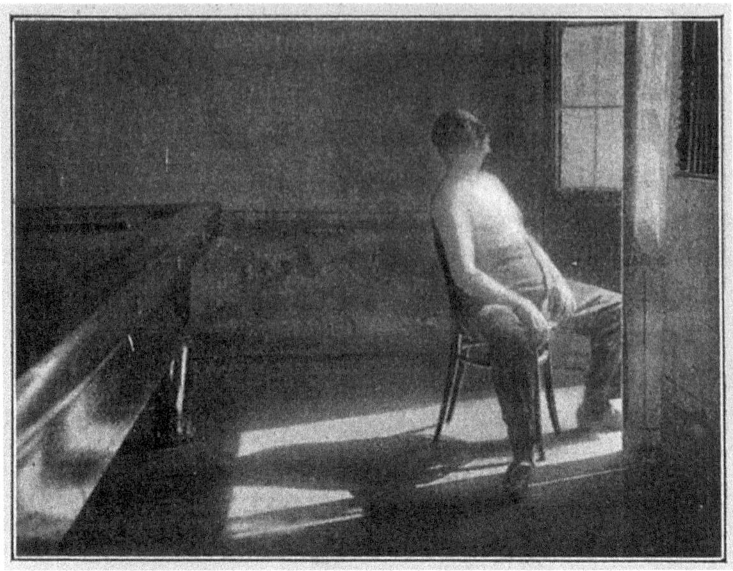

Figure 4.14 Position of pulmonary tubercular patient having an insolation session.
In J. Malgat, *La Cure solaire de la tuberculose pulmonaire chronique* (Paris: J.-B. Baillière et fils, 1911), Figure 2, p. 179. Bibliothèque Nationale de France/Gallica.

(Figs. 3.10–3.11), but when it was first invented some practitioners believed the lamp produced a new kind of ray entirely, termed 'S' rays.[101] Sequeira set out to demonstrate that the lamp produced ordinary actinic light (mainly ultraviolet, though of a richer quantity that the carbon arc) and, like Finsen, used his own forearm as a light register. He even referenced Finsen's experiment by making imprints of his own initials, J. H. S. Unlike Finsen, however, these initials were produced not with India ink but with layers of 'fresh' human skin (J) and frog skin (S) tied to his forearm with string. The 'H' was ordinary paper, and in his reproduced photograph it is clear, despite the lack of clarity, that all three impeded the Simpson lamp's actinic rays to leave distinct, white shapes on his severely burnt arm. Though it may not have been his direct aim, Sequeira showed that human skin was not transparent to ultraviolet light, and went to morbid lengths to prove it.[102]

These differing perceptions of the relative transparency of the body to ultraviolet light were challenged by numerous experiments on the skin's penetrability by different wavelengths.[103] But by the 1920s it was generally understood that ultraviolet radiation only minimally penetrated the skin, and certainly did not enter into the body as infrared radiation did. In 1922, Hill asserted that ultraviolet rays penetrated only 0.1 millimetres, 'being absorbed by the surface film of the skin'.[104] Like X rays and radium, which by now were known to produce varying levels of penetrative rays – some 'soft', others 'hard'[105] – ultraviolet rays had begun to be dissected and analysed in sections, later divided as A, B, and C, and understood for their varying penetrative effects. Yet the myth of the body's transparency to ultraviolet light did not dissipate completely. Reporting on a 1924 accident involving a member of the public who fell asleep under a mercury vapour lamp at home, Drs Henry MacCormac and H. Moreland McCrea described his near-fatal burns and noted that, despite having only exposed his front to the lamp, curiously the man's back was covered with burns as well.[106] Somehow the intense ultraviolet light had penetrated through his body, affecting unexposed body parts – an unintended confirmation of Malgat's earlier theories.

Transillumination had not lost its pull either. Light therapists, including Hill, experimented with electric lamps placed into patients' mouths, noting whether a red glow could be detected through the cheeks.[107] Such an experiment confirmed the penetrability of red light, not ultraviolet, through the skin, blood, and tissues. Hill furthermore used it to prove the relative penetrability and absorptiveness of different racial pigmentations. The skin of white subjects was affected by transillumination but not that of black subjects; the electric light's red glow was impeded by deep pigmentation. (In the next chapter I discuss how often practitioners relied on the evidence of racial variations of pigmentation, especially black skin, to explain therapeutic tanning's action). Hill's colleague at the NIMR, Albert Eidinow, also relied on transillumination during the 1920s. Interestingly, he used it to detect the photosensitivities of patients before commencing light treatment, inserting lights into the sinuses and measuring how intensely red the glow appeared. The redder the effect, the more sensitive the patient would be to ultraviolet light.[108] This practice suggests a fascinating convergence of penetrating illuminations, in which varied methods of bringing light into the patient were relied upon together to ensure sufficient saturation. Practitioners' desires to penetrate bodily orifices, especially those of women, will be discussed at length in Chapter 5 as well, especially in relation to perceptions of light's effect on procreativity and sexuality.

In Hanovia's 'Alpine Sun Lamp' advertisement of 1937 (Fig. 4.6), the layers denoting the emanating invisible light of the ultraviolet and infrared lamps descend onto the figure's body. Like the 'Vi-tan' pamphlet cover (Plate 1), we have little sense of the light's physical penetration into the body: the contours of the light block and those of the figure remain distinct. Is this representation indicative of later views about the relative impenetrability of the body to ultraviolet light, of it remaining only skin-deep? It is tempting to think so, except for the fact that the infrared light, well known to be deeply penetrative, is depicted confusingly in the exact same way.

As viewers we are to assume that direct, beneficial interaction between light and body is taking place in these representations, and that the body is therefore penetrable or, to quote Richardson, to some extent 'translucent', if not transparent, to the rays. Yet the body remains intact and whole, an irony particularly in Figure 4.6 considering its figure is meant to be burnt and wounded as evidenced by the advertisement title. Here the uninterrupted contour of the exposed back and legs is only further emphasised by overdrawing. This occurs invariably in advertisements showing figures exposed to emanating light, the body's contours always remaining sharply delineated to mark out the figure as a separate layer superimposed over or distinct from the light. Their layers are not the physical imprints of shadows left behind by a body's internal tissues, organs, and bones, what Zweifel referred to as literal traces or extensions of the body onto the film of radiographs. Unlike El Lissitzky's montage (Fig. 4.13), which presents misty, translucent layers of overlapping photographs, light therapy's montages have little similarity to a radiograph, even if these images share other techniques of vanguard representation. And, while Moholy-Nagy's montage (Fig. 4.12) includes hard-edged layers of different media, it also presents 'dematerialised' objects, not least a female face that appears to disintegrate in the background of the middle panel. The 'Vi-tan' pamphlet cover and the Hanovia 'Alpine Sun Lamp' advertisement, to the contrary, present bodies and light as overtly materialised, as tangible entities that curiously remain visibly separate and distinct. We see this also in Perihel's advertisement cover (c. late 1940s–50s, Fig. 4.7). Indeed, it visualises the invisible ultraviolet light projecting from its dual-headed lamp (on the right), while the infrared light is absent entirely (on the left). The use of montage in these three instances presents various levels of sophistication, yet it remains a problematic form of representation to accurately disseminate light's specific actions on the body. They confound any clear understanding of the body's penetrability to ultraviolet (or infrared) rays. The models in each of these representations retain his or her cast shadows, of light reflecting off of and not penetrating into or through the body. This conflation, nay collapse, of ultraviolet, visible, and infrared rays exemplifies the clashing beliefs and confusion among practitioners and the public about their uses and differences.

Combining the rays

Hanovia's 'Alpine Sun' montage depicts the emanating, invisible wavelengths of ultraviolet and infrared light as visible, white blocks of negative space (Fig. 4.6). Similarly, the Thermal Syndicate's 'Vi-tan' montage depicts the crepuscular (implicitly ultraviolet) rays of natural sunlight but, by the placement of the lamp within the sun, infers these rays are artificially produced by the 'Vi-tan' (Plate 1). These confounding representations, collapsing distinctions between very different kinds of light and sources, occur again and again in advertisements for lamps.

In fact, the combining of different rays, and different sources, was commonly practised by light therapists and radiotherapists in Britain and abroad. The revered heliotherapist Sir Henry Gauvain, for example, happily combined natural sunlight with artificial light to treat his young patients at Treloar Hospital in Hampshire, and we have already encountered advertisements for home-use lamps in naturist journals like *Sun Bathing Review* (Fig. 4.10), complicating any easy separation between the natural and the artificial.[109] As for the different rays produced by lamps, Beaumont explained that there was no device producing solely ultraviolet light:

> There is no such thing as an ultra-violet lamp, if by that is understood an apparatus which produces a preponderance of ultra-violet radiation. Therefore, to speak of ultra-violet radiotherapy is a misnomer, because in the present state of our knowledge it is not known what results are due to the infra-red, or the visible, or the ultra-violet.[110]

The nurse Myrtle Vaughan-Cowell noted that a variety of lamps were therefore needed, since patients reacted differently to certain types of lamps and their outputs.[111] Surely this only enabled further manufacture and consumption of phototherapy lamps, their sheer variety and patient idiosyncrasy productive forces for the market.

An exemplary case of combining rays in practice was the infrared light specialist Dr William Annandale Troup, practising in the medical district of Wimpole Street, London. Infrared was valuable therapeutically as an analgesic, heat serving this purpose since antiquity. It was used to treat various kinds of aches and pains in the body such as toothaches, earaches, arthritis, neuralgia, and sciatica, in place of drugs. In its ability to increase blood flow, Troup used infrared radiation to treat boils, abscesses, and wounds, irradiating the lesion to increase suppuration, and additionally found it sped healing on fractures.[112] Like many other British practitioners, he also used infrared radiation in combination with ultraviolet radiation, and in some cases with X radiation. Indeed, from their inception during the 1890s, natural light (heliotherapy), artificial light (phototherapy), X rays (diagnostic and therapeutic), and radium (radiotherapy) would be applied, combined, and counteracted in the same department within hospitals, notably the Light Department of the Royal London Hospital and Finsen's Light Institute.[113]

In the literature these rays are explained as interacting in exceptionally complex ways, as both allies and enemies. Troup, for example, used a combination of infrared and ultraviolet rays to treat sinusitis and neuralgia, perceiving the former to aid the latter's penetration into the body.[114] In images we find both kinds of lamps used together, the infrared lamp providing deeply penetrative warmth to assist the 'cold', poorly penetrative light of the mercury vapour lamp. We have already seen their combined use promoted in advertisements (Figs. 4.6–4.7), but clinical photographs exist too (Fig. 4.15). In Figure 4.15, a photograph of goggled child patients receiving phototherapy at the Institute of Ray Therapy, two Jesionek-type mercury vapour lamps irradiated the children while an infrared lamp in the centre provided heat. In fact, the combining of lamps occurred early on, as evidenced by a 1912 catalogue listing by the Cavendish Electrical Company, which promoted combined use of a carbon arc light and an incandescent light 'bath' (made of incandescent light bulbs to provoke intense sweating in the patient).[115]

Though Troup combined infrared and ultraviolet rays, confusingly he also described infrared as *counteracting* the effects of ultraviolet: 'The effects of an overdosage of ultra-violet rays can to a large extent be counteracted by subsequent exposure to infra-red radiation, and the skin effects [solar erythema] can be markedly decreased.'[116] Used before or during treatment, infrared aided ultraviolet radiation's effects on the body. Used afterwards, it apparently decreased them, particularly the severity of solar erythema if overdosed. The confusing love–hate relationship between infrared and ultraviolet radiation in clinical applications occurs between ultraviolet and X radiation as well and is further complicated by the addition of radium's alpha,

Figure 4.15 'Healing Ray' (Institute of Ray Therapy, Camden), 1930.
Hulton Archive, Fox Photos/Getty Images.

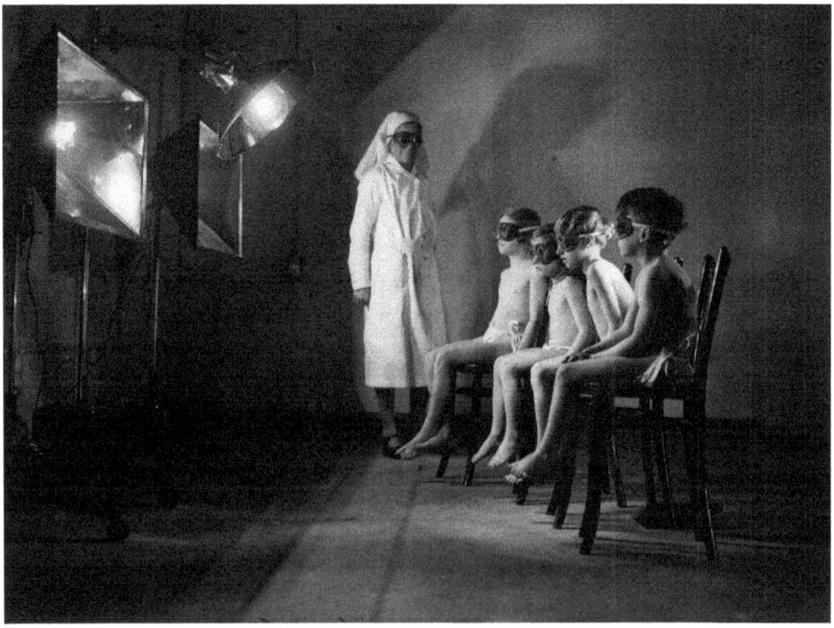

beta, and gamma radiation. For instance, for over forty years ultraviolet light, via carbon arc and mercury vapour lamps, was used to complement X rays and radium, especially when treating lupus vulgaris and other skin diseases.[117] However, physicians also used these ultraviolet lamps and natural sunlight to treat the burns *caused by* X rays and radium, using ultraviolet light to temper or reverse the effects of an X ray or radium overdose – just as Troup advised infrared radiation to counteract ultraviolet overdoses.[118]

Moreover, in the public domain, manufacturers capitalised on the frequent confusion between ultraviolet and violet light. In the words of Drs Eleanor and Kerr Russell, 'At present there is great confusion in the public mind between the two terms "violet rays" and "ultra-violet rays," and they are continually being confounded'.[119] In local and national newspapers, 'violet rays' and 'violet ray apparatus' were commonly used to mean *ultra*violet rays and devices.[120] These may have been innocent slippages, making for short, punchy titles, except that there was also a device widely available known as the 'violet ray machine'. This was an electrical device producing a high frequency current that lit up with a purple-coloured light, which was used to treat hair loss, rheumatism, sciatica, and headaches. Members of the public could access violet-ray treatment in various ways: at beauty salons, from chiropractors, and at home through purchase of units directly from suppliers, including well known, reputable department stores like Selfridges.[121] Advertisements for it were even included in the Sunlight League's journal, *Sunlight*, edited by natural sunlight enthusiast Saleeby (Fig. 4.16). It was popular enough to warrant concern: it was described as a quack device by equally well known, reputable medical men such as Sir Leonard Hill, by manufacturers of 'genuine' light therapy equipment like Hanovia, and in local newspapers.[122] Despite these warnings, the violet-ray machine continued to be produced, marketed, and sold, consumed by a public eager for its stimulating action.

The violet-ray machine shared important similarities with the myriad, contemporaneous products purporting to be enhanced by radium or X rays, advertised in the same venues. In British popular newspapers, radium products were widely advertised in the form of spa waters, like Buxton and Bath, at hotels like Peebles, within illuminated watch dials, pads for gout and rheumatism, skin cosmetics, and via emanators to inhale it directly into the lungs.[123] The actual quantity of radium in these products was questionable, and yet, as Thomas de la Peña argued, the very existence of such a wide variety of radium products suggests that 'consumers sought connections with radium beyond the analytical. They desired to see the element act on the body, to see its invisibility made visible in the form of topical and ingestible products.'[124]

Ultraviolet rays similarly materialised through home-use lamps and were made visible as weighty masses of emanating whiteness in their advertisements. So too were they understood to be ingestible, products to be literally consumed to protect the

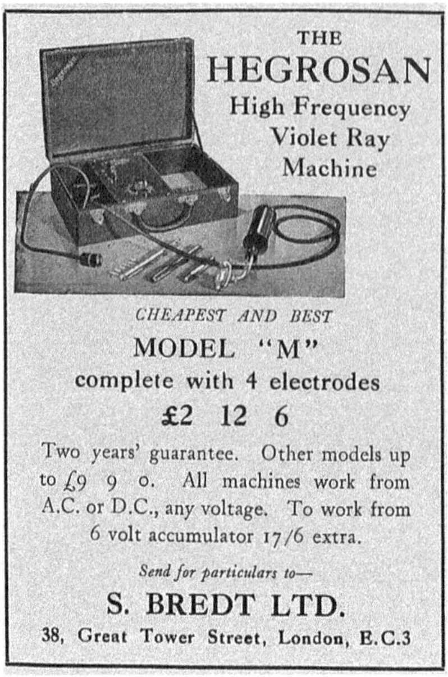

Figure 4.16 Advertisement for the Bredt 'Hegrosan high frequency violet ray machine'. In *Sunlight*, 2:3 (1930), 122. Author's collection.

body from 'sun starvation' (see Chapter 5). Whether as graphic emanating lines that reach out towards the user, as in Figure 4.10, or as solid blocks (Plate 1, Figs. 4.3, 4.6–4.7), in these advertisements the rays are made tangible, graspable, even appetising. To an eager and hungry public, manufacturers encouraged gluttonous consumption of home-use lamps. The 'Vi-tan' lamp's incredible (and incredulous) output of 99 per cent ultraviolet radiation made it a potentially volatile device, yet in its advertising the association between the dynamism of the Art Deco rays and the sexual appeal of their recipient makes them appear less dangerous than delicious (Plate 1). In spite of awareness of the risks, these lamps and their radiation could inflict on patients and members of the public, the 'Vi-tan' pamphlet cover leaves its viewer wanting.

The risky rays

As stated in the last chapter, for Gauvain, therapeutic exposure to sunlight could be understood as a beneficial and stimulating 'light shock' to the body.[125] This notion of the 'light shock' was both metaphorical and unintentionally literal: electric shocks, severe burns, and even death occurred during light-therapy exposures. Practitioners also reported cases of burst bulbs and adverse reactions such as severe burns and blisters, spoke of the eerie, greenish glow of the mercury vapour lamp and the purplish appearance of flesh underneath it, and noted that children were frightened by the carbon arc lamp's spluttering and hissing.[126] Because of this light treatment 'séances' (sittings) had much in common with those involving X-ray machines, which similarly could spark and shock, took place in the dark, frightened patients, and produced noxious ozone.[127] 'Seance' was therefore a fitting description for these treatments, the machines' 'magical' properties less fantastical than dark (Fig. 3.3). When it first emerged in the mid-nineteenth century, photography too was described as form of black magic and one that, until the early twentieth century, retained its associations with the supernatural.[128] Some photographs of phototherapy sessions, such as Figure 3.3, are reminiscent of spiritualist photographs of séances, like those by the noted chemist and physicist Sir William Crookes, which Tom Gunning described as 'oscillating between the amusing and the truly creepy'.[129] Crookes was, like Lodge, a spiritualist, and they both acted as presidents for the Society of Psychical Research (f. 1882).[130] Lodge's foreword in Drs Russells' 1925 book, *Ultra-violet Radiation and Actinotherapy*, in the epigraph above, positions ultraviolet radiation as a mysterious and unknown force not unlike other curious, if not creepy, vibrations and emanations.

Light therapy's literature does not lack for textual descriptions about the dangers and risks of the treatment. From its inception its destructiveness was prized. Finsen considered actinic light's 'injurious' character the very foundation of the treatment's success (see epigraph). Some physicians described the resultant sunburn as a visual sign of the body having received a beneficial 'beating' by radiation.[131] Warnings in the *BMJ* suggest that public sunbathing, with subsequent overexposure, was already a popular practice by the time of the First World War.[132] As early as 1914, an article in *The Times* associated the dangers of ultraviolet light alongside those of X rays and radium:

> While we enjoy the brilliant days that summer may have in store, it is well to realize that light contains dangerous as well as health giving qualities and understand how to use it to the best hygienic advantage [...] These ultra-violet rays are, with the X-rays and radium, among the most remarkable physical phenomena known. They possess the power of destroying animal tissues with great rapidity.[133]

These early examples indicate the openness of sources to discuss light's dangers, much as early reports announced those of X rays and radium, especially latent burns.[134] Though I have found in many of light therapy's images signs of damage, 'burns', and overexposure, its visual culture provides few overt representations of the therapy's risks. In this its history differs significantly from those of radiotherapy, which possesses plenty of visual representations of radiation burns (dermatitis), injuries, and consequent amputations (Fig. 4.17).

Less overt than covert, the visual material communicates light therapy's risks through confounding representations. Let us return to the 'Vi-tan' pamphlet cover

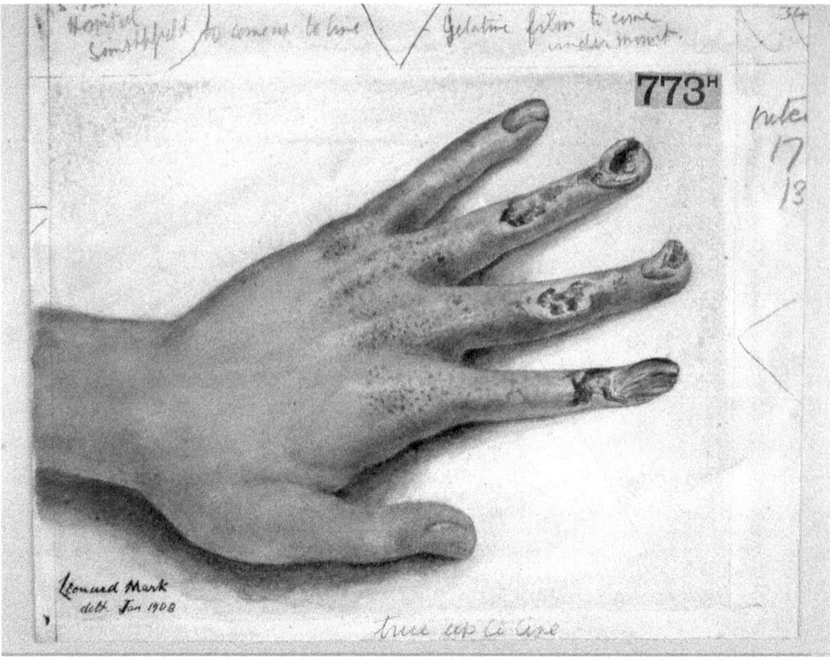

Figure 4.17 Leonard Portal Mark, a patient's left hand affected with chronic dermatitis, the result of exposure to the Röntgen rays, 1908.
Watercolour. Wellcome Library and St Bartholomew's Hospital Archives and Museum, London CC BY-NC 4.0.

as a poignant example (Plate 1). Dressed for the beach, without her requisite pair of goggles, and draped by the lamp's unplugged electrical cord, the woman in the advertisement presents a curious and contradictory set of messages about safe, effective, artificial exposures. Indeed, she is even wearing a swimming cap on her head, making a bold association with the lido or seaside, despite the fact that engaging in any activities involving water while operating these electrical devices was downright dangerous. Reports, for instance, in 1928 of a law student who died by electrocution, operating a lamp while he bathed, were widely circulated in the popular press and commented upon in the *BMJ*.[135] In *The Times*' 'Sunlight and Health' supplement of the same year, Hanovia included a vignette in an advertisement that illustrated two children standing in front of a mercury vapour lamp, placed directly at the edge of a public swimming pool.[136]

A montage from Hanovia's 'Homesun' pamphlet of 1940 is similarly ambiguous about safe exposures (Plate 2). A mother and baby, coloured in a saturated, near-fluorescent orange to represent their glowing tans, are positioned on a bed as they are exposed to the lamp's actinic light. Again note the theatrical hard-edged emanation of white light that splays towards them, like a spotlight on a darkened stage. It is but one of many advertisements featuring users in bed. As mentioned earlier, two London doctors reported a case of overexposure occurring in 1924, which involved a seventy-two-year-old man falling asleep under his mercury vapour lamp at home for over an hour (instead of ten minutes). This resulted in such severe burning, oedema, and heart palpitations over the next two weeks that the man almost died.[137] Inasmuch as the ultraviolet rays were described as vitalising and stimulating, manufacturers warned that using the lamps could soothe users to sleep; this correlates to reports of members of the public severely burnt because they fell asleep in bed under their lamps, alone and unsupervised.[138] One physician even suggested that overuse of a lamp had caused a woman to miscarry.[139]

These accidents only served to confer more authority upon practitioners as the necessary 'expert' administrators and supervisors of patients' treatment, back in the realm of the clinic.[140] While some practitioners celebrated the public's access to artificial light for private use, others anxiously cried out for regulation. In her 1928 book, *Artificial Sunlight*, Vaughan-Cowell, for example, declared:

> The problem of dosage is an extremely complex one, and for this reason all treatments must be carried out strictly under medical supervision, this also is why we must denounce 'home' treatment and the installation of lamps by the lay public. In this respect we must be absolutely loyal, which will not only be the means of protecting our patients and ourselves, but will also be performing a public duty, and prevent what should be purely a medical science from getting into the hands of the 'quack'.[141]

Ironically, in her book the publishers included an advertisement for the 'Home-Sunlight Arc Lamp' by the Westminster Engineering Company (London).

The British Medical Association's 1928 meeting addressed the fact that no law was in place to restrict amateurs and the general public to use ultraviolet rays, in addition to X rays, radium, and electricity.[142] As with these other wild and powerful natural forces, the frequent voicing of concern among practitioners over regulating access to light, especially ultraviolet light, is indicative of underlying anxiety among the medical community about retaining sufficient control over exposures (see Chapter 2). Their aim, Vaughan-Cowell made clear, was to prevent light therapy from losing legitimacy as a valid, successful modern therapeutic in the unqualified hands of the ignorant public or unscrupulous quack. As Thomas de la Peña argued, such declarations were counterproductive, merely reinforcing the products themselves as valid medical devices, whoever owned them.[143]

The attempt to control and manage these wild, natural forces is described by historians as a process of 'domestication'. I find the word's multivalent meanings, as a 'taming' and a 'making suitable for the home', particularly apt in reference to Vaughan-Cowell's book, in which her decidedly anti-'domestic' denouncement of home treatment sits ambiguously alongside Westminster's advertisement. Like electricity entering British households via incandescent lighting, ultraviolet radiation, via home-use lamps, needed to be harnessed to be welcomed into the home (and body). The 'Vi-tan' pamphlet cover's model domesticates its rays by wearing the lamp's cord around her as a fashion accessory. Public displays of female dancers draped in glittering light bulbs achieved the same theatrical and 'magical' effects decades earlier.[144] Yet the 'Vi-tan' lamp is rendered safe not because it has been aestheticised and feminised by the female body but simply because it is not plugged in.[145] If, according to Gooday, 'The taming process involved mitigating the dangers, uncertain behaviour and aesthetic provocations of electricity', then domesticating ultraviolet radiation was doomed to failure from the beginning.[146] That ultraviolet radiation was known to stimulate sexual desire to the point of excess and produce tans inspired by 'primitive' dark bodies would suggest, to the contrary, it rendered its consumers wild and untamed (see Chapter 5).

Light death

The history of home-use lamps in Britain is not a history of the successful 'domestication' of a medical technology, but of the ongoing, unstable character of light therapy and the inability to control a resistant, ephemeral force of nature. Of course, as Rima Apple, Simon Carter, and Matthew Lavine all argued, its instabilities only compelled medical authorities to attempt to intercede more and more, to produce new research and products to counter inaccuracies or unfavourable results, and confer more authority onto medicine and science.[147] This is beautifully illustrated by the following quote by Dr Percy Hall (Mount Vernon Hospital and the Hull Municipal Light Clinic) in a foreword to a 1935 handbook on light treatment for masseuses:

> Probably no new therapeutic method in the history of modern medicine has achieved such widespread use in so short a time as has light treatment. Its apparent simplicity led thousands of doctors, masseuses and others to avail themselves of it in the treatment of various disorders. Hospitals up and down the country opened Light Departments, and clinics for its use sprang up like mushrooms. The trouble was that very few persons had a sufficient knowledge of the subject to enable them to get the desired results. A great many unpleasant and unfortunate consequences occurred which, too often, were blamed on the method rather than the lack of skill and experience of

> the administrator. It was an almost exact repetition of what happened after the discovery of Roentgen was first made public. How, however, the pendulum has begun to swing in the opposite direction, and there is a laudable desire on the part of masseurs and masseuses in particular – who so often, in both hospital and private practice, are entrusted with this treatment without being given precise directions as to technique and dosage – to gain proficient knowledge at the hands of clinicians who are really experienced and competent to impart the necessary instruction.[148]

However much Hall asserted his own superiority as a physician with an expertise in light treatment, his statement betrays certain anxieties over the therapy's rise, fall, resurgence, and widening dissemination to 'lesser' sorts of medical authority (i.e. masseuses). Dependence upon medical authority did not necessarily equate to further control over therapeutic exposures.

The practitioner's need to assert control over the therapy's legitimisation and dissemination went beyond words; it was a bodily commitment. Finsen first understood the penetrative and transforming powers of actinic light by irradiating his own forearm with a carbon arc lamp, not unlike contemporaneous X-ray and radium 'martyrs' whose bodies registered the dangerous effects of radiation exposure in the early days of experimentation.[149] As discussed in Chapter 2, practitioners commonly used their own arms for standardising lamp outputs. This method of self-testing went so far as injecting photo-sensitising chemicals into their bodies. In a 1913 experiment, the German F. Meyer-Betz injected himself with haematoporphyrin, the iron-free derivative of haemoglobin, which made him seriously ill and extremely photosensitive for weeks (Fig. 4.18). No doubt the taking of the photograph was itself an unpleasant experience, requiring exposure to actinic light to be produced. On mice haematoporphyrin produced extreme skin reactions, swelling, convulsions, and shortness of breath, eventually resulting in 'light death'.[150]

The notion of 'death by light' can be correlated to rising awareness during the same period that ultraviolet light was carcinogenic. British researchers began making this connection as early as 1925 and proved by 1928 that ultraviolet light could cause cancer. This began with a report by Dr George William Marshall Findlay, given at the Pathological Section of the Royal Society of Medicine in February 1925.[151] At this time in his long and illustrious career, Findlay was employed in the laboratories of the Imperial Cancer Research Fund in London, and by 1929 with the Wellcome Bureau of Scientific Research.[152] Citing reports from 1896 in Germany, France, America, and Australia, Findlay stated, 'The possibility that the sun's rays may play a part in this excessive production of skin cancer has not lacked supporters.'[153] He admitted, however, that no one had yet definitely reported a case of skin cancer due

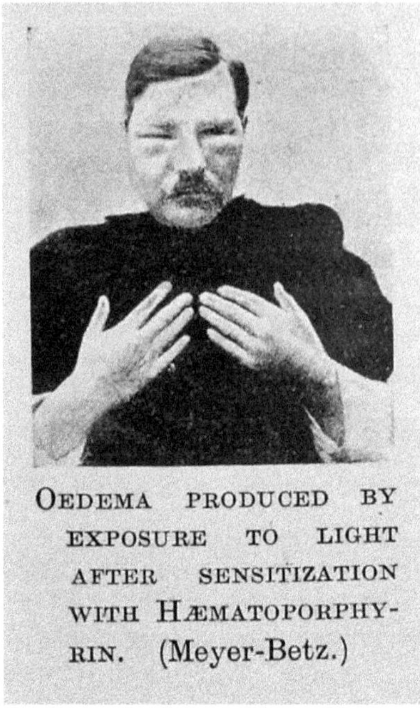

Figure 4.18 Meyer-Betz, 'Oedema produced by exposure to light after sensitisation with haematoporphyrin.' In Leonard Hill, *Sunshine and Open Air: Their Influence on Health, with Special Reference to the Alpine Climate* (London: Edward Arnold, 1925), Plate 7, opposite p. 94. Author's collection.

specifically to ultraviolet light. Findlay's experiments on white mice, reported three years later in the *Lancet* (1928), were the earliest to show the explicitly carcinogenic action of ultraviolet light in the laboratory. Within eight months the rays produced cancerous growths, both 'simple papillomata' and 'malignant epitheliomata', on the mice's backs.

G. Lenthal Cheatle echoed Findlay's initial 1925 report by providing his own opinions about the carcinogenic powers of sunlight, especially ultraviolet light. He cited an article he wrote for the *BMJ* in 1909, on the effects of what he called 'biotripsis' ('life wear') on the hands of elderly countrywomen. He now sought to argue that such 'life wear', resulting in skin cancer lesions (squamous epithelioma) must be due to sunlight, and he furthermore recently witnessed a lesion worsen dramatically following ultraviolet light treatment.[154] Hill responded in the following week's *BMJ* issue by deferring to Bernhard, who had never witnessed epithelioma on the hands or faces (those body parts most exposed to sunlight) of workers regularly out of doors in the intense Alpine sunshine.[155] Hill reasoned that since British sunshine was far less intense than that of the Alps, no danger was to be had there. 'If there were danger of ultra-violet radiation causing cancer, as x rays have done, the operators and patients in such institutes as the Finsen would have shown this by now', he concluded.[156] Edward James Deck, who a year later produced the Sunlight League's popular treatise, *The Sun and How to Use It*, supported Hill's views and added that he, in fact, had successfully treated squamous carcinoma of the hands *with* ultraviolet rays following surgical removal of the growth, and finished his letter: 'In conclusion I would like to refer to the condition of my own hands. After approximately 35,000 administrations of ultra-violet rays I think there is distinctly less sign of "biotripsis" than is customary at the age of 52, though I have never safeguarded my skin in any way.'[157] Deck's concluding remarks were undoubtedly an indirect reference to the hands of X-ray operators, whose gradual destruction – first by X-ray dermatitis, ulcerating lesions, eventual amputation, and finally death – made the medical community fully aware of their lethal power. This connection between the rays would continue well into the 1940s, now further united by their common nature as carcinogens.[158]

When Findlay provided laboratory evidence in 1928 in the *Lancet*, again the responses were swift and sceptical, despite the fact that the journal's editors urged caution in the use of a treatment still 'yet in its infancy'.[159] Findlay's procedure and results were questioned by light therapist and radiologist Dr Maurice Weinbren for their 'incriminating' claims, to which Findlay's pointedly responded with clarity and, in 1930, with further laboratory results, this time using rats.[160] Though British physicians like Findlay were providing laboratory ('controlled') results of ultraviolet light's carcinogenic powers by the mid-1920s, in-depth studies did not occur until the 1940s, due in part to rising interest in radiation research in the forms of radiation biology and nuclear power. As Sally Dunne Romano discussed, it was only in the 1950s and 1960s that the medical community and the public came to fully accept ultraviolet light's carcinogenic power, which grew in part due to larger, generic fears about 'radiation', 'cancer', and their ambiguous meanings.[161]

Conclusion

The 'Vi-tan' lamp and its advertisement (Fig. 4.1, Plate 1) make materially manifest Freund's notion of 'synthetic nature', a fantastical and even 'magical' conceptualisation of modern technology's capacities to perfect the body. Fusing natural and new man-made materials, the lamp is a decorative object offering to beautify the British home and its users by perfecting and exceeding the powers of natural sunlight. Such a promise was further conveyed through the magic of modern advertising. The pamphlet cover presents synthetic nature using the disjunctive layers of montage, which confounds the distinction between the artificial and the natural, the visible and the invisible, reality and fantasy. The lamp's/sun's emanating ultraviolet rays are given visible form as Art Deco sunbeams yet remain the dramatic background for the model, not her cure: this is theatre, not therapy. The montage is beautiful, glamorous, fantastical, and modern, but ultraviolet radiation resisted even vanguard attempts to aestheticise and render safe its dangers. Unlike the incandescent light bulb, the home-use lamp could not be wholly 'domesticated' amidst awareness of its dangerous and even lethal potential to harm members of the public. With its volatile emanating light it could never become 'domestic lighting'.

For manufacturers, selling synthetic nature through 'artificial sunlight' was a risky business. A seductive 'poison', it was equally so for those desiring to consume it.[162] While risk, in medicine and society, is a culturally and historically specific concept, this chapter has focused on the objects and images in terms of risk, danger, and bodily damage to continue exploring the tensions in light therapy's nascent British reception and legitimisation.[163] In focusing on light therapy's risks and technology, my intention has not been to denigrate its successes or historic value but rather to unpick its complicated relationship with other radiation therapies, its public dissemination, and the anxieties of its practitioners concerned about controlling its access. The public received confusing messages about ultraviolet radiation's capabilities from practitioners and manufacturers, not least through the visual. Depicted as razor-edged shafts of light and encroaching masses of negative white space in heavily overworked advertisements, these risky rays transport the user to the realm of science fiction. Indeed, such representations present remarkable similarities to H. G. Wells' lethal 'heat ray' of the Martians in *The War of the Worlds* (1898), in both function and representation. With its destructive white flash, the 'heat ray' was described by Wells as both a 'camera' and a 'searchlight' (carbon arc light), collapsing photographic and phototherapeutic risks alike Meyer-Betz's image (Fig. 4.18).[164] Through the light sensitiser haematoporphyrin, Meyer-Betz had become so saturated by actinic light that he was in danger of 'light death'. A dangerous photogenesis, his bodily state approached the victims of radium poisoning, whose corpses were so saturated that they imprinted themselves onto photographic plates.[165]

By 1914, in *The World Set Free*, Wells predicted the future of atomic warfare in his ongoing fascination with powerful invisible energies, a fascination he shared with scientists like Frederick Soddy as well as members of the public.[166] Indeed, ultraviolet, X, and gamma rays had been seducing professional and lay audiences since the 1890s. For Lavine, 'radiation and radioactivity were not entirely at home in the scientific establishment. They were disruptive; they broke laws and unbalanced equations. They were, as the amused commentary from newspaper editorialists had it, "naughty."'[167] As he made clear, sexual innuendo was part and parcel of radiation's appeal from the outset. Evading practitioners' and manufacturers' attempts to harness it, ultraviolet radiation was similarly risky, untameable, 'naughty'.

The connection between sunlight, sexuality, and death finds an important mediator in the form of the atom bomb. Its nuclear radiation was explained to an international public as artificial sunlight, just as radium had been half a century earlier.[168] An image of actress Rita Hayworth (1918–87) graced the metal shell of bomb 'Able' above Bikini lagoon in July 1946.[169] The 'explosive fashion' of the two-piece swimsuit, the bikini, emerged from Paris four days later.[170] Enabling, nay encouraging, exposure of the bombshell's flesh to the sun's 'kiss' and the admirer's gaze, the bikini cemented associations between light, risk, and sexuality. As evinced in the next chapter, in spite of its risks ultraviolet radiation retained its desirability in the eyes of the public as well as practitioners, government lobbyists, and social campaigners. Its photogenic qualities lent glamour and sex appeal to national interests in regenerating the 'race', saturating the white British body with radiant colour.

Notes

1 Italics mine. Niels R. Finsen, *Phototherapy*, trans. J. H. Sequeira (London: Edward Arnold, 1901), p. 2.

2 Sir Oliver Lodge in Eleanor H. Russell and William K. Russell, *Ultra-violet Radiation and Actinotherapy* (Edinburgh: E. & S. Livingstone, 1925), p. 1.

3 On creating implicit desire and social status in advertising, see Paul Messaris, *Visual Persuasion: The Role of Images in Advertising* (London: Sage, 1997).

4 Based in Northumberland, the Thermal Syndicate specialised in fused quartz silica. In the 1930s it expanded its product offerings by making not just the bulb but an entire lamp. It also supplied materials for the atom bomb's development. See *The Story of the Thermal Syndicate Limited: Commemorating the Jubilee of the Thermal Syndicate Limited, 1906–1956* (Wallsend: N.I., 1956), pp. 38, 41.

5 On the modern look of mixed typefaces, see Paul Jobling, *Man Appeal: Advertising, Modernism and Men's Wear* (New York and Oxford: Berg, 2005).

6 *Actinotherapy Technique* (Slough: Sollux, 1933), p. 13.

7 See Carolyn Thomas de la Peña, *The Body Electric: How Strange Machines Built the Modern American* (New York: New York University Press, 2003), p. 80, in which she described the luxury embellishments of Zander's mechanical horse, *c.* 1892.

8 Graeme Gooday, *Domesticating Electricity: Technology, Uncertainty and Gender, 1880–1914* (London: Pickering & Chatto, 2008), pp. 9, 20. On 'domestication', see also Thomas de la Peña, *Body Electric*, p. 3; Chris Otter, *The Victorian Eye: A Political History of Light and Vision in Britain, 1800–1910* (Chicago, Ill.: University of Chicago Press, 2008), p. 242; Bettyann Holtzmann Kevles, *Naked to the Bone: Medical Imagine in the Twentieth Century* (Reading: Helix Books, 1998), p. 54; Matthew Lavine, *The First Atomic Age: Scientists, Radiations, and the American Public, 1895–1945* (New York: Palgrave Macmillan, 2013), pp. 174, 178; Lisa Cartwright, *Screening the Body: Tracing Medicine's Visual Culture* (Minneapolis, Minn.: University of Minnesota Press, 1995), p. 110.

9 Peter Rowlands, 'Lodge, Sir Oliver Joseph (1851–1940)', *Oxford Dictionary of National Biography*, www.oxforddnb.com/index/101034583/Oliver-Lodge (accessed 16 July 2014).

10 See, for example, the heavily retouched photographs and emanating graphic lines for typewriters and telephones in Ellen Lupton, *Mechanical Brides: Women and Machines from Home to Office* (New York: Cooper-Hewitt National Museum of Design, Smithsonian Institute, and Princeton Architectural Press, 1993), pp. 43, 33.

11 See the patient photographs in Sir Malcolm Morris and S. Ernest Dore, *Light and X-Ray Treatment of Skin Diseases* (New York: Funk & Wagnalls, 1910), and the retouched prints

in the Treloar Archives (e.g., undated photograph taken by the Photo Press [Fleet Street], 47M94/F2/5/4/10).

12 Lavine, *First Atomic Age*, p. 23.

13 Indeed, it was called 'ultraviolet radiotherapy' in W. Annandale Troup, *Therapeutic Uses of Infra-red Rays* (London: Actinic Press, 1936), p. 72. Scholars dismissive of ultraviolet light in radiation histories include Lavine, *First Atomic Age*; Kevles, *Naked to the Bone*; Thomas de la Peña, *Body Electric*; Cartwright, *Screening the Body*; David I. Harvie, *Deadly Sunshine: The History and Fatal Legacy of Radium* (Stroud: Tempus, 2005); Joel D. Howell, *Technology in the Hospital: Transforming Patient Care in the Early Twentieth Century* (Baltimore, Md.: Johns Hopkins University Press, 1996); and Catherine Caufield, *Multiple Exposures: Chronicles of the Radiation Age* (Harmondsworth: Penguin, 1989).

14 See Georg Bröchner, 'An Apostle of Light: Professor Finsen at Home', *Pall Mall Magazine* (June 1904), pp. 202–8, at p. 208; Axel Reyn and Svend Lomholt, *Institut Photothérapique 'Finsen' à Copenhague* (Copenhagen: Dyva & Jeppesen, 1923), p. 7; Axel Reyn, 'Discussion on the Artificial Light Treatment of Lupus and Other Forms of Tuberculosis', *BMJ*, 22 September 1923, pp. 499–503, at p. 499.

15 See Anne Kinloch Jamieson, 'More than Meets the Eye: Revealing the Therapeutic Potential of Light, 1896–1910', *Social History of Medicine*, 26:4 (2013), 715–37; and Anne Kinloch Jamieson, 'An Intolerable Affliction: A History of Lupus Vulgaris in Late Nineteenth- and Early Twentieth-Century Britain' (Ph.D. dissertation, University of Leeds, 2010).

16 Other kinds of rays included René Blondlot's 'N-rays' and Gustave Le Bon's 'black light'. See Harvie, *Deadly Sunshine*, p. 34; and John Gage, 'Matisse's Black Light', in *Colour and Meaning: Art, Science and Symbolism* (London: Thames & Hudson, 1998), pp. 228–40.

17 Lavine, *First Atomic Age*, p. 13. On 'actinic fever', see Simone Natale, 'The Invisible Made Visible: X-Rays as Attraction and Visual Medium at the End of the Nineteenth Century', *Media History*, 17:4 (2011), 345–59.

18 Kelley Wilder, *Photography and Science* (London: Reaktion, 2009), pp. 50, 58–9.

19 See Kelley Wilder, 'Visualizing Radiation: The Photographs of Henri Becquerel', in Lorraine Daston and Elizabeth Lunbeck (eds), *Histories of Scientific Observation* (Chicago, Ill.: University of Chicago Press, 2011), pp. 349–68, at pp. 358, 360; and Antoine-Henri Becquerel, *Rays Emitted from a Radioactive Substance* [Via Uranium Salts] *through a Slitted Screen*, 1901, gelatin silver print, in Corey Keller (ed.), *Brought to Light: Photography and the Invisible, 1840–1900* (New Haven, Conn.: Yale University Press with SFMOMA, 2008), Plate 140.

20 See Richard F. Mould, *A Century of X-rays and Radioactivity in Medicine* (Bristol and Philadelphia, Pa.: Institute of Physics Publishing, 1993), p. 21; Jamieson, 'More than Meets the Eye', pp. 85–95; and Jamieson, 'An Intolerable Affliction', pp. 112–15.

21 Hugh Walsham, 'On the Ultra-violet Light from a Rapid Oscillation High-Tension Arc, for the Treatment of Skin Diseases', *Lancet*, 1 February 1902, pp. 285–8, at p. 287.

22 Mould, *Century of X-rays*, p. 170; and Kevles, *Naked to the Bone*, p. 87.

23 See, for example, J. Alfred Codd, 'Some Results of Treatment by X Rays, High-Frequency Currents, and Ultra-violet Rays', *BMJ*, 23 July 1904, pp. 176–80. See also Jamieson, 'An Intolerable Affliction', pp. 92–3; and Lavine, *First Atomic Age*, p. 14.

24 See Kevles, *Naked to the Bone*, p. 46; Harvie, *Deadly Sunshine*, p. 47; and Georges Chicotot, *The First Attempt of Dr Chicotot to Cure Cancer with X Rays* (Paris: Musée de l'Assistance Publique-Hôpitaux, 1907).

25 See Harvie, *Deadly Sunshine*, p. 82, citing 1914 articles in *The Times*, 24 June, 7 August; and Lavine, *First Atomic Age*, pp. 100–1.

26 See Harvie, *Deadly Sunshine*, p. 120; and Howell, *Technology in the Hospital*, p. 118. See also Chapter 5.

27 Jamieson, 'More than Meets the Eye'.

28 Italics mine. Wilder, *Photography and Science*, p. 53. See also Daniel Bürkner, 'The Chernobyl Landscape and the Aesthetics of Invisibility', *Photography & Culture*, 7:1 (2014), 21–40.

29 *Actinotherapy Technique* (1933), p. 31. Herzig described this as 'suprasensuality' in Rebecca Herzig, 'Removing Roots: "North American Hiroshima Maidens" and the X-Ray', *Technology and Culture*, 40:4 (1999), 723–45, at p. 742.

30 On burns treated by light therapy, see *Actinotherapy Technique* (1933), pp. 67–9; Roditi, *Contribution à l'étude du traitement des brûlures par l'héliothérapie*, and Oskar Bernhard, *Light Treatment in Surgery* (London: Edward Arnold, 1926).

31 See also the photomontage in John Harvey Kellogg, *Light Therapeutics* (Battle Creek, Mich.: Modern Medicine, 1927), opposite p. 108.

32 Miles noted, 'although light is the means by which other things appear it lacks a means of manifesting itself. In other words, light is incapable of announcing its own presence.' Melissa Miles, *The Burning Mirror: Photography in an Ambivalent Light* (North Melbourne: Australian Scholarly Publishing, 2008), p. 37.

33 Shelford Bidwell, *Curiosities of Light and Sight* (London: Swan Sonnenschein & Co., 1899), pp. 18–19.

34 Josh Ellenbogen, *Reasoned and Unreasoned Images: The Photography of Bertillon, Galton, and Marey* (University Park, Pa.: Pennsylvania State University Press, 2012), p. 175. See also Joel Snyder, 'Visualization and Visibility', in Caroline A. Jones and Peter Galison (eds), *Picturing Science, Producing Art* (London and New York: Routledge, 1998), pp. 379–97. On microscopy, see Cartwright, *Screening the Body*, p. 8.

35 See also Elizabeth S. Helfman, *Signs and Symbols of the Sun* (New York: Seabury Press, 1974), pp. 29–31; Richard Hobday, *The Healing Sun: Sunlight and Health in the 21st Century* (Forres: Findhorn Press, 1999, p. 30); and Sut Jhally, 'Advertising as Religion: The Dialectic of Technology and Magic', in Ian Angus and Sut Jhally (eds), *Cultural Politics in Contemporary America* (London and New York: Routledge, 1989), pp. 217–29, at p. 223.

36 Kevles, *Naked to the Bone*, p. 14; and Spencer R. Weart, *Nuclear Fear: A History of Images* (Cambridge, Mass.: Harvard University Press, 1988), p. 41.

37 Combining of ultraviolet and visible light (red to violet rays) was also debated: 'Some evidence has been put forward to show that visible rays interfere with the biological action of ultra-violet rays, and some clinicians therefore exclude daylight from arc lamp rooms. Further and more exact experiment has failed to confirm the existence of such interference.' Leonard Hill, in Leonard Hill, G. B. Dixon, and Dora C. Colebrook, 'Discussion on Influence of Sunlight and Artificial Light on Health', *BMJ*, 12 September 1925, pp. 470–7, at p. 472.

38 Thomas de la Peña, *Body Electric*, p. 114.

39 Thomas de la Peña, *Body Electric*, p. 199. See also Weart, *Nuclear Fear*, p. 42; and Lavine, *First Atomic Age*, p. 221, n. 166.

40 On the connection between the sun and nuclear bombs, see Harvie, *Deadly Sunshine*, pp. 70, 162, 244; Lavine, *First Atomic Age*, pp. 25, 96, 101, 111–12; Thomas de la Peña, *Body Electric*, pp. 183, 188–9, 196, 205; and Sally Dunne Romano, 'The Dark Side of the Sun: Skin Cancer, Sunscreen and Risk in Twentieth-Century America' (Ph.D. dissertation, Yale University, 2006), pp. 142–3.

41 See www.thisismoney.co.uk/money/bills/article-1633409/Historic-inflation-calculator-value-money-changed-1900.html (accessed 11 March 2016).

42 See Gooday, *Domesticating Electricity*, pp. 19, 30, 92; Otter, *The Victorian Eye*, p. 182; and Adrian Forty, *Objects of Desire: Design and Society since 1750* (London: Thames & Hudson, 1995), p. 189.

43 By 1930, appliances and their advertising literature marketed electricity as *the* modern form of energy, coinciding with a price decrease and surge in the mass market. See Forty, *Objects of Desire*, pp. 186–95. Yet these lamp products of the 1920s–40s were electrical devices with a long ancestry: electrotherapy devices were 'standardised', according to Thomas de la Peña (*Body Electric*, p. 95), already by the 1870s. Significantly, she included Finsen's phototherapy as a form of electrotherapy (p. 105).

44 See also a 'Vi-tan' lamp advertisement in *Sunderland Echo and Shipping Gazette*, 25 October 1937, p. 3.

45 See www.thisismoney.co.uk/money/bills/article-1633409/Historic-inflation-calculator-value-money-changed-1900.html (accessed 11 March 2016). See also Jonathan M. Woodham, *Twentieth-Century Design* (Oxford: Oxford University Press, 1997), p. 117.

46 Hanovia, *Get Back in the Sun with a 'Homesun'*, pamphlet, 1940, p. 13. An early plastic, Bakelite was a cast phenolic resin invented in 1907, widely used as a modern material during the early twentieth century.

47 Forty stated, 'Chromed steel and glass were welcomed not just because of their associations with machines, but also because they could easily be kept clean, and, above all, could look absolutely spotless' (*Objects of Desire*, p. 173). See also Woodham, *Twentieth-Century Design*, p. 34. Light bulbs were considered by modernist graphic designers such as Jan Tschichold to be emblematic symbols of contemporary engineering ingenuity. See, for example, Alexander Rodchenko's light-bulb advertisement for GUM (1923) and Francis Picabia's *Américaine* (1917). See Maud Lavin, *Clean New World: Culture, Politics, and Graphic Design* (Cambridge, Mass.: MIT Press, 2001), pp. 32–3; and Caroline A. Jones, 'The Sex of the Machine: Mechanomorphic Art, New Women, and Francis Picabia's Neurasthenic Cure', in Caroline A. Jones and Peter Galison (eds), *Picturing Science, Producing Art* (London and New York: Routledge, 1998), pp. 145–80.

48 Simon Carter, *Rise and Shine: Sunlight, Technology and Health* (New York and Oxford: Berg, 2007), p. 44; Daniel Freund, *American Sunshine: Diseases of Darkness and the Quest for Natural Light* (Chicago, Ill.: University of Chicago Press, 2012), p. 61; and John Stanislav Sadar, 'Unpacking the Latent Bodies of Interwar Ultraviolet Health Glass' (Ph.D. dissertation, University of Pennsylvania, 2010), p. 126.

49 Kendra Smith-Howard, *Pure and Modern Milk: An Environmental History since 1900* (New York and Oxford: Oxford University Press, 2014).

50 Freund, *American Sunshine*, p. 94.

51 Of artificial, man-made light's superiority, even the celebrated heliotherapist Rollier stated, 'Sun and ultra-violet rays bear much the same relation to one another as crude drugs do to their synthetically prepared chemical substitutes' (Russell and Russell, *Ultra-violet Radiation*, p. 41).

52 William Beaumont, *Fundamental Principles of Ray Therapy* (London: H. K. Lewis & Co., 1931), p. 1.

53 My thanks to Dr Anna Lovatt for pointing out the inconsisent use of shadows.

54 See Woodham, *Twentieth-Century Design*, p. 84; and Paul Overy, *Light, Air and Openness: Modern Architecture between the Wars* (London: Thames & Hudson, 2007), p. 16. See also Roger Broders, *Le Soleil toute l'année sur la Côte d'Azur*, poster (colour lithograph), 1931.

55 Sidney Russ, 'The Story of the Rays: The Magnetic Theory of Light', *The Times*, 'Sunlight and Health' special supplement, 22 May 1928 (hereafter *Times* supplement), p. xix. See also Sidney Russ, 'A Broadcast Talk on the Ultra-violet Rays', *Lancet*, 10 November 1928, pp. 1006–7.

56 'Editorial Foreword', *Sunlight*, 1:8 (1929), 6–7, at p. 7.

57 Hanovia, *Homesun* pamphlet, p. 7.

58 Arthur C. Clarke, *Profiles of the Future: An Inquiry into the Limits of the Possible* (London: Pan Books, 1973), p. 39, cited in Sadar, 'Unpacking', p. 141.

59 Charles Bazerman, *The Languages of Edison's Light* (Cambridge, Mass.: MIT Press, 1999), p. 142.

60 See Raymond Williams, 'Advertising: The Magic System', in *Problems of Materialism and Culture: Selected Essays* (London and New York: Verso, 1997), pp. 170–95, at p. 185; and Jhally, 'Advertising as Religion', p. 218.

61 Ernest Turner, *The Shocking History of Advertising* (Harmondsworth: Penguin, 1965), pp. 186, 211–12.

62 Lavine stated, 'Americans did not buy these products because they were simply helpless before the stratagems of manufacturers who cloaked their products in the guise of the new energies, and advertisers who tied the new energies ever more tightly to infallible Science. Rather, they bought them because the claims seemed so plausible in light of the more extravagant claims that had been made in all seriousness by unimpeachably orthodox members of the scientific and medical establishments'. Lavine, *First Atomic Age*, p. 142.

63 Maurice Weinbren, 'The Medical Research Council and Ultra-violet Radiation', *British Journal of Tuberculosis*, 23:3 (1929), 117–22, at p. 117.

64 Kevles, *Naked to the Bone*, p. 2.

65 Sophia Zweifel, 'Pellicular Penetrations: The Skins of the Early X-Ray Image' (MA dissertation, University College London, 2012), pp. 25–6, 29–31.

66 Cartwright, *Screening the Body*, p. 96.

67 Linda Dalrymple Henderson, 'X Rays and the Quest for Invisible Reality in the Art of Kupka, Duchamp, and the Cubists', *Art Journal*, 47:4 (1988), 323–40, at p. 330. See also her *Duchamp in Context: Science and Technology in the* Large Glass *and Related Works* (Princeton, NJ: Princeton University Press, 2005); and 'Francis Picabia, Radiometers, and X-Rays in 1913', *The Art Bulletin*, 71:1 (1989), 114–23.

68 Henderson, 'X Rays and the Quest', p. 325.

69 Matthew Teitelbaum, 'Preface', in Matthew Teitelbaum (ed.), *Montage and Modern Life, 1919–1942* (Cambridge, Mass.: MIT Press with the Boston Institute of Contemporary Art, 1992), pp. 6–18, at p. 8. See also Victor Margolin, *The Struggle for Utopia: Rodchenko, Lissitzky, Moholy-Nagy, 1917–1946* (Chicago, Ill.: University of Chicago Press, 1997); Christina Kiaer, *Imagine No Possessions: The Socialist Objects of Russian Constructivism* (Cambridge, Mass.: MIT Press, 2005); Sally Stein, 'The Composite Photographic Image and the Composition of Consumer Ideology', *Art Journal*, 41:1 (1981), 39–45; and Abigail Solomon-Godeau, 'The Armed Vision Disarmed: Radical Formalism from Weapon to Style', in Richard Bolton (ed.), *The Contest of Meaning: Critical Histories in Photography* (Cambridge, Mass.: MIT Press, 1992), pp. 86–110.

70 Maud Lavin, 'Photomontage, Mass Culture, and Modernity: Utopianism in the Circle of New Advertising Designers', in Matthew Teitelbaum (ed.), *Montage and Modern Life, 1919–1942* (Cambridge, Mass.: MIT Press with the Boston Institute of Contemporary Art, 1992), pp. 36–59, at p. 40. See also Lavin, *Clean New World*, pp. 29–30.

71 Lavin, *Clean New World*, pp. 52–3.
72 Dawn Ades, *Photomontage* (London: Thames & Hudson, 2000), p. 15.
73 Ades, *Photomontage*, p. 13.
74 Ades, *Photomontage*, p. 20.
75 Ades, *Photomontage*, pp. 84, 141.
76 See Duncan Forbes, 'Politics, Photography and Exile in the Life of Edith Tudor-Hart (1908–1973)', in Shulamith Behr and Marian Malet (eds), *Arts in Exile in Britain, 1933–1945: Politics and Cultural Identity* (Amsterdam and New York: Rodopi, 2005), pp. 45–87. Tudor-Hart had impressive connections: the Tudor-Harts were involved in commissioning Wells Coates to design Isokon's Lawn Road Flats (Hampstead, 1934), where Moholy-Nagy, Gropius, and Naum Gabo lived during the mid-1930s. Its roof was designed for nude sunbathing. The Isokon furniture company was run by Coates and Jack Pritchard, who employed his brother, Fleetwood Pritchard, to undertake its marketing. The latter was also heavily involved in the marketing of 'Vita' glass. See Overy, *Light, Air and Openness*, p. 42; Sadar, 'Unpacking', pp. 12, 87–8; Ken Worpole, *Here Comes the Sun: Architecture and Public Space in Twentieth-Century European Culture* (London: Reaktion, 2000), p. 80; Frances Spalding, *British Art since 1900* (London: Thames & Hudson, 1989), p. 112; and Val Williams, *The Other Observers: Women Photographers in Britain, 1900 to the Present* (London: Virago Press, 1994), p. 52.
77 Iria Candela, '"The Only English Periodical of the Avant-Garde": Sidney Hunt and the Journal "Ray"', *The Burlington Magazine* (April 2010), pp. 239–44; and Emma Chambers and Karin Orchard (eds), *Schwitters in Britain* (London: Tate Britain, 2013), p. 7.
78 On Moholy-Nagy's 'New Vision', see Ades, *Photomontage*, p. 148; Wilder, *Photography and Science*, pp. 107–8; Miles, *Burning Mirror*, p. 107; Overy, *Light, Air and Openness*, p. 12; and Eleanor M. Hight, *Picturing Modernism: Moholy-Nagy and Photography in Weimar Germany* (Cambridge, Mass.: MIT Press, 1995), pp. 49, 54.
79 Solomon-Godeau, 'The Armed Vision Disarmed', p. 95; and Hight, *Picturing Modernism*, p. 37.
80 Hight, *Picturing Modernism*, p. 20.
81 Hight, *Picturing Modernism*, p. 188.
82 Worpole, *Here Comes the Sun*, p. 36; Woodham, *Twentieth-Century Design*, p. 23; and Overy, *Light, Air and Openness*, p. 18.
83 See Moholy-Nagy, *The Light-Space Modulator*, 1922–1930, gelatin silver print photograph of the sculpture, Houston, Museum of Fine Arts.
84 Hight, *Picturing Modernism*, p. 142.
85 Christopher Wilk, 'The Healthy Body Culture', in Christopher Wilk (ed.), *Modernism: Designing a New World, 1914–1939* (London: Victoria and Albert, 2006), pp. 248–67, at p. 252.
86 Hight, *Picturing Modernism*, p. 72.
87 Hight, *Picturing Modernism*, pp. 72–3. See also the work of Henderson and Katy Price, *Loving Faster than Light: Romance and Readers in Einstein's Universe* (Chicago, Ill.: University of Chicago Press, 2012).
88 See Hight, *Picturing Modernism*, pp. 56–94; and Ades, *Photomontage*, pp. 148–50.
89 Hight, *Picturing Modernism*, p. 70; and Moholy-Nagy, *Painting, Photography, Film* (London: Lund Humphries, 1969), p. 69, cited in Zweifel, 'Pellicular Penetrations', p. 17.
90 Kevles, *Naked to the Bone*. See also José van Dijck, *The Transparent Body: A Cultural Analysis of Medical Imaging* (Seattle, Wash.: University of Washington Press, 2005).
91 See Jamieson, 'More than Meets the Eye', p. 716; van Dijck, *The Transparent Body*, p. 67; Zweifel, 'Pellicular Penetrations', pp. 7–8; and Cartwright, *Screening the Body*, p. 113.

92 Otter, *The Victorian Eye*, p. 195. See also Stanley Joel Reiser, *Medicine and the Reign of Technology* (Cambridge: Cambridge University Press, 1993), pp. 50–8.

93 Wilder, *Photography and Science*, p. 50. This notion explains the novelty of X-ray goggles, in Britain and abroad. See Caufield, *Multiple Exposures*, pp. 152–3. See also Steven Connor, 'Pregnable of Eye: X-Rays, Vision and Magic', in Phillip Warnell's exhibition catalogue, *The Girl with X-Ray Eyes* (Leamington Spa: Leamington Spa Art Gallery and Museum with the Mead Gallery, 2008), pp. 73–90.

94 'Transmission of Light through Animal Bodies', *Lancet*, 14 March 1896, p. 727.

95 Italics mine. Hermann Vogel, *The Chemistry of Light and Photography* (New York: D. Appleton & Co., 1875), p. 202.

96 See Finsen, *Phototherapy*, p. 69.

97 Finsen, *Phototherapy*, pp. 69–70; and described in Edouard Millioz, *De l'héliothérapie locale comme traitement des tuberculoses articulaires*, medical dissertation (Lyon: Imprimerie L. Bourgeon, 1899), p. 49; and Bröchner, 'An Apostle of Light', p. 208.

98 See Bernhard, *Light Treatment*, p. 73; Margaret Cleaves, *Light Energy: Its Physics, Physiological Action and Therapeutic Applications* (London and New York: Rebman, 1904), pp. 349–50; and Philip E. Hockberger, 'A History of Ultraviolet Photobiology for Humans, Animals and Microorganisms', *Photochemistry and Photobiology*, 76:6 (2002), 561–79.

99 Cited in Albert Robin and Dr H. Bith, 'Biologie de l'héliothérapie', *Congrès de l'Association Internationale de Thalassothérapie de Cannes* (Paris: Éditions de la "Gazette des Eaux", 1914), p. 69. See also 'The "Light Treatment" at the London Hospital', *BMJ*, 30 June 1900, pp. 1595–7, at p. 1595; Valdemar Bie, 'Remarks on Finsen's Phototherapy', *BMJ*, 30 September 1899, pp. 825–30, at p. 825; and Jamieson, 'An Intolerable Affliction', p. 99.

100 Jean-Antoine-Constant Lamaison, *De l'héliothérapie dans la tuberculose*, medical dissertation (Bordeaux: Imprimerie Barthélemy & Clédes, 1913), p. 11. Woodruff reported similar, contemporaneous American experiments in Charles E. Woodruff, *The Effects of Tropical Light on White Men* (London and New York: Rebman, 1905), pp. 83–4.

101 See E. G. Ffrench, 'The Simpson Light in the Treatment of Venereal Lesions', *Lancet*, 29 January 1916, pp. 240–1; 'A New X-Ray', *The Times*, 10 January 1916, p. 5; W. Douglas Harmer and E. P. Cumberbatch, 'The Simpson Light: Its Nature, Mode of Production, and Application, with a Preliminary Note on Its Therapeutic Properties', *Lancet*, 8 January 1916, pp. 76–8; F. Hernaman-Johnson, 'What Is the Simpson Light?' *Lancet*, 11 March 1916, pp. 586–7; Edward J. Deck, 'Heliotherapy and the Wolfram Arc Reactions', *BMJ*, 21 January 1922, p. 124; Bernhard, *Light Treatment*, pp. 113–14; and Russell and Russell, *Ultra-violet Radiation*, p. 54.

102 James H. Sequeira, 'Some Experiments with the Simpson Arc Lamp', *Lancet*, 19 February 1916, pp. 405–7.

103 See Bernhard, *Light Treatment*, pp. 72–4.

104 Leonard Hill and J. Argyll Campbell, 'Metabolism of Children Undergoing Open-Air Treatment, Heliotherapy and Balneotherapy', *BMJ*, 25 February 1922, pp. 301–3, at p. 301.

105 Kevles, *Naked to the Bone*, p. 62.

106 Henry MacCormac and H. Moreland McCrea, 'Severe Dermatitis Following Ultra-violet Light', *BMJ*, 11 April 1925, pp. 693–4, at p. 693.

107 See Walsham, 'On the Ultra-violet Light', p. 286; Bernhard, *Light Treatment*, p. 73; and Leonard Hill, *Sunshine and Open Air: Their Influence on Health, with Special Reference to the Alpine Climate* (London: Edward Arnold, 1925), p. 84.

108 Albert Eidinow, 'Some Observations on the Dosage of Ultra-violet Rays in Artificial Sun Treatment', *Lancet*, 15 August 1925, pp. 317–23, at p. 321.

109 Even earlier, electrotherapeutic devices of the nineteenth century were understood as 'natural', Thomas de la Peña asserting that 'Machines were not to be feared when placed alongside Mother Nature, in a clear continuum of care' (*Body Electric*, p. 83).

110 Beaumont, *Fundamental Principles*, p. 38.

111 Myrtle Vaughan-Cowell, *Artificial Sunlight: Its Use and Application* (London: H. Edgar Smithers, 1928), pp. 49–50.

112 Troup, *Therapeutic Uses of Infrared Rays*. Troup wrote a memoir: *Whimperings from Wimpole Street* (London: Actinic Press, n.d. [1940s]).

113 Jamieson, 'An Intolerable Affliction', p. 51; and Axel Reyn, 'Discussion on the Artificial Light Treatment of Lupus', p. 501.

114 Troup, *Therapeutic Uses of Infrared Rays*, p. 38.

115 See 'Combined Double Light Bath', in the Cavendish Electrical Co. (London), *Catalogue of X-Ray Apparatus, Electro-medical Apparatus and Allied Apparatus of Every Description* (London: Bishopgate Press, 1912), p. 88.

116 Troup, *Therapeutic Uses of Infrared Rays*, p. 38.

117 Jamieson, 'An Intolerable Affliction', pp. 136–7, p. 140.

118 See *Actinotherapy Technique* (1933), p. 159; Bernhard, *Light Treatment*, pp. 185–8; Russell and Russell, *Ultra-violet Radiation*, pp. 178–9; Auguste Rollier, *Le Pansement solaire: héliothérapie de certaines affections chirurgicales et des blessures de guerre* (Lausanne and Paris: Librairie Payot & Cie., 1916), p. 28; and Lavine, *First Atomic Age*, pp. 159–60.

119 Russell and Russell, *Ultra-violet Radiation*, p. 137.

120 See, for example, 'Violet Ray Controversy', *Hull Daily Mail*, 18 November 1929, p. 7; 'Violet Ray Danger', *Yorkshire Post*, 14 January 1929, p. 17; 'Peril of Violet Ray', *Derby Daily Telegraph*, 20 July 1928, p. 8; 'Violet Ray Treatment', *Yorkshire Post*, 25 July 1928, p. 3. In all of these articles the authors mean ultraviolet rays.

121 See the Selfridges advertisement for the 'Ultra Vio' Violet Ray Outfit in *The Times*, 8 December 1924, p. 20. Perihel's home-use lamps could similarly be bought via Boots. For beauty advertisements, see *Devon and Exeter Gazette*, 5 March 1920, p. 4, and *Burnley Express and Advertiser*, 21 April 1928, p. 7; for chiropractors, see *Hastings & St Leonards Observer*, 23 October 1947, p. 7. On violet rays in an American context, see Thomas de la Peña, *Body Electric*, pp. 121–5. Again in America, a useful comparison is the Tricho 'electric wave method' (an X-ray device) for epilation, in which 'deliberate obfuscation of the nature of the epilating rays was pursued seriously and effectively' in the advertising literature (and likely to the beauticians administering treatment), according to Lavine, *First Atomic Age*, p. 157. This continued after the Second World War, the language of commercial X-ray epilation machines described as 'a simple light treatment' (Lavine, *First Atomic Age*, p. 195). See also Herzig, 'Removing Roots'.

122 See Hill, 'Discussion on Influence of Sunlight', pp. 471–2; Hanovia advertisement, *Punch*, 15 February 1928, p. 18; and 'Woman's Ways' in *Nottingham Evening Post*, 22 February 1929, p. 5, and 18 February 1930, p. 3.

123 On spa waters, see *The Times*, 23 October 1916, p. 2, and 26 May 1924, p. 21. Treatments on offer at Peebles included 'radio-active mud packs'; see Scottish Borders Council Archives, Hawick, 210144, *The Peebles Hotel Hydropathic: For Health and Pleasure*, promotional booklet, undated (*c.* 1920s–30s). On painted dials, see *The Times*, 10 August 1914, p. 3, and *Cheltenham Looker-On*, 7 December 1912, p. 10. On radioactive water, see *The Times*, 2 April 1910, p. 7. On 'Radior' pads, see *Daily Mirror*, 16 December 1915, p. 10; and *Nottingham Evening Post*, 2 December 1919, p. 4. On emanators and inhalers, see *The Times*, 24 June 1912, p. 7, and 28 November 1913, p. 11. On radium beauty products, see the advertisement for 'Radium-Vita'

creams in *Aberdeen Press and Journal*, 18 May 1937, p. 2. See, by contrast, 'Radium Perils: Warning against Quack Remedies', *The Times*, 25 April 1914, p. 5. By 1916, the British government officially declared it a hazardous material (Harvie, *Deadly Sunshine*, p. 182).

124 Thomas de la Peña, *Body Electric*, p. 190.

125 Sir Henry Gauvain, 'Discussion on Light Treatment in Surgical Tuberculosis', *Proceedings of the Royal Society of Medicine*, 20:6 (1927), 805–15, at p. 809. See also 'Reflections on Sun Treatment: The Theory of Varying Stimuli and Varying Response', *Practitioner*, 132 (February 1934), 156–65, at pp. 160–2; Hobday, *The Healing Sun*, pp. 109, 154–5; Alexander Cawadias, 'Ultra-violet Irradiation: Technique of Application', *British Journal of Physical Medicine*, 11:12 (1937), 225–9, at p. 228; 'Light Treatment in Hospitals: Finsen Rays and Arc Lamps', *Times* supplement, pp. xxxi–xxxii, at p. xxxii.

126 On burst bulbs and purple flesh, see Russell and Russell, *Ultra-violet Radiation*, pp. 144, 139. On the ghoulish green effects of mercury vapour lamps, see Franz Thedering, *Sunlight as Healer: A Popular Treatise* (Slough: Sollux, 1926), p. 19. On frightened children, see Vaughan-Cowell, *Artificial Sunlight*, p. 66. On spluttering carbon, see Cawadias, 'Ultra-violet Irradiation', p. 228; and Miles, *Burning Mirror*, p. 149.

127 See Lavine, *First Atomic Age*, pp. 71, 77, 80–1, 175; and Howell, *Technology in the Hospital*, pp. 4, 15. Injuries sustained from using X-ray machines also included burns from electrical shocks, imploding tubes, and electrocution; and the film (Eastman Kodak's cellulose nitrate) was so flammable that X-ray rooms frequently caught fire. See Lavine, *First Atomic Age*, pp. 78–7; and Kevles, *Naked to the Bone*, pp. 61, 110. That 'non-flammable' goggles (Portia, *c.* 1940) were made for carbon-arc lamps indicates the spluttering embers even set fire to eye protection (e.g., paper masks, celluloid goggles).

128 Miles, *Burning Mirror*, p. 61; and Patrick Maynard, *The Engine of Visualization: Thinking through Photography* (Ithaca, NY: Cornell University Press, 1997), p. 75.

129 Tom Gunning, 'Invisible Worlds, Visible Media', in Corey Keller (ed.), *Brought to Light: Photography and the Invisible, 1840–1900* (New Haven, Conn.: Yale University Press with SFMOMA, 2008), pp. 51–63, at p. 61.

130 See Renée Haynes, *The Society for Psychical Research, 1882–1982: A History* (London: Macdonald, 1982); William H. Brock, *William Crookes (1832–1919) and the Commercialization of Science* (Aldershot: Ashgate, 2008); and Charles A. Mercier, *Spiritualism and Sir Oliver Lodge* (London: Mental Culture Enterprise, 1917).

131 Beaumont, *Fundamental Principles*, pp. 15–16; and W. Turner Wilson, 'Sun Baths in a Factory', *Times* supplement, p. xxii.

132 'Daylight Treatment', *BMJ*, 29 January 1916, pp. 173–4.

133 'Truth about Sunburn', *The Times*, 18 May 1914, p. 5.

134 See Mould, *Century of X-Rays*, p. 21; and Kevles, *Naked to the Bone*, p. 52.

135 See 'Student's Death in a Bath', *The Times*, 15 December 1928, p. 7; 'Found Dead in Bath: Mystery of Violet Ray Apparatus', *Dundee Courier and Advertiser*, 15 December 1928, p. 6; 'Ultra-violet Ray Apparatus: Student's Death in Bath', *The Times*, 14 January 1929, p. 9; and 'Electrocution from Ultra-violet Ray Lamp', *BMJ*, 26 January 1929, p. 163. See also Martin Edwards, *Control and the Therapeutic Trial: Rhetoric and Experimentation in Britain, 1918–48* (Amsterdam and New York: Rodopi, 2007), pp. 70–1. References to the dangers of using home-use lamps in bathrooms are subtle but common afterwards, see 'Artificial Sunlight: How Treatment Should Be Managed at Home', *The Times*, 13 December 1928, p. 11; and 'Ultra-violet Light and Cancer', *Lancet*, 24 November 1928, pp. 1087–8, at p. 1087.

136 Hanovia advertisement, *Times* supplement, p. xxxiii.

137 MacCormac and McCrea, 'Severe Dermatitis Following Ultra-violet Light'.

138 Russell and Russell, *Ultra-violet Radiation*, p. 140; and Hanovia, *A Short Book of Instructions for Users of the 'Homesun' Sunlamp*, user manual, 1940, p. 5.

139 John H. Tonking, 'Individual Overdose of Ultra-violet Rays', *BMJ*, 6 March 1926, p. 462.

140 See Russell and Russell, *Ultra-violet Radiation*, p. 140; and Thedering, *Sunlight as Healer*, pp. 26, 54.

141 Vaughan-Cowell, *Artificial Sunlight*, p. 65; see also Russ, 'A Broadcast Talk on the Ultra-violet Rays', p. 1007; Leonard Hill, 'The Physiological Effects of Light', *Proceedings of the Royal Society of Medicine*, 17 (1924), 15–21, at p. 21. Indeed, the same concern existed towards heliotherapy, see Victor Dane, *The Sunlight Cure: How to Use the Ultra-violet Rays* (London: Athletic Publications, 1929), p. 5.

142 See 'Peril of Violet Ray: Law Permits Use by Amateurs', *Derby Daily Telegraph*, 20 July 1928, p. 8; 'Dangers of Ultra-violet Light Baths', *BMJ*, 11 April 1925, p. 708; and C. B. Heald, 'The Immediate and Remote Effects of Sunlight', *BMJ*, 11 April 1925, p. 717.

143 Thomas de la Peña, *Body Electric*, p. 96.

144 The use of the female body to display electric 'domestication' in advertising was discussed by Thomas de la Peña, who noted that 'by having a woman's body display electric power as a decoration instead of a man showing electricity's utilitarian function, the technology's inventors positioned electricity as a force compatible with safe domestic consumption'. *Body Electric*, p. 106. See also Gooday, *Domesticating Electricity*, p. 6.

145 On technology and gender, see Margarete Sandelowski, *Devices and Desires: Gender, Technology, and American Nursing* (Chapel Hill, NC: University of North Carolina Press, 2000), pp. 27–8.

146 Gooday, *Domesticating Electricity*, p. 10. See also Bazerman, *Edison's Light*, pp. 294–313, 338.

147 See Rima Apple, *Vitamania: Vitamins in American Culture* (New Brunswick: Rutgers University Press, 1996); Carter, *Rise and Shine*, p. 61; and Lavine, *First Atomic Age*, pp. 153, 179.

148 Percy Hall, in Elizabeth Anderson, *The Essentials of Light Treatment for the Use of Masseuses* (London: Baillière, Tindall & Cox, 1935), p. v.

149 See Cartwright, *Screening the Body*, pp. 125–8; Zweifel, 'Pellicular Penetrations', pp. 38–40; Mould, *Century of X-Rays*, pp. 21–2; Harvie, *Deadly Sunshine*, p. 50; Frederic Lees, 'The Discoverers of Radium', *Pall Mall Magazine* (October 1903), pp. 199–202, at p. 201; and 'Action physiologique des rayons de radium', *Comptes rendus de l'Academie des Sciences*, 132 (1901), 1289–91, reproduced in Pierre Curie (and the Société Française de Physique), *Oeuvres de Pierre Curie* (Paris: Éditions des Archives Contemporaines, 1984), pp. 417–19. On physicians' self-testing, see Susan E. Lederer, *Subjected to Science: Human Experimentation in America before the Second World War* (Baltimore, Md.: Johns Hopkins University Press, 1995), pp. 3, 18.

150 Reported in Hill, *Sunshine and Open Air*, p. 85; Bernhard, *Light Treatment*, pp. 86, 100; and W. E. Dixon, C. E. M. Jones, and G. H. Lancashire, 'Discussion on the Therapeutic Value of Light', *BMJ*, 19 September 1925, pp. 499–504, at p. 499. Certain 'light diseases' (pellagra, beriberi, smallpox, porphyrinuria) could be fatal, and certain medicines could act as dangerous photo-catalysers, not least eosin – a photosensitising substance discovered to excite fluorescence through its use in photography (see Bernhard, *Light Treatment*, pp. 93–9).

151 G. Lenthal Cheatle, 'The Immediate and Remote Effects of Sunlight on the Epidermis', *BMJ*, 28 March 1925, p. 631.

152 See Findlay's obituary, in the *BMJ*, 22 March 1952, pp. 658–60.

153 George M. Findlay, 'Ultra-violet Light and Skin Cancer', *Lancet*, 24 November 1928, pp. 1070–3, at p. 1070.

154 Cheatle, 'The Immediate and Remote Effects', p. 631.

155 Leonard Hill, 'The Immediate and Remote Effects of Sunlight on the Epidermis', *BMJ*, 4 April 1925, p. 679; but see also Bernhard's ambivalent description in full, in *Light Treatment*, pp. 91–2.

156 Hill, 'The Immediate and Remote Effects', p. 679.

157 Edward J. Deck, 'Immediate and Remote Effects of Sunlight on the Epidermis', *BMJ*, 18 April 1925, pp. 761–2, at p. 762.

158 The *Lancet* stated in 1941 that 'in addition to radium and X rays it is now known that ultra-violet light is carcinogenic', in 'Cancer and Ultra-violet Light', *Lancet*, 16 August 1941, pp. 193–4, at p. 193. Dunne Romano provided an in-depth discussion on Harold Blum, who made clear connections and raised awareness, in 'Dark Side of the Sun', pp. 127–33.

159 'Ultra-violet Light and Cancer', *Lancet*, 24 November 1928, pp. 1087–8.

160 See Maurice Weinbren, 'Ultra-violet Light and Cancer', *Lancet*, 8 December 1928, p. 1211; George M. Findlay, 'Ultra-violet Light and Cancer', *Lancet*, 15 December 1928, p. 1263; and 'Cutaneous Papillomata in the Rat Following Exposure to Ultra-violet Light', *Lancet*, 7 June 1930, pp. 1229–31.

161 Dunne Romano, 'Dark Side of the Sun'. Her thesis traced the rising awareness of ultraviolet light's carcinogenic powers alongside the growth of sunscreen development, nuclear warfare, and large-scale cancer research. By the 1940s and 1950s, '"Radiation" became a buzzword among Americans, particularly those concerned with environmental health. The difference between ultraviolet and nuclear radiation was not common knowledge outside of professional medical and scientific circles' (Dunne Romano, 'Dark Side of the Sun', p. 142). The word 'cancer' was similarly ambiguous and unstable. Though the most common types of skin cancer (basal cell and squamous cell) are not malignant, 'the broader term "skin cancer" … leaves the exact type of skin cancer ambiguous, and serves to emphasize the fact that no matter how unlikely to spread or kill the individual, all three types of skin neoplasms were defined as "cancers," a highly loaded and fear-inspiring term' (Dunne Romano, 'Dark Side of the Sun', p. 27). This ambiguity, or instability of definition, is something that Cancer Research UK perpetuates in its campaigns, and it has does so in conjunction with sunscreen manufacturers, who profit from the fear-mongering. Basal-cell carcinoma was known as 'rodent ulcer' a disease that ironically was treated by ultraviolet light (see Bernhard, *Light Treatment*, p. 156). Indeed, non-malignant skin cancers continue to be treated by phototherapy and radiotherapy; see Hobday, *Healing Sun*, pp. 45–6, and the British Association of Dermatologists' website, www.bad.org.uk (accessed 8 February 2017).

162 On ultraviolet light as a 'poison', see 'Light Treatment', *BMJ*, 2 April 1927, p. 630. Radium was also described as a 'cumulative poison'; see R. King Brown, 'Radium by Mouth or Injection', *Lancet*, 28 November 1931, pp. 1212–13, at p. 1212.

163 On the post-Second World War rise of the 'Risk Factor', see Carter, *Rise and Shine*, p. 6.

164 Herbert George Wells, *The War of the Worlds* (1898) (New York: Modern Library, 2002), pp. 24, 27, 57, 62, 64. See Warwick Goble's illustration of the Martians' 'heat ray' in the 1898 version by Harper & Brothers, opposite p. 40. On 'death rays' in stories, comics, and films, see Weart, *Nuclear Fear*, pp. 46–7. He mentions, for instance, the Universal Studios movie,

The Invisible Ray, starring Boris Karloff and released in 1936 (the same year as the 'Vi-tan' pamphlet).

165 See Caufield, *Multiple Exposures*, p. 34, as well as the work of contemporary artist elin O'Hara slavick, and the essay by James Elkins in *After Hiroshima* (Hillsborough: Daylight Community Arts Foundation, 2013).

166 See Lavine, *First Atomic Age*, pp. 67, 126–7; and Gunning, 'Invisible Worlds, Visible Media'.

167 Lavine, *First Atomic Age*, p. 198.

168 Dunne Romano, 'Dark Side of the Sun', pp. 30, 142–3; and Miles, *Burning Mirror*, p. 165.

169 Caufield, *Multiple Exposures*, p. 91.

170 Romano, 'Dark Side of the Sun', p. 98. See also the reference to the 'atomic hair-do' in Christoph Laucht, '"Dawn – or Dusk?" Britain's *Picture Post* Confronts Nuclear Energy', in Dick van Lente (ed.), *The Nuclear Age in Popular Media: A Transnational History, 1945–1965* (New York: Palgrave Macmillan, 2012), pp. 117–48, at p. 124.

5

Photogenic suntans

Ultra-violet radiation puts up the general resistance of the body to disease, and promotes good health and sexual power of citizens who by sedentary indoor lives during the winter have become depressed and out of condition [...] Marasmic and delicate children may be made better, and mothers who cannot nurse their babies may be made more efficient. The general [carbon] arc bath affords a natural, simple, and valuable stimulant of the health functions of the body.[1]

(Leonard Hill, 1925)

Pigmentation is a sign that solar energy has been transformed into human energy. The rays of the sun are very powerful germicides. As the skin imbibes more of these rays, it stores up a great deal of this germ-killing energy ... [and] once pigmentation has taken place, and a nice deep brown skin obtained, any length of exposure can be endured without the slightest feeling of discomfort. Also the body will have stored enough Solar energy ... to fight against any outside disease-bringing influence which may attack him. Therefore, the first goal to be striven for by those who seek regeneration from the sun is, pigmentation. After that, health will come by leaps and bounds.[2]

(Victor Dane, 1929)

Jubilant smiles and radiant tanned skin greet the viewer from a mother and child gracing the cover of Hanovia's 1940 'Homesun' colour pamphlet (Plate 3). With all the warmth and intimacy of a family snapshot taken on a summer's day, the colour photograph skilfully effaces its own careful construction: the precision of its retouching, particularly on the fine hairs of both figures; the familial setting, so far removed from the artifice of the studio; and the masterful capturing of the direct gaze, relaxed pose, and rascally smile of a difficult photographic subject, namely the toddler. Together these effects make for an image so 'natural' and informal as to seem suited equally to the family photo album *or* to the mass-produced advertisement.

As the cover of a pamphlet catering to a middle-class British clientele, it curiously communicates nothing about the actual product, the 'Homesun' mercury vapour lamp (Fig. 4.11). Instead, as with the 'Vi-tan' pamphlet cover we encountered in Chapter 4 (Plate 1), the image conflates natural and artificial exposures, collapsing the distinction between experiences. These include the different outputs of sunshine versus the mercury vapour bulb (the latter considerably higher in ultraviolet radiation), the physical spaces of dark interior versus sunlit exterior, as well as erasing the technological mediation of goggles and electric components required for artificial exposures. This is only further confounded by the caption and the product name itself: 'For health – fitness – beauty – Get back in the sun with a "Homesun."'

Turning the page, contemporary viewers saw this conflation made in an even more overt, visual way (Plate 4). A female sunbather at the beach is stripped, flipped, and transported to the modern boudoir, exchanging the buzzing rays of a highly stylised orange sun for the ruler-edged, white block projecting forth from the lamp's curving, shiny head. What remains of her beach fantasy, back in the drab grey tones of her sophisticated urban dwelling, is *colour*: a saturated, near-fluorescent orange that marks out the ultraviolet rays' good effects in the form of a radiant, glowing tan. It is the same orange colour coating the skin of mother and baby, where it is further offset by the purplish-blues of the mother's flamboyant, floral patterned robe (Plate 3). Elsewhere in the pamphlet are many other partially coloured, heavily retouched photographs, through which the highlighted tans of 'Homesun' users become more and more pronounced, if not outright alien (Plate 5).

This chapter is devoted to the subject of suntan (pigmentation) and the social and political significance of the British public's avid consumption of ultraviolet radiation. There have been frequent references to suntan throughout the book but here it takes centre stage, as it does in the 'Homesun' pamphlet cover. I discussed suntan briefly in Chapter 2 as we waded through the varying, competing definitions of solar erythema (often described as 'sunburn') among light therapists and its ambivalent role in 'dosing' light. Suntan had its part to play as well, some perceiving it a help, others a hindrance, in the healing process. In order to understand the place of suntan in light therapy we must explore how it was defined and conceptualised by physicians and popular promoters, and furthermore how that information was disseminated into the public domain. This is integral to comprehending its *value*, by which I mean its therapeutic and social worth *and* how that worth was bound up with gradations of pigment – with colour values (see Chapter 1). Like solar erythema, pigmentation above all was understood in a visual way; it was a visible marker of changes happening on, and in, the body upon exposure to light, and specifically to ultraviolet radiation.

How is this different from sunburn as a visual 'anchor' (Chapter 2)? Because of their different durations they had different roles to play: if solar erythema was an initial sign of the body's responsiveness to actinic light, pigmentation was a later, more permanent sign of its good effects and thus a gauge of long-term prognosis for the patient. Curiously, unlike solar erythema, pigmentation did not undergo attempts at standardisation. It was not graded, measured, or compartmentalised in charts or through devices like armlets. Albert Eidinow (NIMR) stated outright in 1925 that 'There is no method available at present to determine the degree of pigmentation in any definite units', nor did one develop in subsequent years.[3] The desire for pigmentation manifested differently from that of solar erythema as well, a desire that was explicitly aestheticised, sexualised, and primivitised. It also played a leading role in preventive, public measures.

For Victor Dane, a popular promoter and controversial naturopath, pigmentation was the visible manifestation of 'solar energy' (ultraviolet radiation) stored in the body (see epigraph).[4] He advocated both sunbathing and the use of lamps to poor and rich alike in his 1929 book, *The Sunlight Cure*. As is clear from the first epigraph by Sir Leonard Hill (NIMR), Dane was not alone in encouraging the public. Despite their vastly different credentials, they both perceived ultraviolet radiation as having the capacity to protect the body by stimulating its defensive powers against invading diseases.

Hill may have avoided producing pigmentation in his patients – preferring short, intense doses of ultraviolet light that produced only solar erythema, as we learned in Chapter 2 – but he proudly spoke of taking sunbaths himself and lectured to public audiences that bronzed skin was the marker of an ideal 'A1' citizen.[5] Referencing a 1918 speech by Prime Minister David Lloyd George that 'You cannot maintain an A1 Empire with a C3 nation', military terms of fitness (A1) and unfitness (C3) for combat were extended to the public realm.[6] Raising the standard of health became a national imperative, exacerbated by the catastrophic losses of the First World War. The public were encouraged to build up a 'healthy tan' progressively, avoiding sunburn, as a protective measure in popular newspapers.[7] In Hanovia's 'Homesun' pamphlet, Hill was cited directly as one of many authorities recommending its use, alongside Sir William Arbuthnot Lane (President of the New Health Society), the surgeon Sir Bruce Bruce-Porter, and the eugenicist Dr Caleb Saleeby (President of the Sunlight League).[8] The 'Homesun' might be prescribed for personal curative use by one's physician, but it was primarily designed for preventive use. Indeed, the pamphlet declared that physicians themselves had requested Hanovia invent a home-use lamp for preventive use by the general public, resulting in the first 'Homesun' model of *c.* 1928.[9] Whether Hill invested different values in suntan for the curative versus preventive application of light is not clear, but his ambivalence towards it is indicative of larger conflicting attitudes that have much to do with eugenics, race, and public health at a time of heightened anxieties over Britain as a degenerating 'C3' nation.[10]

This chapter is about bodies of colour, of bodies saturated with radiation and visualised as literally 'photogenic' (light-generating). The words 'radiant', 'glowing', and 'bronzed' remain part of everyday language to describe suntan, they are now naturalised and normalised descriptors, but during the early twentieth century they became powerful, highly aestheticised evocations of the irradiated body's emanating health. References to suntanned skin also as 'bronzed' (metallic, shiny and reflective), in particular, can be found in medical and popular literature alike.[11] As with Chapter 4, this chapter focuses heavily on public advertisements, notably the 'Homesun' colour pamphlet, but also popular photographs in illustrated texts and the nudist magazine, *Sun Bathing Review* (1933–59). Through these images I explore connections between sunlight, sexuality, and tanned skin.

Many practitioners, government officials, and eugenicists greatly desired tanned skin for the British public, and manufacturers and tourist companies offered light for consumption in the battle against 'sun starvation'. This, according to Hanovia's pamphlet, was defined as the 'shortage of ultra-violet rays' marked by 'pallor, sallow skin … combined with loss of "tone," lack of energy, and low resistance to infection'.[12] The 'sun-starved' body was therefore implicitly drained of colour, signalling a body drained of energy. In its many advertisements Hanovia made explicit references to light as a 'food' to be literally consumed, a vital nutrient for the body that the urban-dwelling British population lacked (Fig. 5.1).

As I explain in Section I, rich and poor alike received therapeutic exposures of light in hospitals, health centres, clinics, and at home, and, as they internalised and consumed the light's penetrative rays, their bodies were perceived to gain unparalleled vitality and regenerative force, for the benefit of individual and nation. Natural and artificial light were directed onto mothers' malfunctioning breasts, 'backwards' children, and wounded soldiers. In regenerating these highly valued subjects, practitioners and politicians alike perceived light as an aid to national salvation.[13]

Yet, as we discover in Section II, in encouraging citizens to emulate the dark skins of 'primitive' races, they betray deep-seated and ambivalent attitudes towards the merits of suntanned skin. This ambivalence resided in varying conceptions of suntan's function (as a help or hindrance to bodily health), its duration (relative permanence), and its depth (colour saturation). Even Hanovia's pamphlet expressed doubt towards 'deep' tans: The real value in using the lamp is not for the purpose of tanning; that is only incidental. The deeper the tan, the less benefit obtained'; and, 'Exposures can be increased gradually up to long periods, but they only put more tan on to the skin, not more health into the body.[14]

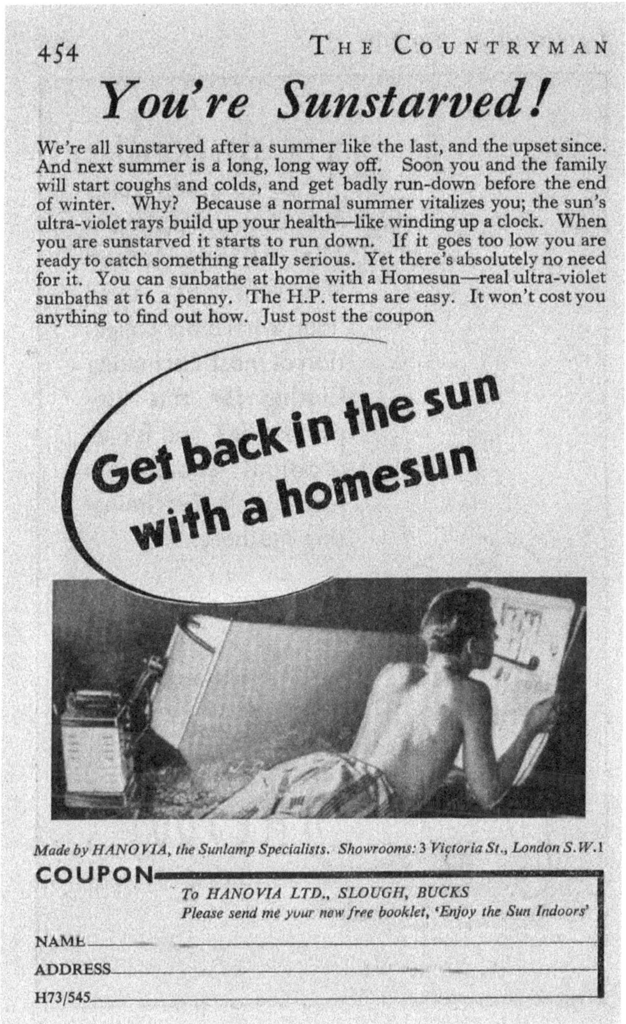

Figure 5.1 Advertisement for the Hanovia 'Homesun' lamp. In *Countryman*, January 1939, p. 454. Author's collection.

The porous boundary between desire and fear towards suntan leaks out in black-and-white too (Fig. 5.2). Lewis Baumer's (1870–1963) 1936 *Punch* cartoon uses close parallel lines to express the darker value of fashionable sunbathers' skin. To the alarm of the uninitiated, their pigment, complemented by slick-backed hair, exposed flesh, and cigarettes in hand, denotes a new and confident sense of 'respectability' that ironically resided in negrophilia. In *Sultry Climates*, Ian Littlewood situated new desires for suntanned skin within the interwar period. He posited that the suntan was, and continues to be, an act of emulation for all things 'black', the pigmentation

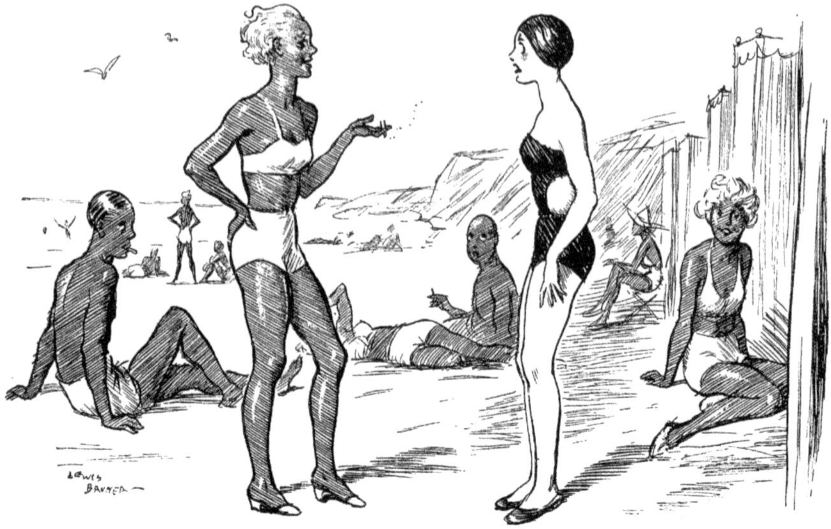

"DON'T WORRY, DARLING, YOU 'LL LOOK QUITE RESPECTABLE IN A DAY OR TWO."

Figure 5.2 Lewis Baumer, 'Don't worry, Darling, you'll look quite respectable in a day or two.' *Punch*, 2 September 1936, p. 266. © Punch Limited.

signifying a newly obtained, 'borrowed' primitivised sexuality. As such the tan was perceived, and perhaps today remains indirectly understood, as an erotic and hedonistic 'cultural sign of the savage and the sensual'.[15] In this context the suntan may have been displayed as a surface 'coat' or mask, a topical coloured *pellicule* (see Chapters 3 and 4) to be worn and shed at will by implicitly white participants, but as a sign, it was always more than skin-deep.[16]

The very legibility of the tan, its colour value and its extent of coverage on the body, could equally be read in terms of regeneration – of healing, adaptation and growth – or degeneration – of primitivism, atavism, and base sexuality. That so many light therapists, who actively encouraged and desired pigmentation as the path to the regeneration of both individual and nation, held eugenic beliefs brings such tensions to the (skin's) surface. With the photogenic bodies of Hanovia's 'Homesun' users guiding my analysis, this chapter investigates suntan as simultaneously a visual marker of recharged health and a troubling act of racial transgression during a period of developing eugenic fervour in Britain and Europe.

I Understanding suntan

The role of suntan (pigmentation) was, like that of solar erythema, hotly debated and ambivalently described by light therapists during the early twentieth century. In the majority, practitioners attributed to suntan a protective function of the skin, in which melanin acted as a natural 'screen' or 'filter' against the excessive action of ultraviolet light. This adaptive process was generally understood to follow after solar erythema had been produced, so that 'sunburn' and 'suntan' were understood as sequential reactions. However, much diversity of opinion existed even on these points, some physicians arguing that different wavelengths were responsible for solar erythema and for pigmentation, others adamant that suntanned patients could still be sunburnt (thus protective only to a certain extent), and still others that pigmentation was not necessarily a reaction only to ultraviolet light since it could be produced by a variety of sources, including chemicals irritants (e.g., mustard plasters) and disease (e.g., body lice, prurigo).[17]

As discussed in Chapter 2, in Britain leading researchers Sir Leonard Hill and Albert Eidinow of the MRC's National Institute of Medical Research (NIMR) considered suntan a hindrance to the therapeutic process because it performed its protective role too well: once pigmentation had been produced, it impeded the penetration of ultraviolet radiation's further beneficial effects into the body, necessitating longer and longer exposures. For this reason they recommended short, intense doses that aimed to produce only mild erythema – a transient, light 'sunburn' that would not result in pigmentation. This method was not only more economical (requiring shorter running times of the lamps), it kept the patient's body in a light-sensitive state and, implicitly, white.

In opposition, other equally well-respected practitioners, such as Britain's leading heliotherapist Sir Henry Gauvain of the Treloar Hospital for Crippled Children in Hampshire, considered pigmentation vital to the cure. They avoided producing solar erythema in favour of pigmentation through careful, graduated acclimation. In doing so Gauvain followed the widespread method of the famous Swiss heliotherapist, Dr Auguste Rollier (Fig. 2.10). For Rollier and his fellow countryman, the surgeon and heliotherapist Oskar Bernhard, as well as many French heliotherapists, pigmentation was celebrated early on as a *gauge*: a key, visual indicator of the therapy's efficacy and thus a sign of prognosis.[18] It was described in the 1910s by Professor Louis Landouzy, the dean of the faculty of medicine in Paris and one of the first vice-presidents of the French Eugenics Society, as a 'barometer' of the cure, a natural instrument with which to forecast therapeutic success or failure.[19] The idea held considerable currency in Britain, in spite of Hill's different method. As the well-known promoter of 'helio-hygiene' and the founder of the Sunlight League, the eugenicist Dr Caleb Saleeby, noted in his 1923 *Sunlight and Health*,

> we must remember that pigmentation of the skin is a marked feature of the sun-cure, and that patients who do not pigment well do not progress well[;] no one who has seen and touched the typical pigmented skin of a

heliotherapeutic patient can doubt that very active chemical processes are there occurring.[20]

By 1929, Dane still described it thusly in his popular treatise to the public:

> Pigmentation is the gauge of the sun cure, and those parts of the body which are well pigmented must be counted as richer in vital energy and in resistance to disease than other parts. Where an invalid does not take to the sun easily it means that progress is slow.[21]

In the previous chapter I explained there was much interest as to the depth of ultraviolet radiation's penetration into the body's interior. As more and more practitioners accepted ultraviolet radiation's relatively minimal depth of penetration, confined to the skin's upper layers, they tried to understand why and how these beneficial wavelengths instigated changes deep within the body, and they looked to pigmentation for an answer. Early on, Rollier argued that pigmentation was a 'transformer' of light wavelengths, converting ultraviolet rays into heat rays, which were known to penetrate deeply into the body.[22] He equally argued that pigmentation naturally inoculated the body from infection, an exterior shield that allowed the body to withstand invading attacks of epidemic fevers, rashes, and acne.[23] Of Rollier's British followers, Gauvain explained the transformative powers of melanin as analogous with those of chlorophyll:

> Pigment once formed appears to have two effects: it has a protective rôle and permits prolonged exposure to light and air without danger, and it has been suggested that it has a transforming faculty, converting the physical energy of sunlight into chemical energy which can be made use of in the body on the analogy of the chlorophyll pigment of the plant.[24]

Others compared chlorophyll with the blood as another sensitised substance with the power to transform light wavelengths.[25] Hill and Eidinow sceptically acknowledged Rollier's conceptions of pigmentation as a 'transformer' and 'sensitiser' but remained ambivalent as to whether melanin could simultaneously enable ('transform') *and* hinder ('protect') ultraviolet radiation's bodily penetration.[26] In *Sunshine and Open Air*, Hill declared: 'In the skin the pigment [like chlorophyll and pigment in the iris] acts as a screen protecting the deeper tissues from excess of radiation, and as a converter of light into heat, also as a sensitizer to the sensory nerves.'[27] Yet, later in the same work, discussing the use of ultraviolet light to fight rickets, he pointed out that,

> Pigmentation hinders the action; longer exposure is needed … [and] negro babies in New York are found to be more susceptible than white babies to

> rickets. This fact is against the view put forward by Rollier, that pigmentation is favourable for heliotherapy, and that the pigment acts as a transformer in the tissues of light rays into some other form of radiation, which has a beneficial effect.[28]

This is but one example of the ambivalent attitudes in Britain towards the role or 'value' of pigmentation to gauge light therapy's efficacies. Further ambivalence existed when it came to different kinds of pigmentation, dependent upon the light source: mercury vapour lamps, carbon arc lamps, and natural sunlight could apparently produce different colour values, densities, and durations of pigmentation. Internationally, physicians cited that natural sunlight produced pigmentation more rapidly, 'denser' and longer lasting than artificial light.[29] Of the latter, Dr James Sequeira noted pigmentation occurred quicker with carbon arc lamps than with mercury vapour lamps, and for Dr John Harvey Kellogg it was more 'pronounced' if produced by carbon arc lamps.[30] Colour values were different too, and inconsistently so. Some described the mercury vapour lamp as producing a 'pale yellowish-brown', others a 'greyish' pigmentation.[31] The 'Homesun', like the 'Vi-tan' and the 'Alpine Sun Lamp' (Chapter 4), was a mercury vapour lamp, yet Hanovia's pamphlet advertised its beneficial effects with a highly saturated orange to denote users' pigmentation (Plates 2–5). On colour variations, Eidinow stated,

> The sun gives rise to a dark brown-black pigmentation. The Finsen [carbon] arc also gives rise to a dark-coloured pigment. The long white flame [carbon] arcs and tungsten arcs give a reddish-brown pigmentation, the mercury vapour lamp a pale yellowish-brown pigmentation. Patients who have been exposed to the sun and are black-skinned gradually lose their pigment, and become a lighter brown on exposure to the mercury vapour lamp or open long flame [carbon] arc.[32]

Just as Hill asserted pigmentation's problematic role as a shield with reference to rickety 'negro babies', so Eidinow explained its curious loss, upon exposure to artificial light, in already black-skinned patients with specific reference to race. Above all, as a form of natural protection – a bodily adaptation – pigmentation was understood in relation to, and explanatory of, racial difference. It continues to do so today, under the politically correct categorisation of six skin 'phototypes', developed from the 1970s by American dermatologist Thomas B. Fitzpatrick.[33]

Thirty years before Hill's and Eidinow's 1925 statements, Finsen pointed out that the distribution of races across the globe could be 'naturally' accounted for by pigment's protective function:

> The colour of peoples and different races is thus easily explained: the nearer we approach the equator the darker the coloration of the skin becomes, and the more remote we go the lighter it is. The red and yellow colours of the Indians and Mongolians present characters of practical value in that they absorb all the chemical rays, but the black skin absorbs the luminous rays still more [...] But, speaking generally a European who lives in tropical countries notices that his skin takes on a darker coloration, while the black colour of negroes who come to Europe is diminished in a sensible degree.[34]

In circular logic, racial differences and distribution played crucial roles for understanding the pigmentation of the (implicitly white) skin of the patient through frequent reference to the naturally dark, protective pigment of the 'negro'.[35] Eidinow's and Finsen's off-handed references to colour loss will crop up later in addressing eugenics, preventive health measures, and the ambivalent aesthetic desirability of 'deep' tans among white European and British citizens.

For now, it is worth noting one further, debated therapeutic function of pigment. The theory belonged to Dr Albert Jesionek, a German light therapist practising in Giessen and namesake of the Jesionek lamp. Attempting to understand how ultraviolet radiation penetrated deeply into the body, he reasoned that unknown substances in pigment itself might be passed into the bloodstream and carried throughout the body. By interrupting the treatment to 'de-pigment' patients – keeping them in the dark for intervals of time – these substances could be released as melanin was absorbed down into the blood.[36] This was not the last time that practitioners toyed with intervals of pigmenting and 'de-pigmenting' patients. Jesionek's theory gave rise to a more general conceptualisation of pigmentation's value; namely, that it physically absorbed and 'stored' ultraviolet radiation. Dr Elizabeth Anderson (Middlesex Hospital) explained in 1935: 'It is possible that pigment also stores up the products of ultra-violet irradiation of the skin, liberating them by degrees, and thereby prolonging and enhancing the chemical effects at a later date.'[37] Like the blood, pigment was perceived to possess key absorptive properties that rendered the body literally photogenic.

Saturated blood

As mentioned above, the analogy of chlorophyll was confusingly applied to explain the functions both of pigment and blood. Sensitised to actinic light and able to 'store' absorbed radiation, pigment and blood fascinated practitioners as the primary carriers of light into the body. If ultraviolet light only minimally penetrated the skin, its internalisation (consumption) was theoretically explained using the laws of physics: Draper's Law (1842) stated that light can only act where it is absorbed, a law that was influential not only to light therapists but to photographers like Hermann Wilhelm Vogel (see Chapter 3), searching for methods to capture light's full spectral range onto sensitised plates – in other words, to the beginnings of colour photography.[38]

That blood absorbed actinic light was known to Finsen: 'no living tissue absorbs so much light as the blood, and, more than that, the blood absorbs a considerable quantity of the [ultra]violet rays'.[39] His method for treating lupus vulgaris with local phototherapy, however, was orientated around blood as a problem, a far too efficient screen that, like pigmentation, hindered light's penetration. Finsen sought to drain blood away from lupus vulgaris lesions by means of compressors, hoping for deeper penetration of the actinic rays to reach the source of tuberculous infection (Fig. 2.7). But his perception of blood as an inhibitor to the internalisation of actinic light gave way to widespread views that blood *enabled* its bodily consumption.

Light absorption of the blood preoccupied British researchers. As Dr William Beaumont, medical director of the Institute of Ray Therapy, succinctly put it: 'It is the absorption of the electro-magnetic waves that is the basis of ray therapy.'[40] At the NIMR, Hill, Eidinow, and Leonard Colebrook analysed irradiated blood samples during the 1920s to investigate light's effects on human physiology. One major find, as stated in Chapter 2, was that ultraviolet light increased the blood's bactericidal powers based on measuring raised haemoglobin levels, and this can account for Hill's and Dane's opening statements that light stimulated bodily 'resistance' to disease.[41] Case studies routinely reported haemoglobin levels before, during, and after light treatment.[42] (It should also be reiterated that Hill's team had discovered that *overdoses* could *lower* the blood's germ-killing powers, necessitating careful dosages of ultraviolet light.)

In popular books for the public, such as Dane's, the language chosen to explain the light's stimulation of the blood and its production of highly desirable pigmentation is significant; it is the textual equivalent of Hanovia's visualisation of saturated, glowing orange suntans (Plates 2–5). Both textually and visually these publicly disseminated representations might seem at first to verge on pure hyperbole. For instance, in the 1926 English translation of Dr Franz Thedering's *Sunlight as Healer: A Popular Treatise*, which notably included a foreword by Lane (the New Health Society's president), light absorption of the blood was conveyed as follows: 'The general effect of light, its influence on the blood and metabolism, is based on the power of the rays to penetrate the tissues and, caught by the blood, to be "absorbed," so that the blood is loaded with irradiative energy.'[43]

What did it mean for the body, and specifically the blood, to be 'loaded with irradiative energy'? *Was* this hyperbolic?

Importantly, it was not. As with electro-therapy and other forms of radiation therapy, the underlying concept here was one of energy transfer.[44] As Rollier stated, 'light absorbed by blood changes it into a receptacle of radiant energy'.[45] Like a battery or solar cell, this energy was absorbed, stored, and then depleted upon use, necessitating further exposures. Hanovia's advertisements recommended ultraviolet light to revitalise the body on the analogy of 'winding up a clock', and advocates of light's health benefits continue today to speak of 'storing' up ultraviolet energy to supply British bodies with vitamin D during the winter months.[46]

Dane explained that 'solar energy' was converted into and stored as 'human energy', externalised by a glowing tan (see epigraph). For Thedering, Dane, and many others the blood, like pigmentation, was fundamental to internalising and 'storing' light rays. Once saturated with irradiative energy, the skin and blood were described internationally by practitioners as having the capability *to produce their own light*. Eidinow wrote in 1925 that, 'When the skin is irradiated with ultraviolet rays it has been shown to demonstrate marked fluorescence', while others reported early experiments that irradiated blood could make impressions on photographic plates by giving off ultraviolet energy.[47] Blood analyses, carried out at the NIMR and in Germany by paediatrician Kurt Huldschinsky, also indicated that light increased the body's production of calcium, closely associated with the discovery of vitamin D and the treatment of rickets. But so too were levels of phosphorus (phosphates) raised in the blood, bringing to mind Sir Arthur Conan Doyle's Sherlock Holmes novel, *The Hound of the Baskervilles* (1901–2), in which the demonic beast glows by means of phosphorus.[48] Like the doomed patients of over-zealous radium experiments, bodies saturated with ultraviolet light were perceived to literally glow.[49]

Punch cartoons played on these associations by conflating child users with the modern and shiny metallic surfaces of home-use technological apparatus, and even with the light itself (Figs. 5.3–5.4): little 'Chromium' and 'Ultra Violet Ray' take their artificial exposures in modern, sophisticated urban dwellings, to the delight of their progressive parents.[50] Note also that Baumer's 1936 *Punch* illustration gives the tanned skin of his hip figures depth and shine with highlighting, achieved through negative white space on their cheeks, necks, arms, and legs (Fig. 5.2). In 1930s posters for Rollier's Leysin sanatoria and the British Wiggleworth's 'Golden Tan' sunscreen (Plates 6–7), the lithe contouring of attractive, healthy bodies is emphasised by bold white outlines.[51] In these representations the 'photogenic' body – beautiful *because* it is irradiative and pigmented – is proudly displayed by means of dynamic colour offset by white contouring: Jacomo Müller's leaping figure is further outlined in bright red, encapsulating an entirely black silhouette, while the 'Golden Tan' users present glowing, rounded forms by means of gradations of dark and light brown highlighting. Returning to the 'Homesun' pamphlet (Plates 2–5), the glowing, saturated suntans of Hanovia's smiling models are equally compelling precisely because they appear to generate their own light. Bordering on fluorescent, the orange pigment coating

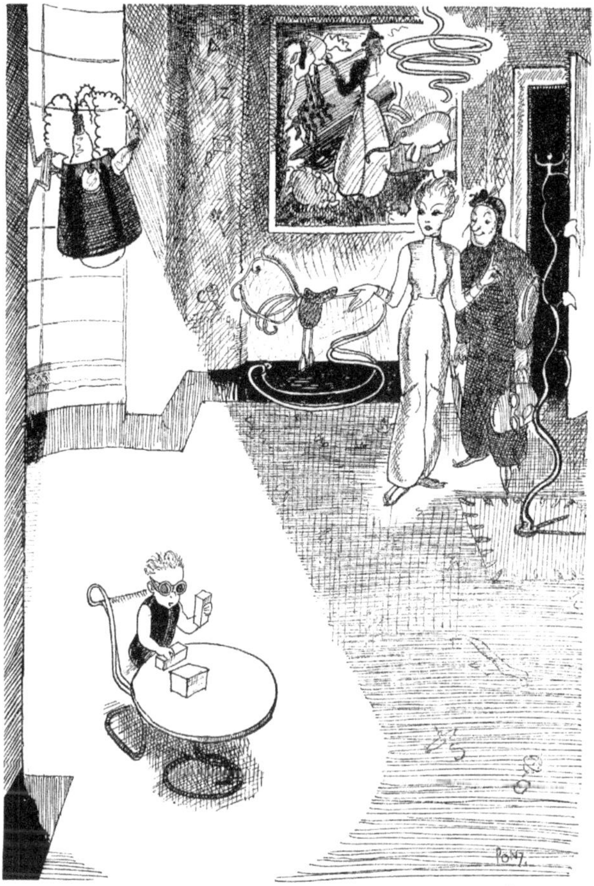

"This is little Chromium, Auntie; but don't disturb him, he's having his hour's recreation."

Figure 5.3 'This is Little Chromium, Auntie; but don't disturb him, he's having his hour's recreation.' *Punch*, 26 September 1934, p. 337. © Punch Limited.

the 'Homesun' users emerges forth from the din of black-and-white surroundings, shocking and delighting the eye.

'Eating' sunshine

Of the varying ways the body could internalise light, so far we have learned that practitioners conceptualised pigmented skin and blood as highly absorptive, photosensitive, and even photogenic upon saturation with ultraviolet radiation. But patients' bodies were also perceived to consume light directly through the orifices: the ears, nose, and throat; the mouth; as well as the vagina, urethra, and anus (Fig. 5.5). Unsettling images of these techniques are confined to irradiation of the mouth,

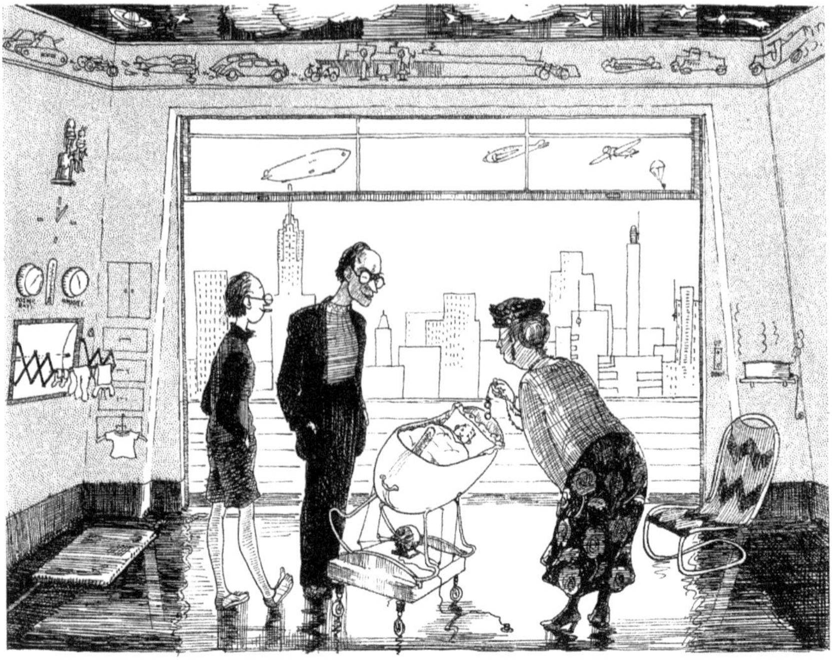

"WELL, AUNT EMILY, AND WHAT DO YOU THINK OF OUR LITTLE ULTRA VIOLET RAY?"

Figure 5.4 'Well, Aunt Emily, and what do you think of our little Ultra Violet Ray?'
Punch, 1 January 1935, p. 23. © Punch Limited.

especially in dental light therapy (Fig. 5.6). In Chapter 4, we encountered experiments to transilluminate and penetrate the body with light by means of applicators, lenses, and mirrors. In the case of Figure 5.6, a 1928 photograph demonstrating treatment of gingivitis by the British dentist Francis Talbot, a patient appears to physically consume or 'eat' the light. It is clear from advertising copy and popular literature that the notion of 'eating' light went beyond convenient metaphor: consumption here was literal, even if Talbot's patient strikes us as an extreme example.

Raymond Williams remarked that 'consumption' is a peculiar bodily metaphor to describe the public use of goods and services, having little relevance to explain how people actually use and engage with the things they buy.[52] However, in the case of light therapy it is vital to understanding how light was 'consumed' by patients and the British public. Just as radium could be ingested in the form of radioactive chocolates and toothpaste, so could ultraviolet radiation enter the body through one's pores by means of impregnated creams and orally via irradiated bread and milk.[53] Interwar advertisements for 'Ultraviolet ray cream', 'Sunshine bread', and 'Ultraviolet ray bread' appear in local newspapers while, more reputably, milk treated by ultraviolet lamps was advocated by leading physicians.[54] Notable among these was (later Sir)

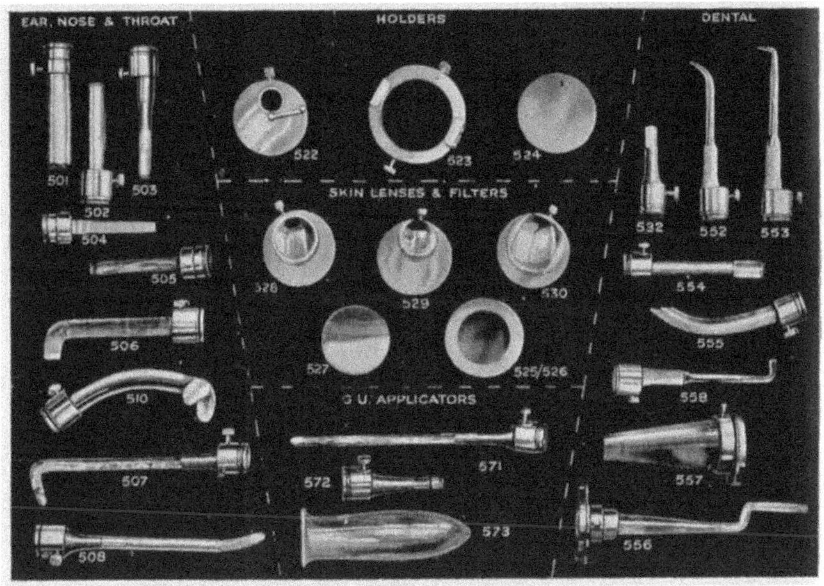

Figure 5.5 'Applicators for the Kromayer (mercury vapour) lamps.' In *Actinotherapy Technique* (Slough: Sollux, 1933), inset between pp. 44–5. Author's collection.

Edward Mellanby, professor of pharmacology at the University of Sheffield and consultant physician at the Royal Sheffield Infirmary, who conducted pioneering research on rickets. At the infirmary, one of Mellanby's colleagues, S. J. Cowell, carried out MRC-funded experiments in which he gave milk exposed to ultraviolet radiation to rickety children and noted marked improvements in bone calcification, in contrast to a control group of children given ordinary milk.[55]

Earlier, Huldschinsky (1919) and American paediatrician Alfred Fabian Hess (1921) both provided evidence that rickets could be treated with artificial or natural sunlight and, along with Mellanby and the American biochemist Elmer Verner McCollum, conducted research that led to the discovery of vitamin D during the 1910s–20s.[56] Hess, as well as Harry Steenbock, professor of biochemistry at the University of Wisconsin-Madison, further showed that irradiating foodstuffs such as milk with ultraviolet light rendered them antirachitic, leading to many experiments from the 1920s onwards in which vegetables, oils, and cereals were exposed to ultraviolet lamps. As Sally Dunne Romano argued, 'Thus, during the 1920s and 1930s the "cutting edge science" of the time, vitamin biochemistry, reaffirmed the health benefits of sunlight … and were well publicized in the popular press, which served to further solidify the popular connection between sunlight and health.'[57]

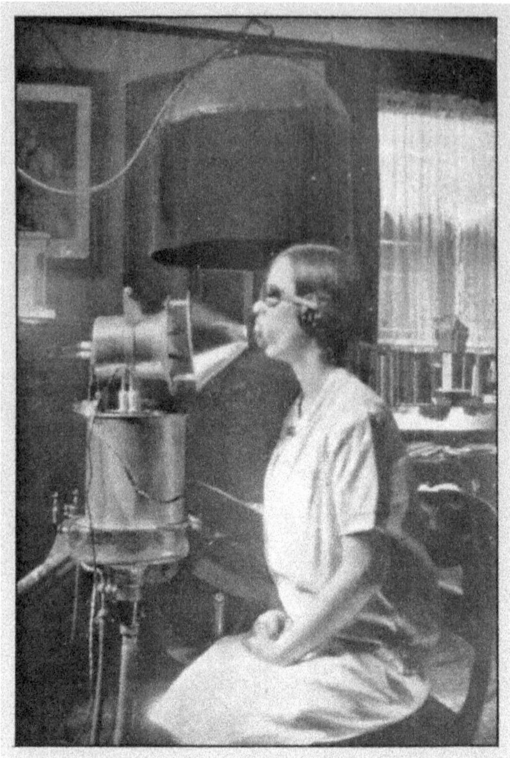

Figure 5.6 'Patient with anterior gingivitis receiving a dose of mixed radiation from an Ajax arc lamp.' In Francis Talbot, *Actinotherapy for Dental Diseases* (London: John Bale, Sons & Danielsson Ltd, 1928), Figure 6, opposite p. 63. Wellcome Library, London.

While many practitioners advocated vitamin D consumption solely through dietary means, such as cod liver oil, others promoted exposure to ultraviolet light as the best means to prevent or cure rickets in children. Some physicians even reported that cod liver oil itself was naturally impregnated with ultraviolet radiation once oxidised, making photographic impressions just as irradiated blood had been shown to do.[58] During a period obsessed with diet, measuring national health, and advancing nutrition research, ultraviolet light was understood as a vital food source for the body.[59]

This notion that light could be 'eaten' occurs surprisingly early on, the French naturist Dr Albert Monteuuis describing sunlight as 'solar nutrition' already by 1911: 'Because of the colouration of their skin and their manner of living semi-nude, Negroes are better adapted to feed directly on the rays of the sun.'[60] Conflating diet and sunshine even further, the famous Danish gymnastics educator, Lieutenant Jørgen Peter Müller, described the process of consuming fresh fruit as 'eating sunshine', a popular way of expressing to the British public the importance of internalising sunlight.[61] Dr Edward J. Deck, of the London Light Clinic (Pimlico), similarly declared in his 1926 populist book for the Sunlight League, *The Sun and How to Use It*:

> It is the action of the Sun which causes the chemical changes that supply the nourishing properties of food [...] The quality of milk is largely affected by the fodder on which the cows feed, and the quality of the fodder depends upon the amount of Sunlight it can absorb. It is essential for good milk that the cows should have a plentiful supply of green leaves which contain the necessary vitalizing properties, and these green leaves are themselves a Sun product. The highest quality of milk can only be produced by cows that are **fed in the Sunlight** on **fodder growing in the Sunlight**.[62]

To that end, pigs and cows were irradiated with lamps at 'electric farms' in Britain to impart the necessary ultraviolet energy to their flesh and milk.[63] An article on 'Vita' glass in *The Times*' 'Sunlight and Health' supplement promoted its use on farms, stating that vegetables ripened quicker and poultry bred and reared their young earlier, with the national implication that British market gardeners and poultry breeders could outstrip foreign competitors.[64] Even cigarettes were irradiated by artificial sunlight; the tobacco 'mellowed' and became less irritable to the throat and lungs by ultraviolet light's action.[65]

In a 1928 advertisement, Hanovia explicitly referred to ultraviolet light as a food to combat 'sun starvation': 'Light is a necessity to life. Where the vital ultra-violet rays are cut off the community suffers. Thousands are only half fit because they are only half fed. It is not solid food they lack – it is *light food*.' By eating sunshine, Britain's restored urban dwellers would become profitable and productive citizens, with Hanovia 'show[ing] the way to an A-I nation'.[66] Invested in regenerating the British race alongside social campaigners like Saleeby and his Sunlight League, Hanovia marketed ultraviolet radiation as an aid to national salvation.[67] The mother and child of its 'Homesun' cover (Plate 3) thus emerge as significant socio-political entities and their pigmentation as a politically loaded marker of citizenship. Put simply, they are model British citizens *because* they are tanned: they are beautiful (photogenic), well-'fed', fully functioning members of society.

II Radiant 'primitives'

The body's internalisation ('consumption') of light was registered by decidedly external signs. This invisible process needed to be assessed on visible changes and, moreover, *visualised* to disseminate its efficacies. Much of this book has concentrated on the reddening or bronzing of the skin. But it also manifested externally through the augmenting of bodily contours, such as improved muscle tone and weight gain, the closing of fetid wounds, and the expelling of necrotic bone and tissue. All of these were imaged in before and after photographs and discussed in case studies. Rollier

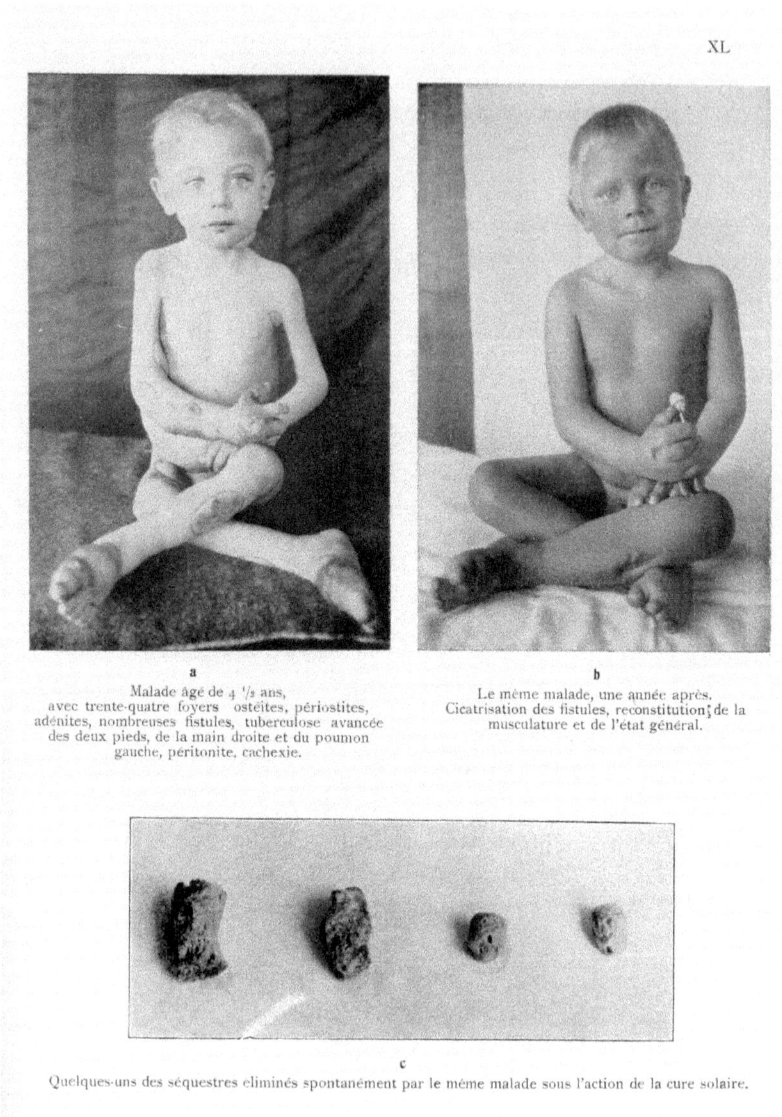

Figure 5.7 [Decaux or Rossier], before and after photographs of a tuberculous child. In Auguste Rollier, *La Cure de soleil* (Lausanne and Paris: Constant Tarin and Baillière & Fils, 1914), Plate 15. Martine Gagnebin and author's collection.

was particularly adept at imaging these bodily alterations, focusing on the plump contours, bronzed skin, and closed tubercular lesions of his healed child patients. He even included photographs of fragments of diseased bone expelled by the body during the cure (Fig. 5.7).[68]

Other bodily products were pulled forth from the interior, notably blood to the surface (hyperaemia) and milk out of the breasts. These last two were particularly valued when it came to treating women's disorders, restoring impaired lactation and menstruation. As a result we find many references to physicians directing artificial sunlight onto women's breasts, abdomens, and genitals, as well as inside the vaginal canal. When Hill spoke of ultraviolet radiation activating the 'sexual power of citizens' (see epigraph), it is clear the citizens he was especially keen to sexually activate were women. Light therapy was strongly centred on women's procreativity and their children in public health measures. Indeed, one of the reasons rickets concerned practitioners so much was that it affected the normal formation of the female pelvis, affecting healthy child-rearing. The British obstetrician Kathleen Vaughan, for instance, argued that particular emphasis should be placed on irradiating future mothers of the race, namely girls fourteen and under, so as to provide sufficient vitamin D to fortify the bones with calcium before their pelvises deformed from rickets, which, she argued, was responsible for high maternal mortality rates.[69] Light-therapy facilities at Labour-driven modern health centres, such as the Bermondsey Public Health Centre (1936, with lamps equipped by Hanovia) and the Finsbury Health Centre (1938, designed by Soviet émigré architect Berthold Lubetkin) were geared especially towards women and children.[70]

Perhaps it is not coincidental that Hanovia disseminated and advertised its products to the public with images of mothers and children (Plates 2–3). In its 1940 'Homesun' pamphlet, expectant and nursing mothers were singled out as especially in need of ultraviolet irradiation due to depleted calcium and phosphorus levels in the blood, lost during pregnancy to support the developing foetus. Hanovia also claimed the 'Homesun' lamp could prevent depression and morning sickness during pregnancy, a notion supported by contemporaneous medical recommendations.[71]

Irradiation of pregnant women occurred throughout Britain at various public health clinics and centres, especially at infant-welfare clinics. As one physician argued,

> If there is a marked ultra-violet light deficiency [during pregnancy] the child will be malformed; great deficiency could produce a monster. If the mother has plenty of ultra-violet light the child starts life with a stored up amount of the products of light and is able to better resist disease.[72]

Again, note the perception that the baby would emerge from the mother's womb already 'charged' with stored light rays, ready to face the world. Nursing mothers experiencing difficulties breastfeeding their newborns were additionally treated at these centres, among them the North Islington Infant Welfare Centre, where Dr Dora Colebrook worked during the mid-1920s. Before her damning reports on light therapy (see Chapter 2), she reported successful cases of working mothers whose failing lactation was restored or improved, particularly those who attended regularly and learned how to weigh their babies before and after feeds so as to track the milk quantities produced and ingested.[73] Surveillance and careful conditioning of 'scientific' habits meant these working women could prove to be productive members of society, in keeping with the cult of 'scientific motherhood' in vogue at the time, and thus ideal 'race mothers'.[74]

Dr Catherine Chisholm, the first woman in Manchester to obtain a medical degree and founder of the Manchester Babies Hospital, similarly conducted a study on the benefits of irradiating nursing mothers at the Manchester Municipal Sun Clinic in 1927.[75] Those mothers with depleted calcium levels – thus endangering themselves and their newborns to rickets – and those experiencing difficulties breastfeeding underwent general phototherapy to the whole body as well as local phototherapy on the abdomen and breasts. Hanovia's 1933 handbook for practitioners, *Actinotherapy Technique*, advised treating impaired lactation locally with the Alpine Sun Lamp, aiming to produce second- or third-degree erythemas on the breasts.[76] Babies already affected by rickets could be cured by irradiating the mother, who would then – 'loaded with irradiative energy' – pass on her antirachitic milk to her infant.[77] The milk supply therefore was not only increased but considered more nutritious. In Hanovia's 'Homesun' pamphlet, both mother and child receive these restorative exposures, their bodies glowing with the saturated radiation impregnated within (Plate 2).

More invasive treatments involved ultraviolet radiation inserted directly into the vagina. British practitioners were guided by German methods, such as those developed by Dr Wilhelm Flaskamp of Erlangen University's Gynaecological Clinic. He spoke at the second International Conference on 'Light and Heat in Medicine and Surgery', held at the University of London in 1928 and organised by Drs William Russell and Richard King-Brown (the latter Bermondsey's medical officer of health and editor of the *British Journal of Actinotherapy and Physiotherapy*). The paper and its responses were published in the conference proceedings, and the comments by British physicians indicate they were particularly receptive and intrigued by Flaskamp's special devices and methods. These included a 'light bidet' and various applicators that were added as extensions onto mercury vapour and carbon arc lamps (Fig. 5.8).[78] With these he treated external genital inflammations (e.g., vulvitis, ulcers and traumas such as tears), internal infections such as thrush and vaginitis, as well as many uterine conditions, including endometritis and even tumours on the fallopian tubes. Gauvain similarly spoke of treating lupus of the vulva with local light treatment at Treloar's.[79]

In this respect, the history of light therapy shares important similarities with those of X-ray and radium therapies, both heavily focused on treating gynaecological disorders and internal cancers, especially of the cervix (see Chapter 4). Radium

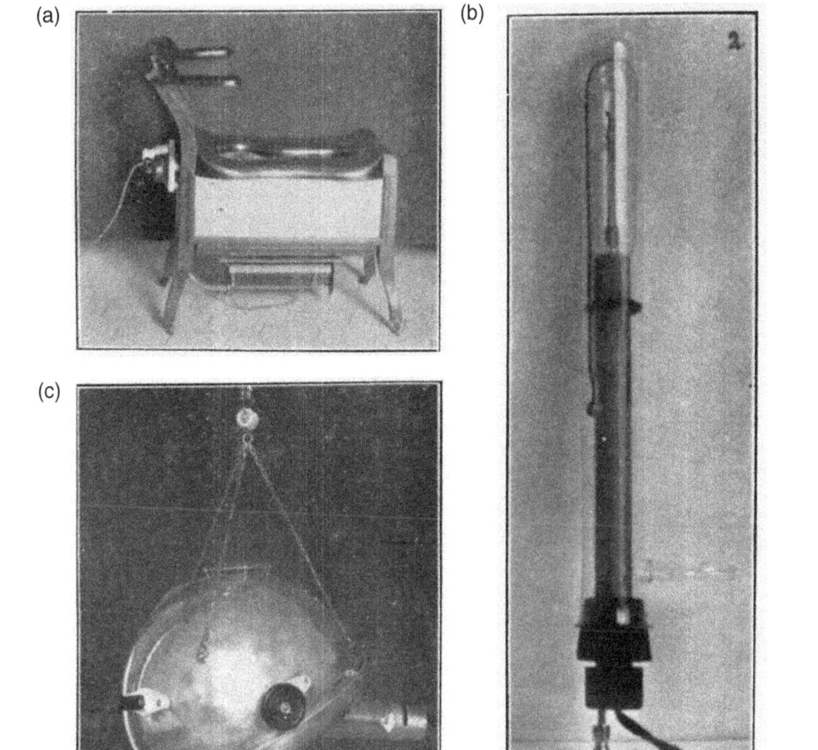

Figure 5.8 Modified lamps and applicators for vaginal irradiation.
In Wilhelm Flaskamp, 'Light and Heat Therapy in Gynaecology', *Light and Heat in Therapy* (London: Actinic Press, 1929), Figure 1–5 between pp. 32–3. Wellcome Library, London.

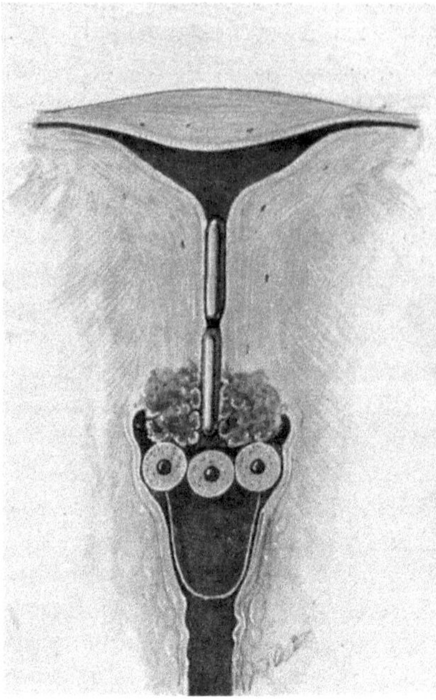

Figure 5.9 George Edmondson Birkett, placement of radium tubes for the treatment of cervical cancer at the Fondation Curie. In G. Dupuy, *Radium Therapy* (London: Cassell & Co., 1931). Wellcome Library, London CC BY-NC 4.0.

tubes, applicators, and needles were 'packed' into the vaginal and uterine canals to treat cancerous growths, known as 'radium bombs' (Fig. 5.9).[80] As Matthew Lavine explained, radiotherapy's intense focus on irradiating the female reproduction system could be viewed

> as a reflection of the persistent sexual undertone that attended discussion of x-rays: 'exposure' suggests voyeurism. Nervous jokes about electrical pepping toms and lead-lined undergarments were a commonplace of nuclear culture, and ubiquitous in its early days. (Radium, too, was sexualized: it was broadly understood to be somehow 'alive', and that vitality quickly became equated with sexual potency via patent medicines aimed at both sexes.)[81]

X-ray proof underwear, for example, was offered to protect women from the rays' penetrative gaze by a London dry goods company during the 1890s at the height of X-ray 'mania'.[82] Female genitalia were thus seen to be especially responsive to these 'exposures', both overtly benefiting from *and* covertly vulnerable to the effects of short-wave radiation. Ultraviolet radiation must be included among this therapeutic group of penetrating rays, desirable for specialised gynaecological use while simultaneously threatening moral and physical harm. Dr William K. Russell, for example, may have welcomed Flaskamp to speak at the 1928 conference, but in his 1925 book, co-authored with his wife and colleague Dr Eleanor Russell, they stated that, 'clothing materials which are partly transparent to ordinary light are also penetrable by ultra-violet rays. This is of importance when children or ladies are being treated, as exposure of surfaces not intended to be irradiated could easily result in the occurrence of erythema in undesired places.'[83] They more explicitly stated that the genital organs should be covered during general treatments.[84] For the Russells, the dangers posed had to do with painful erythema (sunburn) production in sensitive areas, but for others the concern lay with the ultraviolet light's action on menstrual blood. Ultraviolet light was prized for its ability to increase blood flow (hyperaemia) as a way of relieving pain, removing toxins, and carrying light energy to the tissues and organs. When it came to the blood circulating within women's reproductive organs, however, ultraviolet radiation could be both a blessing and a curse. Women suffering from amenorrhoea (the absence of menstruation) or dysmenorrhoea (painful or difficult menstruation) were considered especially suited to light therapy, with Flaskamp and others recommending ultraviolet light to restore proper functioning. But women being treated for other gynaecological conditions – indeed 'normal' women in general, including 'Homesun' users – were told to avoid light exposures during menstruation for fear of excessive blood flow.[85] As stated in the last chapter, one female user apparently suffered a miscarriage through misuse of a home-use lamp.

Sunlight and procreativity

More broadly, such perceptions about ultraviolet radiation's effects on female procreativity are fundamentally intertwined with widely held views that southern, tropical climates accounted for earlier puberty in young girls, especially among Arabic and black African women.[86] Heliotherapists on the Mediterranean coast made specific note of this, and not simply to the climate's heat but to its luminosity as responsible for early menstruation and thus early sexual maturity:

> On the Mediterranean coast and in particular on the Riviera, menstruation is more precocious than in the climates of the North. Young girls in general have regular periods by 10 or 11 years old; and *this is not a fact of atavism*, the same phenomenon is observed amongst other children whose families, originally from the North, come to live on the Côte d'Azur, and it is to the great stupefaction of their parents.[87]

For heliotherapists, the Côte d'Azur's intense luminosity made it especially beneficial to women's 'functional troubles'.[88] In a publication on light and gynaecology, Dr Malvine Brody of Grasse declared that ultraviolet light could even reverse premature menopause, restoring menstruation in mature patients.[89] Hanovia similarly declared in an advert that 'Women undergoing the change of life escape the troubles encountered at this time and enjoy restored health' with the use of their lamps.[90] At a time when France, like Britain, was rife with fears of depopulation, and the French Eugenics Society headed by leading childcare physicians such as obstetrician Adolphe Pinard and paediatrician Eugène Apert, heliotherapists' faith in ultraviolet radiation's procreative powers should not be overlooked.[91]

Beliefs in the rays' stimulating, sexualising powers in warm, sunny climates were not confined to practitioners. Intriguing similarities exist in the realm of popular literature, particularly the work of D. H. Lawrence, who himself had pulmonary tuberculosis and convalesced on the Côte d'Azur, in Bandol and Vence, where he died in 1930.[92] In Lawrence's short story 'Sun' (*c.* 1926), the protagonist, Juliet, is sent to the Italian Riviera for her health. Experiencing fatigue and 'women's troubles', her doctor prescribes sunlight. Lawrence portrayed her prescribed sunbathing as a hedonistic experience by now characteristic of both rivieras:

> Every day, in the morning towards noon, she lay at the foot of the powerful, silver-pawed cypress tree, while the sun strode jovial in heaven. By now she knew the sun in every thread of her body. Her heart of anxiety, that anxious, straining heart, had disappeared altogether, like a flower that falls in the sun, and leaves only a little ripening fruit. And her tense womb, though still closed, was slowly unfolding, slowly, slowly, like a lily bud under water, as the sun mysteriously touched it. Like a lily bud under water it was slowly rising to the sun, to expand at last, to the sun, only to the sun.[93]

In Lawrence's story, Juliet has nothing less than therapeutic sex with the sun. Her ongoing, submissive exposure to the masculine sun's penetrative energies restores her sexual dysfunction, she feels inside 'darker and more savage' and revels in her body's – as well as her exposed infant son's – 'rosy-golden' tan.[94] Again, such representations may strike us as hyperbolic, but Lawrence's sexually charged language can be similarly found in contemporaneous, populist treatises. Influenced by Indian practices, Dane's book recommended, 'Whilst having a sun-bath the vital energy should be visualized, pouring into the system and clearing away disease as a ball knocks over ninepins; man should feel it filling the whole of his being with health, strength and radiant vitality.'[95] The reader addressed here is male, but the book, whose cover features a man, woman, and child facing the piercing graphic rays of the sun, was clearly intended for the whole family. Dane advocated natural and artificial light exposures to both sexes suffering from 'glandular inactivity', which included 'menstrual troubles, difficulties during puberty, and impotency' and echoed the wider medical literature.[96]

While the Russells sought to protect the genitals from ultraviolet radiation with dark fabrics in the vein of X-ray-proof underwear, social-reform groups like the Men's Dress Reform Party, well-known practitioners like Hill, and manufacturers producing ultraviolet-permitting silk fabrics like 'Celanese' lingerie suggest wider initiatives to increase exposures to the reproductive organs rather than limit them.[97] The nudist journal, *Sun Bathing Review: Journal of the Sun Societies* (f. 1933) and its influential founders promoted nude sunbathing with a fascinating mix of highly eroticised images alongside extracts of medical literature by Britain's leading light therapists.

The subject of genitalia, unfettered by fabric and exposed to direct sunlight, was discussed in the journal by physicians and psychologists, among them the highly respected British psychologist, John Carl Flügel. In his 1933 article, extracted from *The Psychology of Clothes* (1930), Flügel spoke of the delights of 'skin eroticism' by the play of air and light on the body's surface.[98] In the same issue, Dr J. A. Braun argued that 'The human body was never meant to be covered with clothes; it is the seat of an intense radio-activity receiving and emitting waves, and this transmission cannot be performed if the body is isolated by clothes from light and air.'[99] He described the unclothed body as emanating or breathing light energy, its vital functions led by the sex glands and craving light's stimulating powers. The nudist's conception of 'sunbathing' was therefore, in practice, quite different from those who flocked to beaches or lidos clothed in swimwear or shielded by parasols. For physicians like Thedering, the nudist's 'natural' lifestyle bordered on 'solar fanaticism'.[100]

Early on, the cover of *Sun Bathing Review* featured an engraving by artist Robert Gibbings, who also helped to found the journal and contributed articles.[101] Post-Cubist maternal bodies, a muscular adult male and a confident, standing child occupy the grassy shores of a secluded pond (Fig. 5.10). Gibbings' economy of line skilfully conveys elegant poses of sun worship in a few key strokes. Within a few years this image was replaced by photographs, in keeping with its interior, which was replete with black-and-white photographs of nude models and lay enthusiasts.

Tentatively hedging the boundary between art and pornography, *Sun Bathing Review* pictured photographs of nude, suntanned skin in a variety of settings and styles, but the full-page spreads feature highly aestheticised photographs in which genitalia, when visible, are ambivalently effaced by means of obvious retouching (Fig. 5.11).[102] Such deliberation and effort indicate a conscious desire to maintain 'decorum' while simultaneously revelling in the glories of exposed, photogenic bodies, no doubt both titillating and reassuring its readership. Indeed, the journal encouraged the public to expose their fully nude bodies not only to natural and artificial light but also to their personal cameras: it ran a competition for readers to send in their own nude sunbathing snapshots, which were judged and reproduced in subsequent issues in

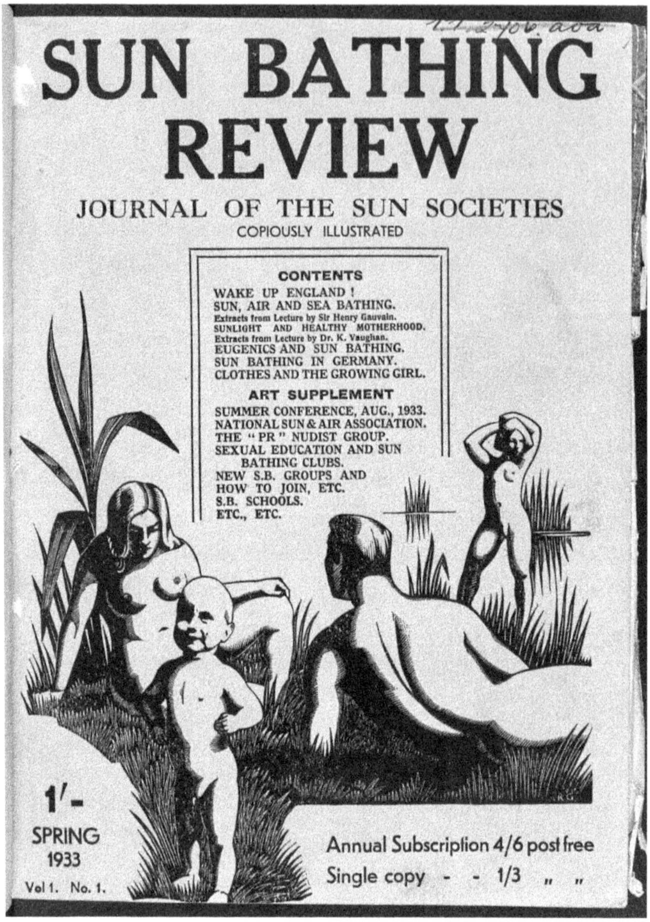

Figure 5.10 Robert Gibbings, *Sun Bathing Review* cover. *Sun Bathing Review*, 1:1 (1933). The British Library and Hawk Editorial, publisher of *H&E Naturist* magazine, www.henaturist.net.

the well-established vein of bodybuilding magazines.[103] This is not surprising when considering that the Health and Strength League, encapsulated by the figure of Eugen Sandow and with Müller as its vice-president, drove public interests in both bodybuilding and sunbathing, and later *Sun Bathing Review* was absorbed by the long-running *Health & Efficiency* magazine (f. 1900).

The journal also included advertisements for discreet photographic development by discerning printing companies, facilitating exposures for the public and journal in equal measure.[104] By these means readers could interact with the journal as active participants in its formation and the naturist movement as a whole. Such interaction was performed through the careful surveillance of the self and others. This 'healthy mode of sexualised looking', to quote Lisa Cartwright, must be understood as being successful precisely because it naturalised medical knowledge about therapeutic

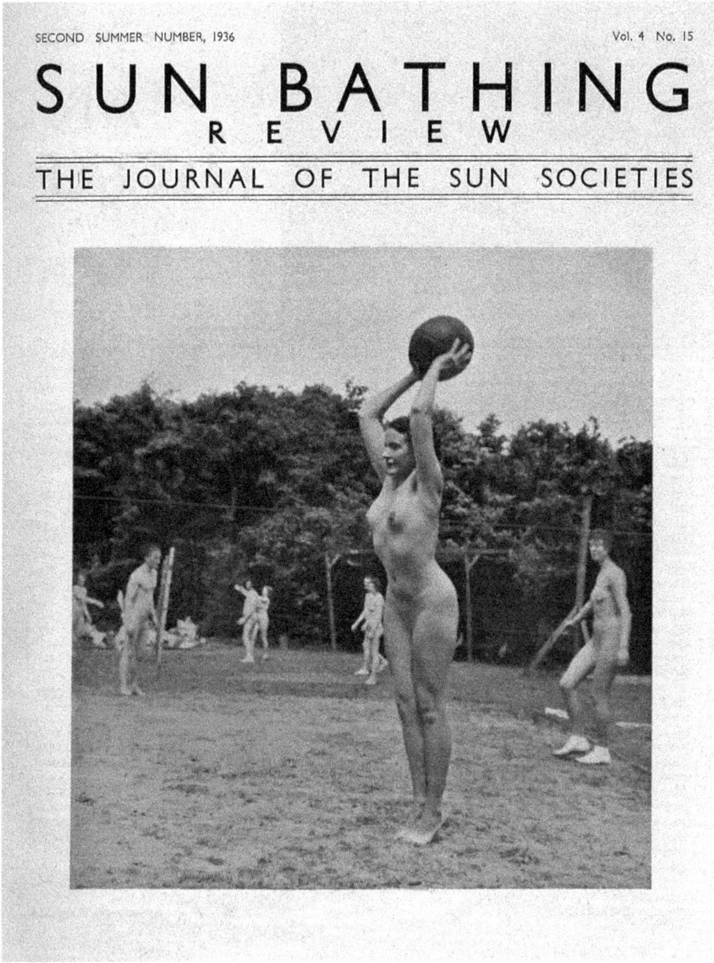

Figure 5.11 'On a summer's day – "somewhere in England".' *Sun Bathing Review*, 4:15 (1936), cover. Hawk Editorial, publisher of *H&E Naturist* magazine, www.henaturist.net.

light and medical practices of looking at the body.[105] After all, the journal included reputable medical literature to support nude sunbathing, in which light therapy was called upon to legitimise naturism, just as it had legitimised large-scale public-health campaigns like those of the Sunlight League.[106] In this way the medical gaze was not 'replaced' by the lay enthusiast's self-reflexive gaze, but rather fully internalised as a normalised way of monitoring one's own health.[107] And, like the physician, the enthusiast's visual gauge of progressing health was the tan.

Natural urges

Though men featured in some photographs, like the 'Homesun' cover the visual focus of *Sun Bathing Review* was overwhelmingly on women and children. One of its primary contributors was photographer Edith Tudor-Hart, whose photograph of general phototherapy at the SLHWC drove Chapter 3 (Fig. 3.1, *c.* 1934). For over a decade Tudor-Hart supplied *Sun Bathing Review* with photographs, predominantly of nude or semi-nude sunbathing children (Fig. 5.12). An early contribution of her photographs appeared in 1935, accompanying the words of none other than Sir Henry Gauvain in an interview on heliotherapy.[108] In these photographs the children were usually shot at close range and appear relaxed, happy and confident – much like the child of the 'Homesun' cover (Plate 3) – and suggest familiarity and intimacy between photographer and subject. In addition to penning articles herself, Tudor-Hart also, less frequently, contributed photographs of nude women for the journal (Fig. 5.13). Notably in her work they are anonymised by artful turns of the head,

Figure 5.12 Edith Tudor-Hart, untitled photograph of a nude sunbathing child.
In *Sun Bathing Review*, 4:13 (1936), p. 5. Wolfgang Suschitzky and Hawk Editorial, publisher of *H&E Naturist* magazine, www.henaturist.net.

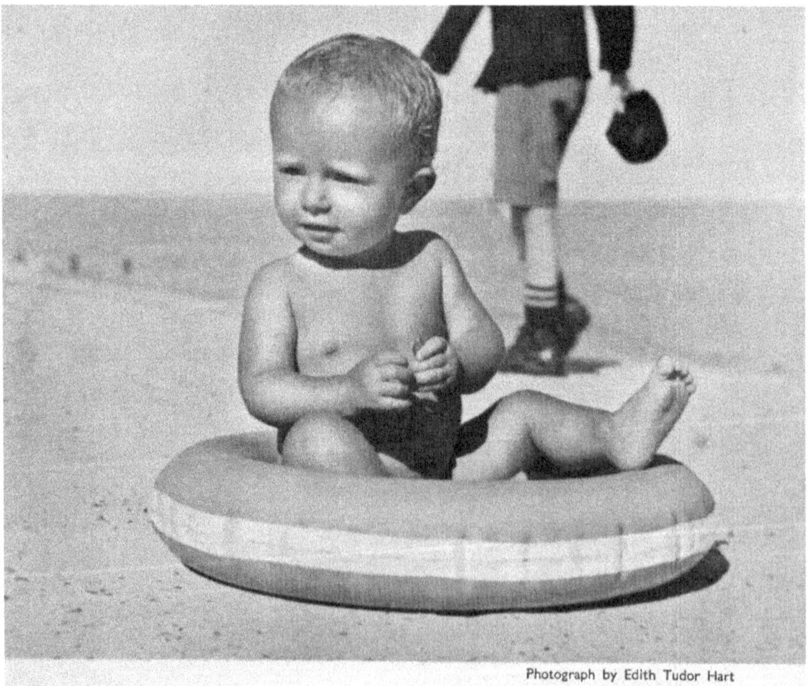

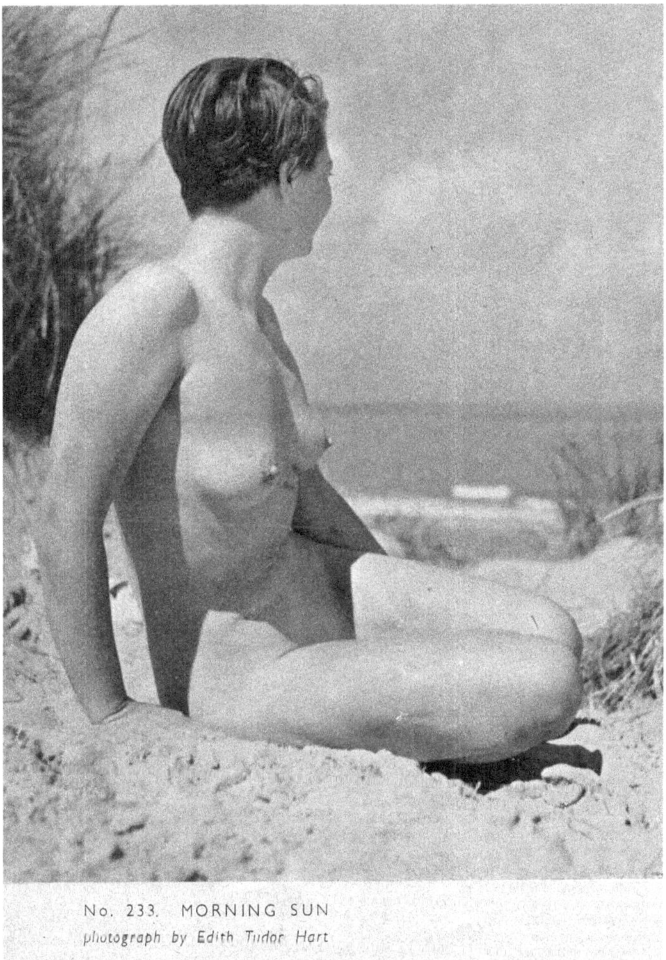

Figure 5.13 Edith Tudor-Hart, *Morning Sun*. In *Sun Bathing Review*, 14:55 (1946), Plate 233, p. 62. Wolfgang Suschitzky and Hawk Editorial, publisher of *H&E Naturist* magazine, www.henaturist.net.

away from the camera. Whether anonymity was deliberately desired by the models or by Tudor-Hart is unclear, but the effect simply facilitates the reader's unobstructed delectation of exposed breasts and skin.

Suntanned skin held significant erotic charge for the photographers of *Sun Bathing Review*. Main contributors Bertram Park (the journal's 'Honorary Art Editor') and Yvonne Gregory expressed intense interest in and preference for tanned models, which they discussed in their 1935 publication, *Sun Bathers*, and in an article for the journal on the difficulties of photographing nude bodies (extracted from a lecture Park gave at the annual congress of the Professional Photographers' Association the same year). In both texts they described the photogenic superiority of 'rich sun bronze' over 'lifeless' and 'colourless' pale skin from the photographer's aesthetic viewpoint. In the opening of *Sun Bathers*, Park and Gregory declared:

> How much more beautiful is the rich sun bronze of many models now to be seen, revelling in the full enjoyment of the freedom and health which the casting off of clothes promotes. True, the joy of colour can only be fully appreciated pictorially with the paint-box, but in translating the colour to monochrome and working with the camera the warm tints of the air-tanned body have infinitely more life and luminosity than the almost dead complexion of a skin that has never really been touched by the light of day.[109]

For these photographers, pale skin proved a resistant subject to the searching eye of the camera and its photosensitive film, frustrating the production of quality, artistic prints. It was, quite simply, not 'photogenic'. It was an aesthetic 'dead' end – an antagonist to the camera set in contrast to the 'lively' and 'warm' values of bronzed skin, which far more willingly complied as a light-generative surface, ripe for photographic capture. This is a curious reversal to the preferences of nineteenth-century photographers, who praised the aesthetic merits of, and ease of capturing, pale skin over darker tones.[110]

Primarily a photographic catalogue of plates, their book is replete with solo and group compositions with female-only nudes. Like Tudor-Hart's photograph (Fig. 5.13), Park and Gregory's plates, such as *Siesta* (Fig. 5.14), represent nude

Figure 5.14 Bertram Park and/or Yvonne Gregory, *Siesta*.
In Bertram Park and Yvonne Gregory, *Sun Bathers* (London: George Routledge & Sons, Ltd, 1935), Plate 35. William Thuillier and author's collection.

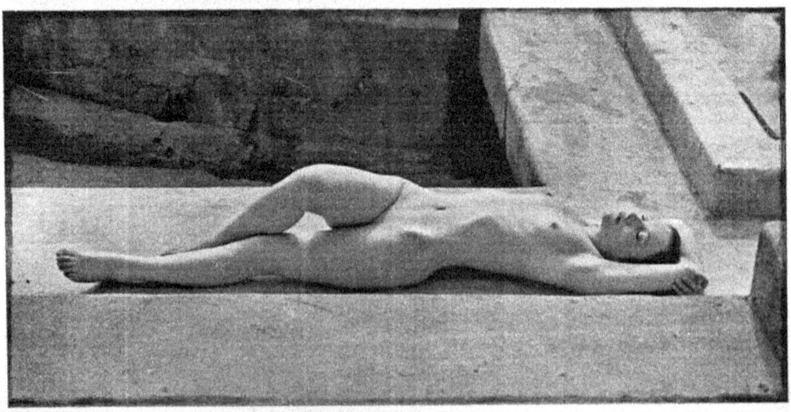

35 SIESTA

women in secluded outdoor settings like contemporary nymphs in their natural environments. The models were situated in either forest settings or against antique backdrops, as in Figure 5.14. The writer and journalist Alan Warwick, in the book's introduction, singled out this plate as 'one of the most beautiful in the book', declaring:

> The truth is that it is representative of woman sleeping naked by an ancient stone bath – sleeping lightly in the mellow sunlight, and as gloriously free and unselfconscious as the faint breeze that caresses her skin. I will go further than that, and say that for every hundred women of which that picture at one time or another is actually representative, it symbolizes the unvoiced longing of thousands of her sisters who, if they had the courage or the opportunity, would embrace the chance to be as free as she of the clothes complex and fear.[111]

For Warwick, the model's photogenic skin, which erotically elicits both gaze and touch, made the photograph as equally titillating to his (male) gaze as to that of a vast female public audience; it provoked envy and didactically spread the naturist's call for unfettered exposure, free of fear, for the greater good.

If we compare these 'artistic' popular photographs with medical photographs of female patients, the boundary demarcating popular from medical photography begins to crumble on aesthetic grounds. Bernhard's 1917 *Sonnenlichtbehandlung in der Chirurgie* and its expanded 1926 English translation, *Light Treatment in Surgery*, included before and after images of graphic war wounds alongside erotically charged images of female patients (Figs. 5.15–5.16). The language of his texts uneasily mixed

Figure 5.15 Twenty-year-old female tuberculous patient. In Oskar Bernhard, *Sonnenlichtbehandlung in der Chirurgie* (Stuttgart: Ferdinand Enke, 1917), Figure 51, p. 163. Author's collection.

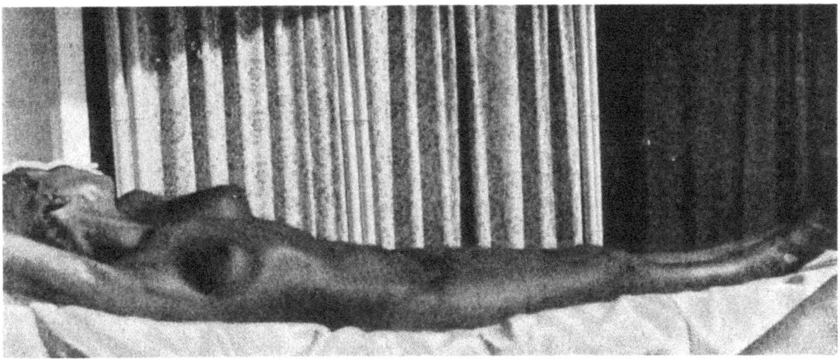

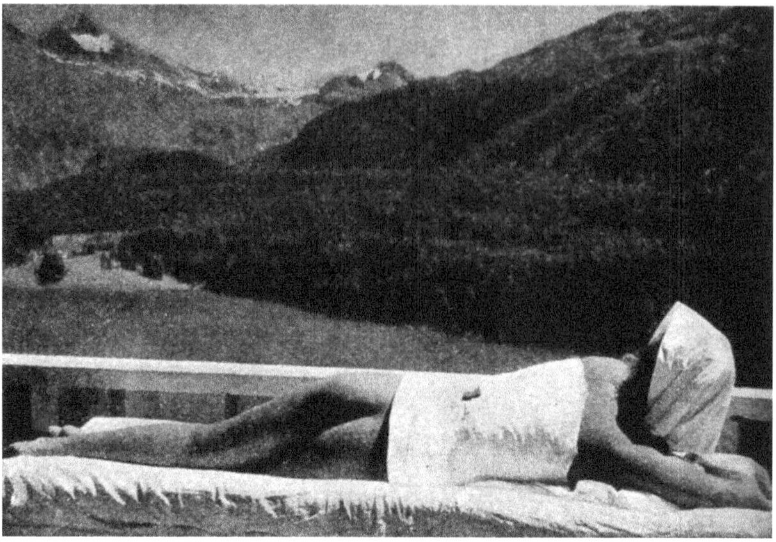

Figure 5.16 Twenty-four-year-old female patient with spondylitis dorsalis. In Oskar Bernhard, *Light Treatment in Surgery* (London: Edward Arnold, 1926), Figure 86, p. 278. Author's collection.

detached, technical, and scientific explanations of the therapy's principles with subjective descriptions of his patients' skin that border on the salacious. Like the editors of *Sun Bathing Review*, Bernhard attempted to take the moral high ground – writing that 'sunning also must never contravene the rules of decorum'[112] – yet images and interjections of deeply sexualised suntanned skin betray his firm conviction.

In Figure 5.15, a healed female patient's bronzed skin positively glistens. At the age of twenty, this patient entered Bernhard's care emaciated and with 'sagging, loose skin', presenting tubercular fistulae of the cervical glands as well as osteitis of the lower jaw and right foot, the latter also resulting in fistulae. Within eight months, she was transformed by heliotherapy; ten kilos heavier and fully healed, the caption proclaimed her in an 'excellent state of health'. It concluded: 'Revel in these recovered lush and beautifully modelled curves of the body and the smooth, stunning bronze-coloured skin.'[113] Bernhard read his patient's health by her aesthetic lines, surface texture, and colouring, like an art connoisseur analysing a painted nude. The figure's position in the photograph allows for both the right side of her lower jaw and her right foot to be visible in one frame, the white markings indicating cicatrised tissue and thus closing of the fistulae. It also retains patient anonymity, her face turned away from the lens, like Tudor-Hart's model. Yet, while composed for clinical observation, as an effective 'after' image, the photograph equally presents to us a modern bronzed odalisque or Venus *au soleil* like Park and Gregory's photograph (Fig. 5.14), the viewer's eye immediately drawn to the figure's pronounced conical breasts and lithe form.

In Figure 5.16, the photographer (perhaps Bernhard himself) artfully arranged a twenty-four-year-old female patient atop a bed on his sanatorium's terrace, with a dramatic backdrop of surrounding mountains and valleys. Turned onto her side, legs crossed, and a scarf over her head that conspicuously ensures anonymity, the patient offers an obscured view of her (unnecessarily) bare buttocks, twisted tantalisingly towards the camera. The point, surely, is to examine the plaster cast containing her back and torso, and the small window cut out from it to allow the sunlight to penetrate a lesion below. The caption explained she suffered from inflammation of the thoracic vertebrae (spondylitis dorsalis) and of the bones (osteitis), presenting fistulae in the sternum and the left clavicle. Bernhard concluded that after two years of heliotherapy, this patient had become the 'mother of healthy children'. Significantly, here he proclaimed her return to health not through the healing of the lesions, weight gain, blood tests, or mobility, but specifically through her ability to procreate.

Like Lawrence's Juliet, Bernhard's patients regenerated their bodies by submission to the sunshine. The intensity of pigmentation in Figure 5.15, whether actual or produced by the lighting techniques, developing process, or retouching, is made extreme. White contouring was added along the figure's face, either to aid anonymity or to heighten the contrast between skin and surroundings – an effect calling to mind the illustrated figures whose pigmented bodies are marked by white contours, in the advertisements by Jacomo and Wigglesworth (Plates 6–7). Like Park and Gregory, Bernhard 'revelled' in this degree of pigmentation, the tone of his language and his photographs suggesting he found heliotherapy's efficacy for his patients aesthetically and even sexually stimulating.

He was not alone among practitioners to do so. Frequent references to suntanned skin as 'beautified', 'delicate', and simultaneously both softer and firmer to the touch occur in physicians' texts internationally.[114] Its appeal to tactility – calling out to the physician to touch it – can also be detected, as Saleeby was wont to do (above). So too was exposure to sunlight conceptualised as an act of being touched, 'massaged' or 'kissed' by the sun.[115] Flügel, quoted earlier, waxed poetic about the erotic pleasure derived from experiencing sunlight upon the skin, and there are references to light therapy instigating not just a sense of well-being but actual *euphoria* in patients.[116] Rollier was compelled to warn his medical colleagues by 1916 that patients had to be monitored to curb their 'zeal'. The intense joy was so seductive that, left unsupervised, they exposed themselves for dangerously long time periods.[117] But under appropriate surveillance, patients submissive to treatment – to the authority of physician and to the stimulating light itself – were rendered happy, compliant, and prone. The visual complements of Lawrence's Juliet, the nudes in Bernhard's and Park and Gregory's photographs undergo the act of heliotherapy as one of willing receptivity to the sun's penetrating touch and procreative energy, to be *impregnated* with and by light (Figs. 5.14–5.16).

'Bright' babies and virile soldiers

Up to this point I have concentrated on light therapy's engagement with women and its visual and literary rhetoric of producing healthy mother-citizens – exposing its deeply sexualised undertones in the process – to begin contextualising the therapy's larger social aims and proclaimed national usefulness.

But let us not forget the toddlers and babies imaged in the 'Homesun' pamphlet (Plates 2–3, 5). The sheer quantity of visual and textual material about child patients evinces that they were the therapy's major target group.[118] Children were the subjects of, and subject to, multiple large-scale trials about light therapy, carried out by Hill, Gauvain, Colebrook, and many others, during its early development and heyday.[119] Rollier's Leysin sanatoria, Gauvain's sanatoria in Hampshire, and the numerous infant-welfare clinics in urban areas throughout Britain (and internationally) – these institutions first and foremost treated children, curatively and preventively, especially for forms of tuberculosis and for rickets.[120]

Mental health was also believed to benefit from light treatment. Practitioners spoke of restored 'brightness' in children's dispositions and cognitive functioning, and young children were irradiated, in clinics and at home, to treat 'backwardness'.[121] Dora Colebrook, undertaking research at the North Islington Infant Welfare Centre supported by the London County Council, mentioned 'brighter' babies and children as but one beneficial side effect of irradiation.[122] A trial on child patients at Treloar's showed their advanced mental activity in comparison to 'physically defective' London children, and Gauvain suggested this could be attributed to ultraviolet radiation's improvement of 'the nutrition of the grey matter of the brain'.[123] 'The bright eyes, bronzed skin, and firm flesh' of Gauvain's child patients were remarked upon by visitors.[124] These valuable future citizens externalised their 'brightness' by being happier *and* smarter following irradiation. It makes the representation of the toddler in the 'Homesun' pamphlet especially poignant, with his rascally smile and engaging, direct gaze with the viewer: his photogenic body, his 'glow' or 'brightness', is a sign of both mental and physical health (Plate 3).

Like women, children were considered to be particularly responsive to ultraviolet radiation. In this respect they were frequently compared to plants and animals, finding their natural home outdoors in the fresh air and sunlight.[125] Treloar's ambulant child patients were commonly photographed in the Hampshire countryside and coast (Figs. 1.9–1.11, 5.17). Figure 5.17 depicts children undergoing heliotherapy while picking flowers, making an overt association between the tanned skin of Treloar's young patients and the lush green vegetation surrounding them. The children were

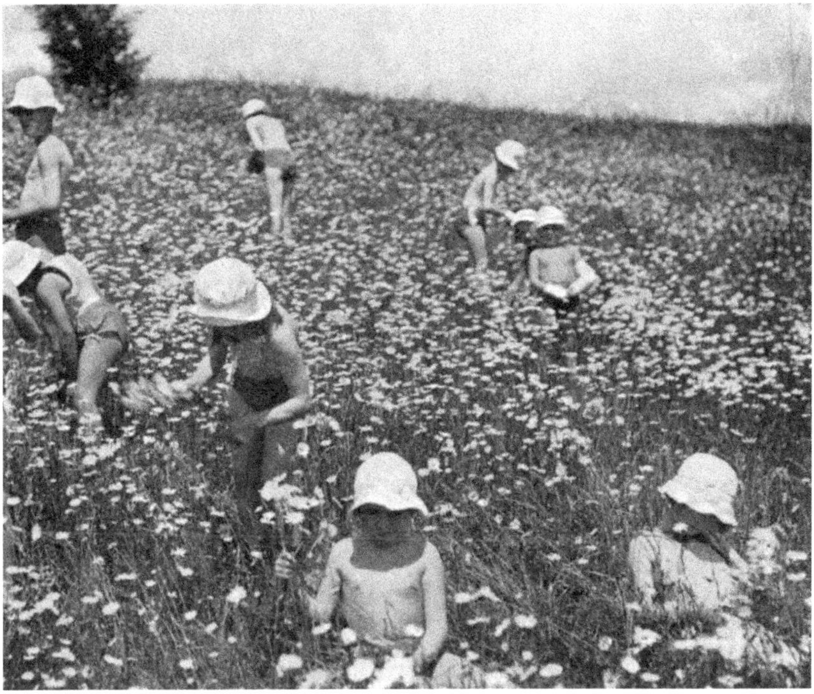

Figure 5.17 'Some of Sir Henry Gauvain's little patients at Alton, Hants.'
In Katherine Gamgee, *The Artificial Light Treatment of Children in Rickets, Anaemia and Malnutrition* (London: H. K. Lewis and Co., 1927), Figure 10, p. 33.
Wellcome Library, London.

here in their 'natural' place, healing and growing in the sunshine like Alton's wild flowers. The image is reminiscent of Frances Hodgson Burnett's *The Secret Garden* (1911): the protagonists Mary and Colin, once ill-tempered and sickly-looking children, gradually regain their health as they experience the rejuvenating powers of fresh air and sunlight. The vital connections made throughout the novel between the health and growth of the children and the secret garden find significant resonance within light therapy as well as naturist literature.[126]

Yet there was controversy over the particular photosensitivity of children's skin. Such authorities as Hill, Eidinow, and Hamilton reported in the mid-1920s that children under three were apparently *less* sensitive to ultraviolet light than adults, showing milder erythematic reactions.[127] Other contemporaries, like the Russells, stated the opposite, and significantly this was the medical opinion disseminated to the public.[128] Articles in *The Times* and *Sunlight* warned parents of the dangers of exposing their children to the sunshine – not with intention of stopping them from doing it, however, only advocating that adults and children alike do so gradually, building up a 'healthy tanned skin' incrementally, in the manner of Rollier's method (see Chapter 2).[129]

All of these benefits, physical, and mental, held political significance for a nation desirous of producing future 'A1' citizens from a current 'C3' population during the interwar period. As Roger Cooter explained, 'by the 1920s child health and welfare was not only medicalized, it was serving as a powerful argument for extending the role of the state in health and welfare generally'.[130] In Deck's 1926 popular treatise (itself intended to promote and solicit funds for the Sunlight League), Colebrook's North Islington Infant Welfare Centre was praised exuberantly for its targeted treatment of 'thousands of slum children', transforming each one into an 'entirely new being':

> Cases of malnutrition, rickets, general debility and many forms of – so-called – nervous diseases have been treated in this way and the result is an immediate improvement in appearance, activity, appetite, weight, etc., and instead of these children becoming chronic invalids and filling our hospitals and institutions, they have a chance of developing into strong, healthy boys and girls, capable of employment and able to play their part in the battle of life.[131]

Three years later, Dane echoed that it was a parental responsibility to expose children, both curatively and preventively, to the sunlight on behalf of the degenerating, 'C3' nation: 'Decide that you will be part of this scheme, that your children will be A1 specimens.'[132] In clinics, young children were first introduced to lamps by being placed on their mothers' laps to help allay fears, gain confidence, and ensure compliance.[133] Mothers thus continued to play a central role in the treatment of children, nurturing and guiding these young, valuable citizens towards the light.

One of the first acts of the Sunlight League (f. 1924) was the organisation of heliotherapy facilities for children at Kenwood (Hampstead). Over the summer, thirty-five children, sent from 'schools for the physically defective' and from hospitals, were monitored by a medical committee and photographed.[134] Before opening the Institute of Ray Therapy in 1930, Beaumont oversaw the children here. By 1925, he was also the honorary medical superintendent of another Sunlight League project, the Municipal Sunlight Clinic in St Pancras. The latter, when it opened its doors in March 1925, was partly funded by the Save the Children Fund and was enthusiastically described in *The Times* as London's first clinic for artificial light therapy, operating out of an infant-welfare centre in Highgate. The child patients were referred for treatment via the ten infant-welfare centres in the borough of St Pancras, under the authority of its medical officer of health.[135] Other boroughs quickly followed suit, and by 1931 Beaumont declared that 'now clinics are springing up all over the country'.[136]

Many of the leading members of the league and the New Health Society (formed out of the People's League of Health), including Sir Alfred Fripp and Hill, wanted natural and artificial light-therapy facilities available not only in clinics or in hospitals, but in every school. Hill suggested that carbon arc lamps be operated in schools by teachers, nurses, or other suitably 'skilled attendants', while ultraviolet-permitting 'Vita' glass replaced the school's ordinary glass windows.[137] Like the animals at the London Zoo, where lamps and 'Vita' glass windows were first experimentally installed, the children received natural and artificial exposures to vitalising ultraviolet rays, safely housed and supervised. As John Stanislav Sadar argued, by installing ultraviolet-permitting glass into British homes, zoos, and schools, these structures were themselves transformed, becoming 'heliotherapeutic devices'.[138] 'Vita' glass is but one example of new material products, alongside Celanese fabric, sunscreen, and home-use lamps (termed 'socio-technical artefacts' by Simon Carter) that facilitated public access to ultraviolet radiation beyond the light clinic or the trip to the beach or lido. Carter, Sadar, and Ina Zweiniger-Bargielowska also made clear that these public measures, driven by groups like the Sunlight League, altered widespread attitudes towards ultraviolet radiation (and sunlight generally) during the 1920s into a natural, powerful source of preventive care for the individual and nation.[139] As Deck described, ultraviolet radiation was producing 'entirely new beings', resistant to the degenerative influences and diseases of modern life, and was thus a weapon of social hygiene. It cut across class lines too: natural and artificial sunlight was enthusiastically aimed onto rich and poor alike, curatively and preventively, via local free and private clinics, hospitals, schools (especially open-air schools, enthusiastically promoted by the National Association for the Prevention of Tuberculosis), outdoor parks and lidos, beaches, and home-use lamps.[140]

In the words of Bernhard, reflecting on his extensive experience utilising natural sunlight: 'Air and sun had not only strengthened the body and provided it with weapons for a victorious fight with the infecting organism, but in this victory had armed it with immune bodies for future protection.'[141] To this end, alongside mothers and children, soldiers and athletes were further target groups for curative and preventive exposures, couched in a rhetoric of sexualised potency and military efficiency. Both heliotherapy and phototherapy were used during the First World War, especially to treat wounds, by British, French, Swiss, and German physicians. Ultraviolet light was additionally relied upon to sterilise water and for signalling purposes.[142] The war proved an unparalleled testing ground for applications of light, just as it did for other forms of modern medicine, and this was surely one of the reasons why light therapy emerged with such force during the 1920s and why it continued to be valued as a treatment during the Second World War.[143] Beaumont reported an enthusiastic new influx of relatively healthy young men at the Institute for Ray Therapy in the summer of 1939, seeking to fix minor pains, acne, and low energy levels so as to avoid any chance of being turned down for service.[144]

The Swiss physicians Bernhard and Rollier undertook pioneering work during the First World War and wrote about their experiences, no doubt facilitated by their nation's neutrality. In their publications they deferred to the work of French and German colleagues in equal measure.[145] Bernhard used natural and artificial light to treat wounded German soldiers in 1914–15, then from 1916–17 acted as Swiss military surgeon to war prisoners' camps in Germany, Britain, and northern France. Like Rollier, he brought back cases to intern in Switzerland at his facilities, which occurred until the end of the war and beyond it. Rollier discussed heliotherapy for war wounds in *Le Pansement solaire* (1916). He argued that heliotherapy healed wounds and maintained joint and muscle functions to the affected areas, rendering injured soldiers once again fit for work and ready for the 'battle for existence'. This is why he described heliotherapy as a 'conservative' treatment, which avoided unnecessary amputations. He also cited it could aid surgical and orthopaedic therapy as well as plastic surgery.[146] Rollier concluded the text by discussing the preventive use of heliotherapy in future military training, arming young soldiers with additional resistance to infections, chief among them tuberculosis.[147]

In Britain, phototherapy was used to treat wounded soldiers in Oxford, Newcastle, and London and at naval hospitals in Chatham and Haslar, while heliotherapy was used in Maidenhead under the direction of the Canadian Red Cross.[148] The Simpson lamp, discussed in Chapter 4, was one particular model used to treat soldiers at London hospitals such as St Bartholomew's, not only for wounds but also for venereal lesions. Ultraviolet light was particularly prized as a bactericide, naturally disinfecting wounds, as well as for its ability to induce suppuration, expel necrotic bone and tissue, and increase blood flow to speed healing. It also produced much more aesthetically appealing scar tissue (cicatrisation). Soldiers' bodies were not only healed, they remained whole by avoiding the surgeon's knife, and thus they could retain their status as valued and productive citizens during and after the war.

Like the soldier, the athlete found his body – and his masculinity – a special target of ultraviolet radiation. Athletes were advised to expose themselves to the 'Homesun' lamp in Hanovia's pamphlet to counter 'staleness' through over-training, recharging lost energy and increasing 'vital capacity'. Hanovia also boasted its lamps were used by professional footballers, a practice that was reported in local and national newspapers to improve athletic performance by means of increased stamina and general health. Among the clubs who used the technology were Northampton, Hull City, Chelsea, West Ham, Leicester City, Sunderland, and Glasgow Rangers.[149] Hanovia included an image of champion boxer Jack Petersen receiving a vitalising exposure, his skin tinted a saturated orange like the other models' and his contours crisply outlined from heavy retouching. A 'hardy' tan, as Carter explained, made for a virile man, representing 'a visible link between the body, ideals of nature and masculinity'.[150] Part of this process involved 'training' the skin to ultraviolet radiation and all manner of climatic conditions.

Hardening the body ensured increased virility for the truly fit man. Those who worked sedentary occupations and stayed chiefly indoors were, according to Hill, doomed to a 'loss of breeding power'.[151] The statement is not surprising. As we have seen already, one of Hill's major arguments for regular exposures to ultraviolet radiation was that it increased the sexual power of citizens (see epigraph). This overt sexualisation of ultraviolet radiation, of its procreative powers and production of aesthetically desirable pigmentation, appears on the surface to have had overt eugenic ends: photogenic, procreative, and physically fit women and men meant ideal 'race mothers', A1 soldiers, and resultant 'bright', healthy babies. Significantly, Hill lectured widely throughout Britain using visual aids to make direct contrasts between sun-fed and sun-starved bodies to public audiences. In one lecture given in Leeds in 1926, he showed an image of a Graeco-Roman statue and contrasted the 'almost perfect body' – achieved through bodily exposure to fresh air and sunlight by practising sport in the open – to that of a 'C3 man of today' with a 'malformed chest', 'contracted jaws', and a 'badly developed' nose. Hill then further contrasted the image of the 'C3' individual to that of a contemporary young German, bronzed like a statue through naked outdoor exercise.[152] During a time of heightened eugenic fervour, the suntan gained unparalleled social and political value in Britain and abroad. It is no coincidence, in other words, that during the first forty years of the twentieth century, when eugenics developed as a legitimate study of racial improvement throughout the globe, the suntan was celebrated as a sign of health and beauty. Indeed, it is precisely *as* an aesthetic that the suntanned body held value, particularly for eugenicists like Saleeby. That the 'Homesun' pamphlet was produced at the opening of the Second World War *in colour* is significant; its representations of coated, smiling models have (socio-political) *value* by virtue of being coloured.[153] But equally important here is the *colour value*, the use of a highly saturated orange that borders on Technicolor. The values of suntan in eugenicists' minds were slippery at best, positioned precariously on what might be understood as a sliding (colour) scale, (evolutionary) ladder, or (moral) compass. Suntan's function, duration, and depth could simultaneously signal the white, British body's renewed racial health *and* its impending degeneration.

Saturated colour

Compare the 'Homesun' cover, a colour photograph (Plate 3), to the retouched and tinted black-and-white images in the rest of the pamphlet (Plates 2, 4–5). It is clear that, in the printing process, Hanovia tried very hard to replicate the colour tones of the models' tanned skin in Plate 3 to represent users' skin in the black-and-white images, however non-naturalistic the end results. Are we to read these coatings of colour as 'bronzed', 'golden brown' tans? The fluorescent colour value borders on the radioactive. Despite the use of highlighting in some of the figures' bodies (e.g., Plate 4), we have less sense that it is an externalised reflection ('shine') than an interiorised projection of light ('glow').[154] The common description of a 'glowing' or 'radiant' tan is fitting; pigmentation was perceived to be a manifestation of bodily photogenesis. Visually the colour orange is used consistently, and uniquely, throughout the pamphlet. In varying values it is used along the borders, for the titles of sub-sections, behind offset text as image captions, and most importantly to represent highly stylised suns. In Plate 4, for example, the bold orange of the sun (used also for the model's hair and swimsuit in the 'outdoor' scene) is echoed in subdued values for skin, towel, and sand, then transported and mimicked below in the tanned skin of the model taking her 'Homesun' bath. A connection is made visually between the photogenic sun and the photogenic body, through colour alone. The sun's vital energy is transferred to, consumed, and stored by the model, and likewise the lamp's ultraviolet emanations are meant to impart equal, if not superior, power. The models are saturated by ultraviolet radiation, and this is expressed through saturated colour reminiscent of contemporaneous Technicolor films – representations that, according to Sarah Street and Tom Gunning, likewise struggled to successfully exploit colour as simultaneously naturalistic, or true to nature, *and* spectacular.[155]

An extreme colour choice, the orange in the 'Homesun' pamphlet is applied as a top coat to black-and-white skin, overlaid in the final stages of the printing process. It appears more like the artifice of make-up (Plate 5) than the deeply ingrained pigment embedded in the colour photograph (Plate 3). We might today liken it to the orange disaster that is the fake tan, an obvious, applied surface coat or mask that is not easily confused with the natural pigmentation of 'black' skin. It is a borrowing, mimicry, or even attempt at racial 'passing' gone wrong, provoking anxiety or ridicule.[156]

For early twentieth-century practitioners, patients, and naturists, similar anxiety resided in uneven colour complexion, especially the tanning of the face; in other words, in an even, convincing and total coverage that could enable – or disrupt – racial categorisation.[157] In Baumer's 1936 *Punch* cartoon, the alarm we are meant to read humorously on the face of the sunbathing initiate as she stares at her dark companion is significant (Fig. 5.2). She is alarmed because she witnesses a disruption of racial difference in her companions, in spite of the fact that their dark bodies retain the physiognomic facial characteristics of ideal British 'whiteness': pert nose, thin lips, small chin, and high cheekbones and forehead. The viewer *knows* the tanned bodies are 'white' but *sees* them as 'black'. Furthermore, her alarm can be read as fear for her own body, her own sense of self. As the caption stated, the same transformation would soon happen to the initiate's own white skin, and rapidly so, should she conquer her fears and give in to the pressure from her fashionable peers.

For David Batchelor, colour itself is feared and marginalised as trivial, as artifice, as 'other', and has been so throughout the history of Western civilisation, particularly in relation to art and architecture. He termed this 'chromophobia', describing the prejudice against colour as operating in two ways:

> In the first, colour is made out to be the property of some 'foreign' body – usually the feminine, the oriental, the primitive, the infantile, the vulgar, the queer or the pathological. In the second, colour is relegated to the realm of the superficial, the supplementary, the inessential or the cosmetic. In one, colour is regarded as alien and therefore dangerous; in the other, it is perceived merely as a secondary quality of experience, and thus unworthy of serious consideration. Colour is dangerous, or it is trivial, or it is both.[158]

Significantly, Batchelor argued its opposite, 'chromophilia', simply celebrates and even heightens these perceptions, much as early twentieth-century primitivism and 'negrophilia' revelled in so-called 'primitive' or 'black' aesthetics, fundamentally fuelling, rather than challenging, normalised perceptions of racial difference.[159] In Baumer's cartoon, the tan is simultaneously the source of negrophilic desire *and* negrophobic alarm. He playfully references the contemporaneous comedy of 'blackface' minstrelsy, yet takes a step too far – the pigmentation is too totalising, too deep. It is acquired pigmentation (colour) that curiously is represented as trendy, sexualising, trivial (hence humorous), and dangerous, all at the same time.

Such ambivalence resides in medical and popular understandings of suntan with respect to its depth and its permanence. Descriptions of suntan as a mere surface marker, residing only temporarily on the surface, occur frequently. A 'coat' or 'mask' to be worn and shed at will by white patients and enthusiasts, the tan finds analogy with cosmetics and clothing, and certainly as a shield or 'screen' demonstrated its protective function. Thedering described the tan as a 'coat of armour' for the body, for instance, while the National Association for the Prevention of Tuberculosis described children's bronzed skin as a 'natural clothing' in their 1921 film, *Air and Sun*.[160] Beyond the pith helmet (solar topi), clothing designed specially for British travellers to the tropics mimicked 'black' skin. Ryan Johnson pointed out that, paradoxically, in doing so:

> 'Black' skin, the very characteristic that most obviously marked difference between colonizers and colonized and which was a source of so much racist commentary in the late nineteenth and early twentieth centuries, was also

the very quality that British men and women sought to imitate while living in the tropical colonies.[161]

Adopting the natural state of the 'savage', colonisers wrapped themselves in manufactured tropical 'skin' as a means of protecting their vulnerable bodies against disease, degeneration, and the descent towards savagery itself. For Johnson, this paradox 'unmasks the close connections that still existed between colonizers [white] and colonized [coloured], rather than a growing divide between the two'.[162] Carter likewise pointed out the transgressing of boundaries between the two was carried out physically through their perceived 'deviant' sexual contact; that is, through racial miscegenation.[163]

Far more radically than in Baumer's cartoon, the collapsing of distinction between 'white' and 'coloured', light and dark, takes place in the case of solarised photographs (Chapter 3). By the 1930s, infrared photography opened up another world, a world of strange reversals of light and dark in which pale skin appeared 'black' and vice versa, reminiscent of Man Ray's positive and negative versions of *Noire et blanche (Kiki [Alice Prin] with an African mask)* (1926).[164] It is, by means of multiple light exposures, saturation gone too deep, confounding the racialised distinctions between 'white' model and 'primitive' mask, and furthermore rendering Kiki as dangerously seductive as Baumer's smoking negrophiliac (Fig. 5.2).

Transgressive tans

Discussing the tensions between 'racial colour' and 'tanned colour', Sarah Ahmed asserted that, in early twentieth-century tourism literature, 'The perfectibility of "tanned skin" remains bound up with notions of hygiene. Tanned colour is clean colour and is hence immediately distinguished from the infectability of being-Black'.[165] Along with fresh air, clean water, and open spaces, sunlight was promoted by advocates as part of a natural regime for bodily health and social hygiene. Saleeby and his Sunlight League perceived sunlight, and ultraviolet light specifically, as a disinfecting agent with which to rid the masses of 'diseases of darkness', notably tuberculosis and rickets. He lobbied for strict smoke abatement laws to reduce the fog and grime hanging over London and other major British industrial cities, seeking to exchange the nation's dependence upon coal for electricity. Eradicating slums, building lidos, and irradiating children were Saleeby's aims, in keeping with his belief in positive eugenics.[166] Ahmed's framing of the tan and race in relation to hygiene is therefore apt since, for promoters like Saleeby, ultraviolet light acted not unlike soap as a weapon for racial health. Advertisements for 'ultraviolet ray soap' present a fascinating fusion of these two consumable products.[167] As Anne McClintock so convincingly argued, the promise of racial regeneration, maintenance, and cleansing through the fetishistic use of soap was part and parcel of the Empire's civilising mission. Yet in Victorian and Edwardian advertisements of 'blacks' turned 'white' through its miraculous cleansing action, soap, like ultraviolet light, could be perceived as an agent actively maintaining *or* disrupting racial difference.[168]

Sally Dunne Romano asserted that, 'At the start of the twentieth century, the healthy suntan did not endanger native-born, white skinned Americans' racial identity because, as opposed to the permanency of race, a suntan was temporary.'[169] Anxieties over the 'infectability' (to quote Ahmed) of racial transformation through light exposure apparently did not threaten predominant, Darwinist understandings of 'fixed' characteristics of race and identity in twentieth-century America. Yet Man Ray's 1926 photograph of Kiki and the controversial book, *The Effects of Tropical Light on White Men*, by Major Charles Woodruff of 1905, complicate Dunne Romano's argument.[170] However much some practitioners viewed the tan as 'merely' a temporary surface coat, there were others not entirely certain of its latent effects on the body and the psyche. We find them in Britain as well as America, Denmark, France, Germany, and Switzerland. As discussed earlier, the depth and function of the tan were perceived to reach well into the body's interior by many international practitioners. They were also unclear just how temporary the tan was. Again, explanation resided in the skin of the 'coloured' body, Müller writing:

> If during summer you have acquired a pretty tanned skin all over, it will almost fade before next season, though not quite. You will keep a light shade of tanning, and when you again start sun-bathing, you will find that now you can stand practically any amount of sunshine without the ill-effects [e.g., erythema] so characteristic for beginners. The cause is that your skin has formed its own means of protection by creating a sort of pigment. We find similar pigments as an inherited gift in most other human races, from the light yellow of the Japanese to the ebony black of the real Negro.[171]

For Müller, retaining pigment, described here as a process of *adaptation* more in keeping with Neo-Lamarckian thought, was considered a positive outcome of regular exposure to the natural environment. But he too expressed concern over sunlight's lasting effects, especially on young, impressionable bodies. Müller's English version of *My Sun-Bathing and Fresh Air System* (1927) included warnings about sunbathing being dangerous if overdone. His reason was that 'the sex life is awakened too soon in children by too much sun-bathing'.[172] This is reminiscent of Revillet's comment, stated above, when he discussed young females induced into early puberty by the Côte d'Azur's sunlight and felt the need to stress this was not an 'atavistic' phenomenon. The tanned body's perceived descent towards atavism, immorality, and base sexuality correlated with the colour depth (value) of pigmentation: the 'deeper' the tan, the greater the possibility of irreversibly crossing racial lines. But even here light therapists, many of them eugenicists, sought out extreme pigmentation for their weakly, white-skinned patients.

Of the many foreign physicians visiting Rollier's facilities in Leysin, the French Dr Renon commented in 1913 that,

> I was extremely impressed to see patients as *black* as Negroes, with considerable and multiple healed tubercular wounds and with healed white tumours [tumours of chronic tubercular arthritis]; without the photographs of the lesions before the treatment, never would it have been possible to believe that the same disorders existed beforehand.[173]

For Renon, the confounding of patients' racial identity through intense heliotherapy was impressive work indeed. The American Dr Otis similarly commented, upon visiting Rollier's facilities in 1912 that, 'It was difficult to tell to what race they [the children] belonged, they were so pigmented, the majority being a mahogany or chocolate colour.'[174] In Britain, Dane commented in his 1929 popular book that 'a [naturally] dark Englishman will soon become quite as dark as an Arab and even darker in many cases.'[175]

As Maren Möhring discussed, in Germany extreme pigmentation was discussed at length by sunbathers ascribing to the *Nachtkultur* (naked culture) movement. In the process of bronzing one's skin:

> The ideal skin color was a nevertheless a moderate bronze, for the sunbather was warned against excessive tanning that might make his or her body 'look like a Hottentot's body'. The dark skin of the 'Hottentot' was considered as the embodiment of the ugly and as the effect of layers of dirt. Since skin color was one of the most important racial signifiers in theories of race circulating in the early twentieth century, the shade of one's tan became a controversial point. Ongoing efforts to define a 'healthy brown' or a 'natural white' make apparent the ambiguity and permeability of the category of whiteness.[176]

Here then was that tricky border between *looking like* an 'Arab', 'Negro', or 'Hottentot' – for the white, sick patient or lay enthusiast an act of emulation through which to regain vigour, health, and sexual function – and *becoming* one, namely an act of total racial transformation. Bernard attempted to stabilise these fears by arguing that the differences lay within the minute depths of the skin's physiological make-up: 'Acquired pigment is extracellular, as opposed to the normal pigment, which is intracellular, as for example the colouring matter of the negro, which must afford constant protection against light.'[177] Awash with uncertainty and contradiction, he also stated in the same work that racial colour was not fixed, or even inherited. Rather, it was his view that the *ability* to 'manufacture and store pigment in the skin under the influence of light' was passed on from generation to generation, not the pigment itself.[178]

Under the seductive pull of negrophilia, others collapsed the distinction between acquired and inherited pigment altogether, speaking of the black body as representative of the healthy, deep tan. In *The Times*' 'Sunlight and Health' supplement of 1928, for instance, one correspondent stated:

> From the earliest times Africa has been for the people of Europe a synonym for sunshine. Everything and everybody African were sunburned till they were black; and by the mere action of the sun life there bred innumerably; a land of mystery and multitudinous strange gods all drawing their own existences from the life-given power of the supreme sun-god himself.[179]

Such conflations fed back into light-therapy practice, driving some to alter their methods. By the late 1930s, the issue of excessive pigmentation led Dr Charles Brody, the husband of Dr Malvine Brody, to address the matter directly and methodically in his practice. In his massive, internationally authored edited series, *Traité d'hélio- et d'actinologie* (1938), he included an essay on a new method to *de*pigment his patients. He began by complaining that tanning had become too fashionable among tourists as well as patients in heliotherapeutic sanatoria on the Côte d'Azur, an indirect reference perhaps to the sudden rise in numbers to the region as a result of the newly instigated law that allocated paid holiday leave for workers in 1936, *les congés payés*. For these tourists, Brody wrote, tanning had become the goal of sun treatment rather than merely a product of it.[180] He promoted a new method of his design involving a depigmentation process at certain intervals during heliotherapy treatment so that his patients slowly weaned themselves off of sunshine. The reason, he stated, was that long, uninterrupted sunbathing, with the intention of producing extreme tans, was unnecessary to the healing process and even dangerous:

> It can even happen that the appearance of a sudden and intense pigmentation is the element of a severe prognosis and, sometimes even, the prodrome of a fatal, short-term outcome. Such is the case with sufferers of cachexia [general wasting disease]. Here we have noted that after a short exposure, even in an insignificant dose, a sudden and intense pigmentation of chocolate colour appears. Far from being a good omen, here this rapid and dark pigmentation signifies a tissular disintegration of the organism on the path to destruction and is comparable, for us, to a warning sign.[181]

In fact, he described pigmentation as a skin 'allergy', and viewed excessive tanning as the body overdosed and saturated by the sun; he wrote of '*surpigmentation, surdosage, sursaturation solaire*' necessitating not simply depigmentation but *désaccoutumance*, the word *accoutumance* significantly meaning either 'adaptation' or 'addiction'.[182] By shortening exposure times and assuring the well-being of his patients, Brody insisted that the advantages would be economic as well as social and moral.[183]

Already by the 1920s, however, Thedering described a similar method designed to overcome what he termed the 'dead end' of light treatment on patients. Intense, continuous exposures produced excessive pigmentation – Thedering's 'coat of armour' – and inhibited further progress. The practitioner could deliberately choose to expose his patients until this plateau was reached, followed by several weeks without treatment for the body to 'rid itself of the excess pigment', then start again, creating cycles of 'dead ends' and recoveries.[184] In Beaumont's 1931 handbook, he called this the 'dead point' method, a particularly fitting phrase that, as I discuss in Chapter 6, aligned excessive light exposure with the dangers of racial degeneration, damage, and death.[185]

Conclusion

Though Thedering attempted intensely pigmenting, then depigmenting, his patients, he noted that a much preferred method was to give shorter exposures throughout the cure, avoiding pigmentation altogether and ensuring the skin's receptivity to the light. As discussed in Chapter 2, this was the method advocated by Hill and Eidinow at the MRC-funded NIMR, at least for patients when curatively applied. Yet, when it came to the tan's preventive merits on the British population at large, Hill simultaneously praised the nudist practices made so well known by Müller and his rival, the German Hans Surén. The latter's book, *Man and Sunlight* (*Der Mensch und die Sonne* of 1924, with a 1927 English translation for which Saleeby wrote the foreword), promoted intense sunbathing as part of the physical-culture movement and was later accepted party propaganda during the Nazi regime (see Fig. 1.1).[186]

Earlier, it inspired British poet and writer Alfred Noyes' playful novel, *The Return of the Scare-Crow* (*The Sun Cure*; 1929). Noyes' novel addressed the joys, and ridiculousness, of the cult of nudity through the story of a normally straight-laced pastor who accidentally loses his clothing during a spontaneous sunbathing session along the Sussex coast. As a result he spends several days in hiding to avoid the scandal of being seen while simultaneously revelling in the delights of his new-found freedom, constantly nude in the sunshine. Describing Surén's book as replete with photographs of Germans so tanned they appeared to be 'South Sea Islanders', the novel makes explicit connections between the act of sunbathing and primitivist longings for exotic islands, jungles, and childhood innocence.[187] Most of all, Noyes' protagonist, the reverend Basil Strode, experiences the pleasures and perils of loosening moral standards accompanying the invigorating sun cure.

If tanned skin was, according to Ahmed, historically perceived as 'clean colour', we must recognise that the 'infectability' of blackness – of degenerative racial 'contagion' or transgression – was uncomfortably close on the colour scale, always threatening to bleed. It is perhaps deliberate that Hanovia sought to represent its photogenic, 'bronzed' models using gradations of orange rather than brown, signalling the transference of solar energy instead of race (Plates 2–5). Health, happiness, and procreativity sought after by saturating the body with ultraviolet radiation could easily descend into the realm of disease, deviance, and degeneration. The value that Hill attributed to ultraviolet radiation, and its resultant tan, to stimulate the 'sexual power of citizens' (see epigraph), was thus at once eugenically desirable and dangerous.[188]

Practitioners' perceptions about the ultraviolet rays' sexually activating powers set it apart from X rays and radium, known by contrast for their sterilising action on the reproductive organs – used to horrific, eugenic effect on so-called 'degenerative' groups around the globe.[189] But the investment in ultraviolet radiation to produce photogenic bodies, however promising, was never uniformly understood as a 'positive' eugenic measure. It is crucial we recognise that, first, the matter was never fully resolved and, second, this ambivalence towards the tan was bound up with sex, race, and national health.

Lastly, to view the tan as 'only' an aesthetic is to overlook the power of the visual. It was precisely on the surface that its 'value' was, however ambivalently, understood. Even when conceptualised as a surface layer or coating of colour, its meaning was always more than skin-deep. In early twentieth-century Britain and abroad, the tan was perceived as the externalisation of stored solar energy in the body, of vital energy radiant and glowing. Presented in the full glory of saturated colour, the smiling mother and child in the 'Homesun' cover delight and disarm us (Plate 3). Yet their curious pigmentation remains unfixed along a slippery colour scale, revealing that seeking a suntan could go either way on the evolutionary ladder.

Notes

1 Leonard Hill, in Leonard Hill, G. B. Dixon, and Dora C. Colebrook, 'Discussion on Influence of Sunlight and Artificial Light on Health', *BMJ*, 12 September 1925, pp. 470–7, at p. 472.

2 Victor Dane, *The Sunlight Cure: How to Use the Ultra-violet Rays* (London: Athletic Publications, 1929), p. 9.

3 Albert Eidinow, 'Some Observations on the Dosage of Ultra-violet Rays in Artificial Sun Treatment', *Lancet*, 15 August 1925, pp. 317–23, at p. 321.

4 Dane's credentials were suspect, being implicated in a patient's death; see 'Jury and Nature Cure Practitioner', *The Times*, 14 March 1931, p. 3; and 'Fatal Nature Cure', *Western Morning News and Mercury*, 14 March 1931, p. 9.

5 Leonard Hill, *Sunshine and Open Air: Their Influence on Health, with Special Reference to the Alpine Climate* (London: Edward Arnold, 1925), pp. 124–5, and 'Let Children Live in Sunshine! (By a Woman Doctor)', *Yorkshire Evening Post*, 28 May 1926, p. 5. See also Ina Zweiniger-Bargielowska, *Managing the Body: Beauty, Health, and Fitness in Britain, 1880–1939* (Oxford: Oxford University Press, 2010), especially pp. 151–92.

6 'The War and After', *The Times*, 13 September 1918, pp. 7–8.

7 See Charles Corfield, 'Sun-Bathing', *The Times*, 10 July 1935, p. 10.

8 On the New Health Society and the Sunlight League, see Chapter 1, and John Stanislav Sadar, 'Unpacking the Latent Bodies of Interwar Ultraviolet Health Glass' (Ph.D. dissertation, University of Pennsylvania, 2010), pp. 108–10.

9 Hanovia, *Get Back in the Sun with a 'Homesun'*, pamphlet, 1940 (Thackray Medical Museum, CAT HAN 1940 1088, S.2434/240), pp. 6–7. See also the 'Homesun' advertisement in *The Times*, 12 October 1928, p. 9.

10 Britain's Eugenics Society included such illustrious members as the biologist and eugenicist (later Sir) Julian Sorell Huxley (son of the staunch Darwinist Thomas Henry Huxley and brother of novelist Aldous Huxley), Leonard Darwin (Charles Darwin's son), and Prime Minister Neville Chamberlain. Sadar, 'Unpacking', p. 107.

11 See, for example, Myrtle Vaughan-Cowell, *Artificial Sunlight: Its Use and Application* (London: H. Edgar Smithers, 1928), p. 18; Franz Thedering, *Sunlight as Healer: A Popular Treatise* (Slough: Sollux, 1926), p. 24; Auguste Rollier, *Le Pansement solaire: héliothérapie de certaines affections chirurgicales et des blessures de guerre* (Lausanne and Paris: Librairie Payot & Cie., 1916), p. 67; and Jørgen Peter Müller, *My Sun-Bathing and Fresh-Air System* (London: Athletic Publications, *c.* 1927), p. 42.

12 Hanovia, *Homesun* pamphlet, p. 10.

13 See Roger Cooter and John Pickstone (eds), *Medicine in the Twentieth Century* (Amsterdam: Harwood Academic Publishers, 2000), pp. xiii–xix, at p. xvii, and John Pickstone's 'Production, Community and Consumption: The Political Economy of Twentieth-Century Medicine', in Roger Cooter and John Pickstone (eds), *Medicine in the Twentieth Century* (Amsterdam: Harwood Academic Publishers, 2000), pp. 1–19.

14 Hanovia, *Homesun* pamphlet, both p. 11.

15 Ian Littlewood, *Sultry Climates: Travel and Sex since the Grand Tour* (London: John Murray, 2001), p. 194. Popular histories of tanning tell us that pale, lily-white skin was highly prized by Victorians and Edwardians, to be swiftly replaced during the 1920s by a new vogue for suntanned skin. See Littlewood, *Sultry Climates*; Mary Blume, *Côte d'Azur: Inventing the French Riviera* (London: Thames & Hudson, 1992); Richard Dyer, *White* (London and New York: Routledge, 1997); Pascal Ory, *L'Invention du bronzage* (Paris: Éditions Complexe, 2008); Bernard Andrieu, *Bronzage: une petite histoire du soleil et de la peau* (Paris: CNRS Éditions, 2008); Bill Cormack, *A History of Holidays, 1812–1990* (London: Routledge and Thomas Cook Archives, 1998); and Keith Dutton, *The Perfectible Body: The Western Ideal of Physical Development* (London: Cassell, 1995). Primary medical literature, however, suggests there was no easily demarcated time period during which suntanned skin replaced pale skin as a beauty fad, no resolute shift in aesthetics. See my articles, '*Le Pays du soleil*: The Art of Heliotherapy on the Côte d'Azur', *Social History of Medicine*, 26:1 (2013),

74–93; and '"Kissed by the Sun": Tanning the Skin of the Sick with Light Therapeutics, *c.* 1890–1930', in Kevin Siena and Jonathan Reinarz (eds), *A Medical History of Skin: Scratching the Surface* (London: Pickering & Chatto, 2013), pp. 181–94. See also Simon Carter, *Rise and Shine: Sunlight, Technology and Health* (New York and Oxford: Berg, 2007), pp. 18–28; and Sally Dunne Romano, 'The Dark Side of the Sun: Skin Cancer, Sunscreen and Risk in Twentieth-Century America' (Ph.D. dissertation, Yale University, 2006), pp. 37–45.

16 As Sir Clifford Allbutt, speaking at the Lord Mayor Treloar Cripples' Hospital and College, stated, 'far more than a superficial varnish, [suntan] signified a profound alteration within'. In 'The Sun Cure for Surgical Tuberculosis', *BMJ*, 21 July 1923, pp. 111–12, at p. 111.

17 See, respectively: *Actinotherapy Technique* (Slough: Sollux, 1933), pp. 22–3; Albert Eidinow, 'A Note on Phototherapy', *Lancet*, 25 September 1926, pp. 645–8, at p. 647; John Harvey Kellogg, *Light Therapeutics* (Battle Creek, Mich.: Modern Medicine, 1927), p. 38; Oskar Bernhard, *Light Treatment in Surgery* (London: Edward Arnold, 1926), p. 89; and W. E. Dixon, in W. E. Dixon, C. E. M. Jones, and G. H. Lancashire, 'Discussion on the Therapeutic Value of Light', *BMJ*, 19 September 1925, pp. 499–504, at p. 499.

18 Bernhard, *Light Treatment*, p. 65. See also Elizabeth Anderson, *The Essentials of Light Treatment for the Use of Masseuses* (London: Baillière, Tindall & Cox, 1935), p. 16; and Auguste Rollier, *Heliotherapy* (London: Henry Frowde and Hodder & Stoughton, 1923), pp. 10, 24.

19 Jean-Antoine-Constant Lamaison, *De l'héliothérapie dans la tuberculose*, medical dissertation (Bordeaux: Imprimerie Barthélemy & Clédes, 1913), p. 25. On the French Eugenics Society, see William Schneider, 'Towards the Improvement of the Human Race: The History of Eugenics in France', *Journal of Modern History*, 54:2 (1982), 268–91; and William Schneider, 'The Eugenics Movement in France, 1890–1940', in Mark B. Adams (ed.), *The Wellborn Science: Eugenics in Germany, France, Brazil, and Russia* (Oxford: Oxford University Press, 1990), pp. 69–109.

20 Caleb W. Saleeby, *Sunlight and Health* (London: Nisbet & Co., 1923), pp. 20–1. Schneider stated Saleeby was a neo-Lamarckian; see 'Eugenics Movement in France', p. 75. Carter described Saleeby as 'a "reformist" rather than a "conservative" eugenicist' because he did not subscribe to the 'better dead' school of negative eugenics promoted by Sir Francis Galton; see Carter, *Rise and Shine*, p. 73.

21 Dane, *Sunlight Cure*, p. 10.

22 See Rollier, *Heliotherapy*, pp. 205–6; Kellogg, *Light Therapeutics*, p. 39; Bernhard, *Light Treatment*, p. 67; Anderson, *Essentials of Light Treatment*, p. 17; and Eleanor H. Russell and William K. Russell, *Ultra-violet Radiation and Actinotherapy* (Edinburgh: E. & S. Livingstone, 1925), p. 120.

23 See Rollier, *Pansement solaire*, p. 67; and Rollier, *Heliotherapy*, pp. 10–11.

24 Henry Gauvain, 'The General Principles of Treatment in Tuberculous Disease of the Bones and Joints in Children', *BMJ*, 26 November 1921, pp. 876–84, at p. 878.

25 Hanovia's *Homesun* pamphlet described chlorophyll as the 'green blood' of plants, p. 4. See also Thedering, *Sunlight as Healer*, pp. 22–3.

26 See Albert Eidinow, 'Observations on Some of the Principles of Artificial Sun Treatment', *British Journal of Tuberculosis*, 19:3 (1925), 113–26, at p. 121; Eidinow, 'Some Observations', p. 322; Steven Connor, 'Integuments: The Scar, the Sheen, the Screen', *New Formations*, 39 (winter 1999), 32–54, at p. 50; and Hill, *Sunshine and Open Air*, p. 84.

27 Hill, *Sunshine and Open Air*, p. 85.

28 Hill, *Sunshine and Open Air*, pp. 98–9.

29 See Kellogg, *Light Therapeutics*, p. 38; Anderson, *Essentials of Light Treatment*, p. 16; Bernhard, *Light Treatment*, p. 59.

30 Kellogg, *Light Therapeutics*, p. 38.

31 Russell and Russell, *Ultra-violet Radiation*, p. 119.

32 Eidinow, 'Observations on Some of the Principles', p. 122.

33 T. B. Fitzpatrick, 'Soleil et peau', *Journal de Médecine Esthétique*, 2 (1975), 33–4; and T. B. Fitzpatrick, 'The Validity and Practicality of Sun Reactive Skin Types I through VI', *Archives of Dermatology*, 124:6 (1988), 869–71. Types I–III are variations of white skin, IV is 'Mediterranean', V is 'Middle Eastern', and VI 'dark brown to black' skin tones. See also Richard Hobday, *The Healing Sun: Sunlight and Health in the 21st Century* (Forres: Findhorn Press, 1999), pp. 24–5. On race and pigmentation more broadly, see Nina Jablonski, *Skin: A Natural History* (Berkeley, Calif.: University of California Press, 2006); and Nina Jablonski, *Living Color: The Biological and Social Meaning of Skin Color* (Berkeley, Calif.: University of California Press, 2012); Roberta Bivins, 'Ideology and Disease Identity: The Politics of Rickets, 1929–1982', *Medical Humanities*, 40:1 (2014), 3–10. On race and photography, see Tanya Sheehan, *Doctored: The Medicine of Photography in Nineteenth-Century America* (University Park, Pa.: Pennsylvania State University Press, 2011), pp. 89–105; and Melissa Miles, 'Out of the Shadows: on Light, Darkness and Race in Australian Photography', *History of Photography [P]*, 36:3 (2012), 337–52.

34 Niels R. Finsen, *Phototherapy*, trans. J. H. Sequeira (London: Edward Arnold, 1901), p. 9.

35 See Hill, *Sunshine and Open Air*, pp. 83–4; Russell and Russell, *Ultra-violet Radiation*, p. 119; and Vaughan-Cowell, *Artificial Sunlight*, pp. 18–19. As Ahmed stated, 'Race has a cause/effect relation to pigmentation: race causes colour which is then read as a sign of race.' Sarah Ahmed, 'Animated Borders: Skin, Colour and Tanning', in Margrit Shildrick and Janet Price (eds), *Vital Signs: Feminist Reconfigurations of the Bio/Logical Body* (Edinburgh: Edinburgh University Press, 1998), pp. 45–65, at p. 53.

36 Bernhard, *Light Treatment*, p. 68.

37 Anderson, *Essentials of Light Treatment*, p. 17.

38 On citations to Draper's Law, see, for example, Finsen, *Phototherapy*, pp. 17–18; and *Actinotherapy Technique* (Slough: Sollux, 1943), p. 20. See also Klaus Hentschel, *Mapping the Spectrum: Techniques of Visual Representation in Research and Teaching* (Oxford: Oxford University Press, 2002), p. 250.

39 Finsen, *Phototherapy*, p. 18.

40 William Beaumont, *Fundamental Principles of Ray Therapy* (London: H. K. Lewis & Co., 1931), pp. 13–14.

41 See Chapter 2 as well as Thedering, *Sunlight as Healer*, pp. 29–30; Russell and Russell, *Ultra-violet Radiation*, p. 127; *Actinotherapy Technique* (1933), p. 24; Dane, *Sunlight Cure*, pp. 12–13; and Albert Eidinow, 'The Action of Ultra-violet Rays on the Skin', *British Journal of Tuberculosis*, 22:3 (1928), 136–9.

42 For example, see the many case studies in Rollier, *Heliotherapy*.

43 Thedering, *Sunlight as Healer*, p. 29. Bernhard used almost identical language in *Light Treatment*, p. 48.

44 Carolyn Thomas de la Peña, *The Body Electric: How Strange Machines Built the Modern American* (New York: New York University Press, 2003). See also Wolfgang Schivelbusch, *Disenchanted Night: The Industrialization of Light in the Nineteenth Century*, trans. A. Davies (Berkeley, Calif.: University of California Press, 1995), p. 71; and Anson Rabinbach, *The Human Motor: Energy, Fatigue, and the Origins of Modernity* (Berkeley, Calif.: University of California Press, 1990).

45 Auguste Rollier, 'The Share of the Sun in the Prevention and Treatment of Tuberculosis', *BMJ*, 21 October 1922, pp. 741–5, at p. 742.

46 Hanovia advertisement in *Countryman* (January 1939), p. 454; Hobday, *Healing Sun*, p. 19.

47 Eidinow, 'Observations on Some of the Principles', p. 117. See Bernhard, *Light Treatment*, p. 48; Russell and Russell, *Ultra-violet Radiation*, p. 127; and Rollier, *Heliotherapy*, pp. 212–13.

48 On raised phosphorus levels, see Allan G. Hamilton, 'Light Treatment at an Infant Welfare Centre', *Public Health* (February 1927), 144–9, at p. 149; and Russell and Russell, *Ultra-violet Radiation*, pp. 126–7.

49 The glowing corpses of patients succumbing to radiation overexposure are poignant examples of bodily photogenesis: on the dial painters of the US Radium Corporation, see David I. Harvie, *Deadly Sunshine: The History and Fatal Legacy of Radium* (Stroud: Tempus, 2005), p. 172; on Radiothor patients, see Matthew Lavine, *The First Atomic Age: Scientists, Radiations, and the American Public, 1895–1945* (New York: Palgrave Macmillan, 2013), p. 150; on 'Radiogenol' patients, see Richard F. Mould, *A Century of X-Rays and Radioactivity in Medicine* (Bristol and Philadelphia, Pa.: Institute of Physics Publishing, 1993), p. 22; and on Thorotrast patients, see Bettyann Holtzmann Kevles, *Naked to the Bone: Medical Imaging in the Twentieth Century* (Reading: Helix Books, 1998), p. 105. See also Chapter 4.

50 Paul Overy, *Light, Air and Openness: Modern Architecture between the Wars* (London: Thames & Hudson, 2007), p. 80.

51 For an in-depth history of sunscreen development in America, see Dunne Romano, 'Dark Side of the Sun'. For its European context, see Carter, *Rise and Shine*, pp. 101–2; Andrieu, *Bronzage*, pp. 87–99; and Ory, *L'Invention du bronzage*, pp. 46–57. Other filters and screens included various interposing fabrics – sunshades or veils of muslin, dark paper, and even 'thin lead-foil' – and greasy substances such as olive oil, lanolin, pigmented soap, and Vaseline. See Bernhard, *Light Treatment*, pp. 90–1, 244; Vaughan-Cowell, *Artificial Sunlight*, p. 59; Russell and Russell, *Ultra-violet Radiation*, p. 157; Dane, *Sunlight Cure*, p. 18. Vaseline in particular fascinated because it fluoresced upon irradiation, taking on a bluish colour: Beaumont, *Fundamental Principles*, p. 14.

52 Raymond Williams, 'Advertising: The Magic System', in *Problems of Materialism and Culture: Selected Essays* (London and New York: Verso, 1997), pp. 170–95, at p. 187. Metaphors of eating light still occur today: Hobday discusses 'light hunger', light 'cravings', 'bingeing' on sunlight, and the 'vitamin D famine' in his books; see *Healing Sun*, p. 35, and *The Light Revolution: Health, Architecture and the Sun* (Forres: Findhorn Press, 2006), pp. 23–4. Woodruff references a Dr R. A. Katz using the phrase 'light hunger' in 1902, in Charles E. Woodruff, *The Effects of Tropical Light on White Men* (London and New York: Rebman, 1905), p. 95.

53 On ingestible radium products, see Thomas de la Peña, *Body Electric*, pp. xi–xii; and Spencer R. Weart, *Nuclear Fear: A History of Images* (Cambridge, Mass.: Harvard University Press, 1988), p. 50.

54 See Gladys Cooper's advertisement, *Pall Mall Magazine* (June 1934), p. 91; 'Ultra-violet ray bread' advertisement, *Derby Daily Telegraph*, 13 August 1927, p. 5; and Robert & Sons' advertisement, *Hereford Times*, 2 February 1935, p. 12. On 'Vitamilk', see Hanovia's advertisement in *The Times*, 'Sunlight and Health' special supplement, 22 May 1928 (hereafter *Times* supplement), p. xxxiii. On irradiating cereals, see Leonard Hill, 'Light against Disease', *The Times*, 4 July 1925, p. 10; and Bernhard, *Light Treatment*, pp. 102–3. On irradiating milk, beer and bread in America, see Daniel Freund, *American Sunshine: Diseases of Darkness and the Quest for Natural Light* (Chicago, Ill.: University of Chicago Press, 2012), pp. 135–63.

55 S. J. Cowell, 'Irradiation of Milk and the Healing of Rickets', *BMJ*, 28 March 1925, pp. 594–5.

56 See Dunne Romano, 'Dark Side of the Sun', pp. 64–6; Carter, *Rise and Shine*, pp. 42–3; and Alfred F. Hess, 'The Prevention and Cure of Rickets by Sunlight', *American Journal of Public Health*, 12:2 (1922), 104–7.

57 Dunne Romano, 'Dark Side of the Sun', p. 66.

58 Russell and Russell, *Ultra-violet Radiation*, pp. 131, 214–15.

59 On nutrition science, vegetarianism, and state interest in the national diet, see Zweiniger-Bargielowska, *Managing the Body*.

60 'À cause de la coloration de leur peau et de leur habitude de vivre demi-nus, les nègres sont plus aptes à se nourrir directement des rayons du soleil.' Albert Monteuuis, *L'Usage chez soi des bains d'air, de lumière et de soleil* (Nice: Librairie Visconti, 1911), p. 124.

61 Müller, *Sun-Bathing*, p. 67.

62 Bold original. Edward J. Deck, *The Sun and How to Use It* (London: Sunlight League, 1926), pp. 10–11. Hanovia's *Homesun* pamphlet similarly stated, 'We feed on plants raised in sunlight, or on animals reared on them – for all flesh is grass, and all grass is sunlight' (p. 2).

63 'All-electric farm', *Sunday Post*, 4 September 1927, p. 17. Vegetables, fruits, and plants grown underground with 'huge ultra-violet ray lamps' were reported to have grown better and quicker than in natural sunlight in an underground garden at Cumberland Lodge, Windsor Great Park, to the king and queen's amazement. See 'Nature Cheated by the Ultra-violet Ray', *Western Daily Press*, 26 May 1930, p. 7.

64 '"Vita" Glass: Value to Animal and Plant Life', *Times* supplement, p. xvii.

65 Jenkyn's 'Kensitas' cigarettes, *Yorkshire Evening Post*, 25 February 1931, p. 4. In America, Lucky Strike did the same; see Freund, *American Sunshine*, p. 143.

66 'Ultra-violet light: the need of a fit nation', Hanovia advertisement, *Punch*, 11 January 1928, p. x.

67 'The fight for sunlight, indeed, is a fight for humanity in the broadest sense of that term.' 'League of Nations and Health: New Study of Rickets', *Times* supplement, p. xxxi.

68 See Tania Woloshyn, 'Patients Rebuilt: Dr Auguste Rollier's Heliotherapeutic Portraits, *c*. 1903–1944', *Medical Humanities*, 39:1 (2013), 38–46.

69 Kathleen Vaughan, 'Three Reasons for Our Increasing Maternal Mortality', *Sunlight*, 2:7 (1932), 201–3. On Vaughan (d. 1957), see Carter, *Rise and Shine*, pp. 77–8; and Ornella Moscucci, 'Holistic Obstetrics: The Origins of "Natural Childbirth" in Britain', *Postgraduate Medical Journal*, 79:929 (2003), 168–73. Vaughan regularly contributed articles on emulating 'primitive' practices of outdoor living for healthy motherhood for *Sunlight*: 'Open-Air Life and Healthy Motherhood', *Sunlight*, 1:10 (1929), 21–2 and 'Three Reasons for Our Increasing Maternal Mortality', *Sunlight*, 2:7 (1932), 201–3.

70 See Carter, *Rise and Shine*, pp. 90–1; Ken Worpole, *Here Comes the Sun: Architecture and Public Space in Twentieth-Century European Culture* (London: Reaktion, 2000), pp. 57–9, 64–5; Esyllt Jones, 'Nothing Too Good for the People: Local Labour and London's Interwar Health Centre Movement', *Social History of Medicine*, 25:1 (2012), 84–102; and Hanovia, *The New Light Treatment Department (Solarium) in the Public Health Centre, Bermondsey* (Slough: Hanovia, 1936), p. 19.

71 Hanovia, *Homesun* pamphlet, pp. 7–8. See also *Actinotherapy Technique* (1933), pp. 110–12.

72 Dr L. C. Donnelly (1925), cited in *Actinotherapy Technique* (1933), p. 111.

73 Dora Colebrook, in Hill et al., 'Discussion on Influence of Sunlight', p. 476. On this clinic, see also Deck, *The Sun*, pp. 12–14.

74 On 'scientific motherhood', see Rima Apple, *Perfect Motherhood: Science and Childrearing in America* (New Brunswick: Rutgers University Press, 2006). On 'race mothers', see Zweiniger-Bargielowska, *Managing the Body*, pp. 105–48.

75 Catherine Chisholm and Margaret McKillop, 'Notes on Treatment of Nursing Mothers with Ultra-violet Rays', *Lancet*, 30 July 1927, p. 227. On Chisholm, see Mary Ann Elston, '"Run by Women (Mainly) for Women": Medical Women's Hospitals in Britain, 1866–1948', in Lawrence Conrad and Anne Hardy (eds), *Women and Modern Medicine* (Amsterdam and New York: Rodopi, 2001), pp. 73–107, at pp. 89–90.

76 *Actinotherapy Technique* (1933), pp. 111–12.

77 *Actinotherapy Technique* (1933), pp. 112, 172. See also Dr Harriette Chick, 'Cure of Rickets: Pioneer Work in Vienna', *Times* supplement, p. xxx; and Hobday, *Light Revolution*, pp. 55–6.

78 Wilhelm Flaskamp, 'Light and Heat Therapy in Gynaecology', *Light and Heat in Therapy: The Proceedings of the 2nd International Conference on Light and Heat in Medicine and Surgery, University of London, October–November 1928* (London: Actinic Press, 1929), pp. 20–37. On p. 27 he also cited a precursor to the electric lamps by Engelhorn known as the 'vaginal lamp', by which light, concentrated by lenses, was brought into the vagina through a speculum – a literal 'burning mirror'/speculum as theorised by Luce Irigaray. See Melissa Miles, *The Burning Mirror: Photography in an Ambivalent Light* (North Melbourne: Australian Scholarly Publishing, 2008).

79 Sir Henry Gauvain, 'Organisation and Work of a Light Department in a Hospital for Surgical Tuberculosis', *Lancet*, 4 July 1925, pp. 10–16, at p. 14.

80 See Mould, *Century of X-Rays*, pp. 120–6; Weart, *Nuclear Fear*, p. 48; Joel D. Howell, *Technology in the Hospital: Transforming Patient Care in the Early Twentieth Century* (Baltimore, Md.: Johns Hopkins University Press, 1996), pp. 146–50; Catherine Caufield, *Multiple Exposures: Chronicles of the Radiation Age* (London: Penguin, 1989), p. 17. Lavine noted, 'any bodily orifice might be exploited to help localize the irradiation, [and] patients might have wondered whether x-rays were really any less invasive than surgery', *First Atomic Age*, p. 83.

81 Lavine, *First Atomic Age*, p. 10. Howell also explained that physicians perceived women and babies easier to radiograph than men since they had less blood circulating in their bodies, and were thus easier to penetrate: Howell, *Technology in the Hospital*, p. 146.

82 Kevles, *Naked to the Bone*, p. 27.

83 Russell and Russell, *Ultra-violet Radiation*, pp. 157–8.

84 Russell and Russell, *Ultra-violet Radiation*, p. 158.

85 See Flaskamp, 'Light and Heat Therapy in Gynaecology', pp. 29, 35–7; W. Turner Wilson, 'Sun Baths in a Factory', *Times* supplement, p. xxii; Hanovia, *Homesun* pamphlet, p. 5; and Woodruff, *Effects of Tropical Light*, pp. 107, 120–1.

86 Dane, *Sunlight Cure*, p. 40; Thomas Nogier, *La Lumière et la vie* (Lyon: Imprimerie Waltener, 1904), p. 317; L. Revillet, 'De l'héliothérapie marine dans les tuberculoses abdominales, organes génito-urinaires', *Congrès de l'Association Internationale de Thalassothérapie de Cannes* (Paris: Éditions de la 'Gazette des eaux', 1914), p. 20. In the light's absence, the reverse took effect: 'It is also reported of Eskimo women that, during the polar night, their "periods" stop', Bernhard, *Light Treatment*, p. 51.

87 My emphasis. 'Sur le littoral méditerranéen et en particulier sur la Riviera, la menstruation est bien plus précoce que dans les climats du Nord. Les fillettes sont en général réglées de 10 à 11 ans; et ce n'est pas un fait d'atavisme, le même phénomène s'observe chez les enfants, dont les familles, originaires du Nord, viennent habiter la Côte d'Azur, et cela à

la grande stupéfaction de leurs parents.' Revillet, 'De l'héliothérapie marine', pp. 19–20. Carter has importantly noted that in the tropics white female colonisers were considered to be at particular risk, experiencing irregular menstruation, see *Rise and Shine*, p. 17.

88 Revillet, 'De l'héliothérapie marine', p. 17. On the Côte d'Azur's therapeutic climate, see Woloshyn, 'La Côte d'Azur: The *Terre Privilégié* of Invalids and Artists, *c.* 1860–1900', *French Cultural Studies*, 20:4 (2009), 383–402. On British attitudes to southern bodies and climates generally, see Carter, *Rise and Shine*, pp. 20–3; Littlewood, *Sultry Climates*; and John Pemble, *The Mediterranean Passion: Victorians and Edwardians in the South* (Oxford: Clarendon Press, 1987).

89 Marvine Brody, 'Gynécologie et la lumière', in Charles Brody (ed.), *Traité d'hélio- et d'actinologie: physique – biologie – thérapeutique*, 2 vols. (Paris: Maloine, 1938), vol. II, pp. 1463–73, at p. 1466.

90 Hanovia advertisement, *Sunlight*, 1:8 (1929), p. ii.

91 Schneider, 'Towards the Improvement of the Human Race', p. 278. See also Tania Woloshyn, 'Regenerative Tanning: Pigmentation, Neo-Lamarckian Eugenics and the Visual Culture of the *Cure de Soleil*', in Fae Brauer and Serena Keshavjee (eds), *Picturing Evolution and Extinction: Regeneration and Degeneration in Modern Visual Culture* (Newcastle upon Tyne: Cambridge Scholars Publishing, 2015), pp. 193–216.

92 Patrick Howarth, *When the Riviera Was Ours* (London: Routledge & Kegan Paul, 1977), p. 125.

93 D. H. Lawrence, 'Sun' (*c.* 1926) in Brian Finney (ed.), *D. H. Lawrence: Selected Short Stories* (Harmondsworth: Penguin, 1985), pp. 424–43, at p. 428. There are similar, overtly sexualised descriptions of sunbathing in André Gide's *L'Immoraliste* (1902). See Woloshyn, '"Kissed by the Sun"'; Carter also mentions Ernest Hemingway's *The Garden of Eden* (begun 1946) and F. Scott Fitzgerald's *Tender Is the Night* (1934), in *Rise and Shine*, p. 104.

94 Lawrence, 'Sun', p. 431. On gendered representations of the sun, see Melissa Miles, 'Sun-Pictures and Shadow-Play: Untangling the Web of Gendered Metaphors in Lady Elizabeth Eastlake's "Photography"', *Word & Image*, 24:1 (2008), 42–50.

95 Dane, *Sunlight Cure*, p. 16. Thomas de la Peña declared, 'We know that the terms "vim, vigor, virility, and vitality," when used between 1850 and 1930, almost always referred to sexual power', *Body Electric*, p. 140.

96 Dane, *Sunlight Cure*, pp. 12, 40. On ultraviolet light's effects on endocrine function, see Beaumont, *Fundamental Principles*, p. 80; and A. P. Cawadias, 'Ultra-violet Irradiation: Technique of Application', *British Journal of Physical Medicine*, 11:12 (1937), 225–9, at p. 227.

97 'Celanese' was an expensive artificial cellulose silk, or rayon, developed in 1905. See Paul Jobling, *Man Appeal: Advertising, Modernism and Men's Wear* (New York and Oxford: Berg, 2005), pp. 124–30. On 'Celanese' and other ultraviolet-permitting fabrics, see Hill, 'Discussion on Influence of Sunlight', 473; Hill, *Sunshine and Open Air*, pp. 124–5; Vaughan-Cowell, *Artificial Sunlight*, p. 58; Bernhard, *Light Treatment*, p. 75; 'Maternity and Child Welfare Conference in London (by a Woman Doctor)', *Yorkshire Evening Post*, 9 July 1926, p. 4. See also a 'Celanese' underwear advertisement in *Nash's and Pall Mall Magazine* (October 1925), p. 121.

98 J. C. Flügel, 'The Psychology of Clothes', *Sun Bathing Review*, 1:2 (1933), 14–15; and Graham Richards, 'Flügel, John Carl (1884–1955)', *Oxford Dictionary of National Biography*, www.oxforddnb.com/view/article/60995 (accessed 20 November 2014). Flügel was one of many diverse luminaries who penned a letter to *The Times* about nude sunbathing: The

other signatories included Rollier, Gibbings, Julian Huxley, George Bernard Shaw, writer and pacifist Vera Brittain, feminist and socialist campaigner Countess Dora Russell (wife of philosopher Bertrand Russell), and radiologist Alfred C. Jordan (founder of the Men's Dress Reform Party, a branch of the New Health Society and Sunlight League; see Carter, *Rise and Shine*, pp. 78–9). See 'Sun Bathing: Benefits of Light and Air [letter to the Editor]', *The Times*, 18 March 1932, p. 10.

99 J. A. Braun, 'The Need for Full Exposure of the Body', *Sun Bathing Review*, 1:2 (1933), 16.

100 On 'true' sunbathing, in the eyes of the nudist, versus 'popular' (partially clothed) sunbathing, see Alan Warwick's introduction in Bertram Park and Yvonne Gregory, *Sun Bathers* (London: George Routledge & Sons, Ltd, 1935), pp. vii–viii; and Thedering, *Sunlight as Healer*, p. 54. On the naturist's engagement with the environment, see Nina J. Morris, 'Naked in Nature: Naturism, Nature and the Senses in Early 20th Century Britain', *Cultural Geographies*, 16:3 (2009), 283–308.

101 Gibbings' cover was used for the first eight issues. For an example of his written contributions, see 'An Artist Speaks on Sun Bathing', *Sun Bathing Review*, 2:5 (1934), p. 10. See also Martin J. Andrews, *The Life and Work of Robert Gibbings* (Bicester: Primrose Hill Press, 2003), pp. 176–8. Gibbings was cited briefly for taking over the Golden Cockerel Press, in collaboration with Eric Gill (who also contributed to the journal), in Frances Spalding, *British Art since 1900* (London: Thames & Hudson, 1989), p. 71.

102 I wish to explore these images, and the magazine as a whole, in a future research project on naturism, natural therapies, and notions of 'exposure'. In some cases genitalia is violently scratched out in the reprinting process, presumably in order to be 'fit' for view, necessitating lines be literally drawn to distinguish 'art' from 'pornography'. The cover models were retouched/covered from winter 1943 (10:40). See also Shaffer, 'On the Environmental Nude', pp. 131–2.

103 On Sandow, see Ellery Foutch, 'Arresting Beauty: The Perfectionist Impulse of Peale's Butterflies, Heade's Hummingbirds, Blaschka's Flowers, and Sandow's Body' (Ph.D. dissertation, University of Pennsylvania, 2011). See also Tamar Garb, 'Modelling the Male Body: Physical Culture, Photography and the Classical Ideal', *Bodies of Modernity: Figure and Flesh in Fin-de-Siècle France* (London: Thames & Hudson, 1998), pp. 55–79.

104 See, for example, 2:5 (1934), which advertised services by George Gregory (Norwich) and Boutalls Ltd (London).

105 Cartwright, *Screening the Body*, p. 154.

106 Saleeby's writings were also included in *Sun Bathing Review*: e.g., 'Spreading the Light', 2:5 (1934), 1–2; and he provided the foreword for Hans Surén's *Man and Sunlight* (Slough: Sollux, 1927). However, as editor of the Sunlight League's journal, *Sunlight*, Saleeby spoke of disassociating the league's aims from those of the 'cult of nudity' (*Sunlight*, 1:8 [1929], 7). Nonetheless, an advertisement and enthusiastic article by Jordan about the Sun Bathing Society's activities were included in *Sunlight* (2:6 [1932], frontispiece and pp. 187–91). See also Zweiniger-Bargielowska, *Managing the Body*, pp. 168, 300; Morris, 'Naked in Nature'; and Worpole, *Here Comes the Sun*, pp. 47–8.

107 Carter wrote, 'the suntan is a visual symbol for the consumption of others and is acquired within the gaze of others. Originally the gaze was that of the approving medical professional but now this medical gaze has been replaced with the self-reflexive tourist's own gaze.' *Rise and Shine*, p. 103.

108 See the anonymous article on Gauvain, 'Sunlight Treatment', *Sun Bathing Review*, 3:11 (1935), 90–3. Contributing to diverse venues, Tudor-Hart produced photographs for

Pears Soap, 'Humanised Trufood', and Ovaltine Rusks, as well as for photo-essays in *Picture Post* and politically radical exhibitions such as the AIA (Artists International Association, founded in 1933). See Val Williams, *The Other Observers: Women Photographers in Britain, 1900 to the Present* (London: Virago Press, 1994), p. 129. For an example, see the Trufood Ltd advertisement in *The Times*, 14 February 1936, p. 6.

109 Park and Gregory, *Sun Bathers*, p. v. See also Bertram Park, 'Photography of the Nude', *Sun Bathing Review*, 3:10 (1935), 54–6, at p. 55.

110 Sheehan, *Doctored*, p. 96. Just like light therapy, exposure times for nineteenth-century photographs were similarly calculated according to the sitter's colouring: the lighter the skin, the shorter the exposure.

111 Warwick in Park and Gregory, *Sun Bathers*, p. xii. Warwick was friends with Gibbings, the two sunbathing together in Gibbings' garden; see Andrews, *Robert Gibbings*, p. 178.

112 Bernhard, *Light Treatment*, p. 244.

113 'Man beachte die wieder gewonnenen vollen und schön modellierten Körperformen und die glatte, prächtige Bronzehaut'. Bernhard, *Sonnenlichtbehandlung in der Chirurgie* (Stuttgart: Ferdinand Enke, 1917), p. 163. My thanks to Gabriele Neher for this translation.

114 See, for example, Kellogg, *Light Therapeutics*, p. 43; Bernhard, *Light Treatment*, p. 67; Flügel, 'The Psychology of Clothes', p. 14. It occurred in populist texts as well, Müller describing the suntanning process as one of 'hardening' the skin yet rendering it as 'soft as velvet' (*Sun-Bathing*, p. 42).

115 See Russell and Russell, *Ultra-violet Radiation*, p. 113. Part of light therapy's appeal for lupus vulgaris patients was its aesthetic effects, resulting in excellent scar tissue, unlike previous treatments. See Finsen, *Phototherapy*, p. 71. Jamieson explained that lupus vulgaris was often confused with syphilis, a disease known to be sexually transmitted and thus morally charged; Anne Kinloch Jamieson, 'An Intolerable Affliction: A History of Lupus Vulgaris in Late Nineteenth- and Early Twentieth-Century Britain' (Ph.D. dissertation, University of Leeds, 2010), p. 47. Dane stated that sunlight was used to treat syphilis in *Sunlight Cure*, pp. 40–1, suggesting light could be both a source of sexual health and sexual danger.

116 Flügel, 'The Psychology of Clothes', p. 14. On light's euphoric effects, see Woloshyn, '*Le Pays du soleil*'.

117 Rollier, *Pansement solaire*, p. 72. The addictive nature of actinic light has been described more recently as 'tanorexia', stimulating the body's endorphins, dopamine, and testosterone in men. See Hobday, *Light Revolution*, p. 35.

118 I discuss the subject of 'exposing' children in light therapy's history in a forthcoming publication with Natasha McEnroe, associated with the Wellcome Trust-funded exhibition, 'The Kiss of Light' (Florence Nightingale Museum, 2015). See also Chapter 1.

119 Regarding Hill, see 'The Ultra-violet Ray … 400 Children in Test', *Nottingham Evening Post*, 9 February 1931, p. 1; and Leonard Hill and J. Argyll Campbell, 'Metabolism of Children Undergoing Open-Air Treatment, Heliotherapy and Balneotherapy', *BMJ*, 25 February 1922, pp. 301–3. Regarding Colebrook, see Hill et al., 'Discussion on Influence of Sunlight'. Several trials involving children are listed in *Actinotherapy Technique* (1943), pp. 96–8. See also the work of Lederer: *Subjected to Science: Human Experimentation in America before the Second World War* (Baltimore, Md.: Johns Hopkins University Press, 1995); 'Orphans as Guinea Pigs: American Children and Medical Experimenters, 1890–1930', in Roger Cooter (ed.), *In the Name of the Child: Health and Welfare, 1880–1940* (London

and New York: Routledge, 1992), pp. 96–123; and 'Children as Guinea Pigs: Historical Perspectives', *Accountability in Research: Policies and Quality Assurance*, 10:1 (2003), 1–16.

120 Public-health clinics using light therapy treated infants, pre-school and school-age children suffering from rickets and vitamin deficiencies, malnutrition, anaemia, 'functional nerve troubles', catarrh, and the 'pre-tuberculous'. Katherine Gamgee, 'The Child's Heritage of Health', *Sunlight*, 1:8 (1929), 26–7.

121 See Hanovia, *Homesun* pamphlet, p. 8; G. B. Dixon, in Hill et al., 'Discussion on Influence of Sunlight', 474; Beaumont, *Fundamental Principles*, p. 108; Russell and Russell, *Ultra-violet Radiation*, pp. 134, 222–3; and Bernhard, *Light Treatment*, p. 50.

122 Colebrook, in Hill et al., 'Discussion on Influence of Sunlight', p. 476.

123 See Dixon et al., 'Discussion on the Therapeutic Value of Light', p. 501. See also 'Light as Brain Food', *The Times*, 29 May 1925, p. 5.

124 'The Sun Cure for Surgical Tuberculosis', *BMJ*, 21 July 1923, pp. 111–12, at p. 112.

125 See also Linda Bryder, '"Wonderlands of Buttercup, Clover and Daisies": Tuberculosis and the Open-Air School Movement in Britain, 1907–39', in Roger Cooter (ed.), *In the Name of the Child*, pp. 72–95, at p. 79.

126 Frances Hodgson Burnett, *The Secret Garden* (London: William Heinemann, 1911). Many contemporaneous children's novels celebrate children growing in the fresh air and sunlight, including the early and influential *Heidi* (1880). My thanks to Natasha McEnroe for this.

127 See Eidinow, 'A Note on Phototherapy', pp. 647–8; Hamilton, 'Infant Welfare Centre', p. 148; and Katherine Gamgee, *The Artificial Light Treatment of Children* (London: H. K. Lewis & Co., 1927), pp. 38–9.

128 Russell and Russell, *Ultra-violet Radiation*, p. 116. They specified: 'Children can stand about half the dose of an adult male of a similar type, and infants about half that of children. Women are as a rule more sensitive than men, and sensitiveness decreases as age increases' (p. 150).

129 See Stella Churchill, 'The Care of Children when Sun-Bathing', *Sunlight*, 1:8 (1929), 8–9; Charles Corfield, 'Sun-Bathing', *The Times*, 10 July 1935, p. 10; and 'Sunbathing: Liberty and Precaution', *The Times*, 6 July 1938, p. 21.

130 Cooter, *In the Name of the Child*, p. 12.

131 Deck, *The Sun*, p. 13. He further singled out Treloar's branches, the London Hospital, and the Heritage Craft Schools at Chailey (about which the Wellcome Library has a rare photographic album marking Rollier's visit in 1924, ref. 680190i). Vaughan-Cowell, who worked under Deck, reported he treated 400 patients daily at the London Light Clinic. Deck stated it had the capacity to treat 1,000 patients daily. See Vaughan-Cowell, *Artificial Sunlight*, p. 50; and Edward J. Deck, 'The London Clinic', *Sunlight*, 1:10 (1929), 32.

132 Dane, *Sunlight Cure*, p. 79. Thedering also appealed directly to mothers (*Sunlight as Healer*, p. 54). Even in 1890 Palm urged mothers to systematically expose their children, and themselves, as a preventive public-health measure against rickets: Theobald A. Palm, 'The Geographical Distribution and Aetiology of Rickets', *Practitioner*, 45:4 (1890), 270–9, and 45:5 (1890), 321–42, at p. 342.

133 Russell and Russell, *Ultra-violet Radiation*, p. 140. See also the photograph included in Gamgee, *Children*, p. 11.

134 On the Sunlight League's facilities at Kenwood (1924), see *Sunlight*, 1:10 (1929), 3–5. In 1930, it also created a sunbathing centre in Regent's Park, treating 148 children, see *Sunlight*, 2:7 (1932), 200.

135 'Artificial Sunlight Treatment', *The Times*, 19 March 1925, p. 11.

136 Beaumont, *Fundamental Principles*, p. 7.

137 Hill, 'Discussion on Influence of Sunlight', p. 471. See also Vaughan-Cowell, *Artificial Sunlight*, pp. 36, 38, 51; and Russell and Russell, *Ultra-violet Radiation*, p. 102.

138 John Stanislav Sadar, '"Vita" Glass and the Discourse of Modern Culture', in Grace Lees-Maffei (ed.), *Writing Design: Words and Objects* (London and New York: Berg, 2012), pp. 103–17, at p. 111. See also Sadar, 'Unpacking'; Carter, *Rise and Shine*, p. 68; and Hobday, *Light Revolution*, p. 121. On the London Zoo's installation of lamps and 'Vita' glass, animals, and children, see G. M. Vevers, 'Fresh Air and Sunlight at the Zoo', *Sunlight*, 1:8 (1929), 21–3.

139 Carter, *Rise and Shine*, p. 64. On eugenics, social hygiene, and nationhood specifically, see pp. 24–8, 66–7, 71–2, and Zweiniger-Bargielowska, *Managing the Body*, p. 166.

140 See Linda Bryder, 'Wonderlands of Buttercup'; and Overy, *Light, Air and Openness*, p. 127.

141 Bernhard, *Light Treatment*, p. 236.

142 'The Sterilisation of Water by Ultra-violet Rays', *Lancet*, 5 February 1916, p. 310; 'Military Hygiene and the Efficiency of the Soldier', *BMJ*, 27 March 1915, pp. 553–4; and 'Medical Arrangement of the British Expeditionary Forces', *BMJ*, 6 February 1915, pp. 264–5; and Russell and Russell, *Ultra-violet Radiation*, p. 105.

143 See Rabinbach, *Human Motor*, p. 260.

144 See William Beaumont, 'The Timbre of the Twenties', *The Times*, 8 July 1939, p. 13.

145 See Rollier, *Pansement solaire*; and Bernhard, *Light Treatment*, pp. 164–76. See also Hobday, *Healing Sun*, pp. 95–9. French sources include Gontrand Léo, *Trois mois de chirurgie de guerre* (Paris: Maloine, 1915); and Gontrand Léo, 'Héliothérapie et plaies traumatiques ou chirurgicales (non tuberculeuses)', in Charles Brody (ed.), *Traité d'hélio- et d'actinologie: physique – biologie – thérapeutique*, 2 vols. (Paris: Maloine, 1938), vol. II, pp. 1257–86; Maurice Cazin, *La Cure solaire des blessures de guerre (méthode Rollier)* (Paris: Maloine, 1917).

146 Rollier, *Pansement solaire*, pp. 5, 7.

147 Rollier, *Pansement solaire*, pp. 85–7.

148 See Hill, 'Discussion on Influence of Sunlight', p. 473; W. J. Turrell, *The Principles of Electrotherapy and their Practical Application* (Oxford: Oxford University Press, 1929), frontispiece; 'Physical Therapy in the Navy', *BMJ*, 15 May 1920, pp. 683–4; Maurice Weinbren, 'A Chronic War Wound Treated by Ultra-violet Radiation', *British Journal of Actinotherapy*, 1:9 (October 1926), 16–19; *Actinotherapy Technique* (1933), pp. 203–4, and (1943), pp. 200–10; Deck, *The Sun*, p. 14; Russell and Russell, *Ultra-violet Radiation*, pp. 13–14; and Bernhard, *Light Treatment* (p. 174).

149 See Hanovia, *Homesun* pamphlet, p. 8; 'Rays – then Hoorays', *Derby Daily Telegraph*, 4 January 1929, p. 4; 'Two of the Hull City Football Players Receiving Artificial Sunlight Treatment', *Hull Daily Mail*, 3 March 1930, p. 2; and *Leicester City Is the First Team to Adopt the Electric Sun Treatment for Their Players*, Greater Manchester County Archives, GB124.DPA/1129/30, photograph.

150 Carter, *Rise and Shine*, p. 34. He addressed the scouting movement, muscular Christianity, the growth of camping, and pastorialism, pp. 33–6.

151 Hill, 'Discussion on Influence of Sunlight', p. 473; and *Sunshine and Open Air*, p. 93.

152 See 'Let Children Live in Sunshine!' *Yorkshire Evening Post*, 28 May 1926, p. 5.

153 Colour photography became available on the market in the mid-1930s; see Hentschel, *Mapping the Spectrum*, p. 208; and Kelley Wilder, *Photography and Science* (London: Reaktion, 2009), pp. 69–71.

154 In *White*, Dyer argued that 'shine' is aligned with sweat, dirt, and 'non-white people' (p. 78) and 'glow' with 'idealised white women' (p. 122). See also Connor, 'Integuments', p. 50. In the figures throughout this chapter, figures display both 'shine' and 'glow', exemplifying the collapse of racial distinctions.

155 See Sarah Street, *Colour Films in Britain: The Negotiation of Innovation, 1900–55* (Houndmills: Palgrave Macmillan on behalf of the British Film Institute, 2012), p. 60; and Tom Gunning, 'Colorful Metaphors: The Attraction of Color in Early Silent Cinema', *Living Pictures*, 2:2 (2003), 4–13. Intriguingly, the technical guidelines for using Technicolor, as designed by Natalie Kalmus, were premised upon intense lighting conditions using arc lamps, see Street, *Colour Films in Britain*, p. 54; and Dyer, *White*, pp. 89–93.

156 See Sander Gilman, *Making the Body Beautiful: A Cultural History of Aesthetic Surgery* (Princeton, NJ: Princeton University Press, 1999); Carter, *Rise and Shine*, p. 110; Sheehan, *Doctored*, pp. 93–5. As Batchelor noted, 'If colour is cosmetic, it is added to the surface of things, and probably at the last moment. It does not have a place *within* things; it is an after-thought; it can be rubbed off'. David Batchelor, *Chromophobia* (London: Reaktion, 2005), p. 52.

157 Müller wrote, 'an unclean, white-grey skin, with black spots, red blotches and yellow patches is repulsive to all healthy minds' (*Sun-Bathing*, p. 99). Most suspect was the face, the physiognomic seat of beauty and character. Contemporaneous advertisements selling 'whitening' beauty products to remove freckles, suntan, and sunburn – described as 'ugly' and unwanted – were specifically targeted for facial use. Regarding concerns over tanned faces, see Vaughan-Cowell, *Artificial Sunlight*, p. 59; and Hanovia, *Homesun* pamphlet, p. 7.

158 Batchelor, *Chromophobia*, pp. 22–3. See also Roland Barthes, *Camera Lucida: Reflections on Photography* (London: Vintage, 2000), p. 81; and W. J. T. Mitchell, *What Do Pictures Want? The Lives and Loves of Images* (Chicago, Ill.: University of Chicago Press, 2005), p. 308.

159 Batchelor, *Chromophobia*, p. 71. On British artists and negrophilia, see Spalding, *British Art since 1900*, p. 96; Overy, *Light, Air and Openness*, p. 188; and Dyer, *White*, p. 49. More generally, see Petrine Archer-Straw, *Negrophilia: Avant-Garde Paris and Black Culture in the 1920s* (London: Thames & Hudson, 2000); Susan Guber, *Racechanges: White Skin, Black Face in American Culture* (Oxford: Oxford University Press, 1997); Jan Nederveen Pieterse, *White on Black: Images of Africa and Blacks in Western Popular Culture* (New Haven, Conn.: Yale University Press, 1992); and Marianna Torgovnick, *Gone Primitive: Savage Intellects, Modern Lives* (Chicago, Ill.: University of Chicago Press, 1991).

160 Thedering, *Sunlight as Healer*, pp. 24, 28; and Bryder, 'Wonderlands of Buttercup', p. 80. For naturists such as Warwick, light itself 'clothed' the body (Park and Gregory, *Sun Bathers*, p. xiii). See also Dunne Romano, 'Dark Side of the Sun', pp. 51–2; and Connor, 'Integuments', p. 50.

161 Ryan Johnson, 'European Cloth and "Tropical" Skin: Clothing Material and British Ideas of Health and Hygiene in Tropical Climates', *Bulletin of the History of Medicine*, 83:3 (2009), 530–60, at p. 559. See also Woodruff, *Effects of Tropical Light*; and 'Coloured Clothing for Tropics', *The Times*, 20 June 1922, p. 12.

162 Johnson, 'European Cloth and "Tropical" Skin', p. 555.

163 Carter, *Rise and Shine*, pp. 17–18. See also Dan Stone, *Breeding Superman: Nietzsche, Race and Eugenics in Edwardian and Interwar Britain* (Liverpool: Liverpool University Press, 2002), p. 107.

164 See Miles, *Burning Mirror*, pp. 43–4, 68–9. Interestingly, in Troup's third edition of *Therapeutic Uses of Infra-Red Rays* (1936), he included an appendix on infrared photography (pp. 142–7). He discussed an infrared photograph of a 'negro' that showed the subject's

skin as light but concluded this only enabled easier reading of his racial origin: 'The photograph showed the racial characteristics far better than a normal photograph. In this case a strain of Mongoloid descent was at once perceived by ethnologists' (pp. 146–7). The disconcerting reversal occurred when viewing negatives too, Vogel writing, 'The white face is made black, and the black coat, light. No one would hang up on his wall a picture representing him as a Moor.' Hermann Vogel, *The Chemistry of Light and Photography* (New York: D. Appleton & Co., 1875), p. 46.

165 Ahmed, 'Animated Borders', p. 58. Müller wrote, 'It is a curious fact, that not all white men can obtain the shining golden-brown colour. A few get a *dirty* dark-brown, some others a yellowish colour, and some – in most cases the red-haired – get only freckles' (my italics, *Sun-Bathing*, p. 46).

166 See Caleb Saleeby, *Sunlight and Health, Parenthood and Race-Culture* (New York: Moffat, Yard & Co., 1909); and Caleb Saleeby, *The Progress of Eugenics* (London: Cassell & Co., 1914).

167 'Ava' ultraviolet soap advertisement, *Devon and Exeter Gazette*, 12 August 1932, p. 3.

168 Anne McClintock, *Imperial Leather: Race, Gender and Sexuality in the Colonial Contest* (London and New York: Routledge, 1995), especially her discussion of the 'Chlorinol' advertisement, pp. 220–1. See also Rebecca Herzig, 'Removing Roots: "North American Hiroshima Maidens" and the X-Ray', *Technology and Culture*, 40 (1999), 723–45; Amina Mire, '"Skin Trade": Genealogy of Anti-Ageing "Whiteness Therapy" in Colonial Medicine', *Medicine Studies*, 4:1–4 (2014), 119–29; Claudia Benthien, *Skin: On the Cultural Border between Self and the World*, trans. T. Dunlap (New York: Columbia University Press, 2002), p. 148; Sheehan, *Doctored*, pp. 89–90; and Thomas de la Peña on radium and X-ray experiments of *c.* 1903–4 to turn 'Negroes' white in *Body Electric*, pp. 171–2; and 'Bleaching the Ethiopian: Desegregating Race and Technology through Early X-Ray Experiments', *Technology and Culture*, 47:1 (2006), 27–55. Fascinatingly, one well-known radiologist believed to have taken part in the experiments was Dr Henry Pancoast, the son of Dr Seth Pancoast, who wrote about the merits of blue-light therapy (1877) as discussed by Sheehan. Ultraviolet radiation has the ability to both produce colour and remove it; it can pigment skin and bleach the pigment out of fabrics. Hanovia's user manual warned that the 'Homesun' would fade the carpets like sunshine (*A Short Book of Instructions for Users of the 'Homesun' Sunlamp*, user manual, 1940, p. 5). This bleaching effect is encapsulated in the French word, *décoloration*, a phenomenon that intrigued and perplexed artists encountering the intense Mediterranean sun and its 'blanching' of local colour. See Woloshyn, 'Aesthetic and Therapeutic Imprints: Artists and Invalids on the Côte d'Azur, *c.* 1890–1910', *Nineteenth-Century Art Worldwide*, 11:1 (2012).

169 Dunne Romano, 'Dark Side of the Sun', pp. 50–1. She noted this was in contrast to contemporaneous Australian fears over the instability of 'whiteness', as discussed by Warwick Anderson, *The Cultivation of Whiteness: Science, Health and Racial Destiny in Australia* (New York: Basic Books, 2003). See also Dyer, *White*, pp. 49, 57; and Freund, *American Sunshine*, p. 106.

170 For Woodruff, acclimatisation was ultimately impossible (*Effects of Tropical Light*, pp. 271, 321). He considered that each race, based on degrees of pigmentation, belonged to particular environmental zones according to sunshine levels, and that racial stock eventually deteriorated as a result (p. 216). See also Sheehan, *Doctored*, pp. 90–4, 104; Carter, *Rise and Shine*, pp. 13–16; and Johnson, 'European Cloth and "Tropical" Skin', p. 548.

171 Müller, *Sun-Bathing*, p. 46.

172 Müller, *Sun-Bathing*, pp. 21–2. In this he attempted to distance himself from Surén's *Nachtkultur* movement. Woodruff believed excessive light exposure accounted for immorality, crime, drunkenness, suicide, and disease in America; see *Effects of Tropical Light*, pp. 217–23. Curiously, others noted the moralising (as opposed to immoralising) effect of sunbathing; see, for example, Deck, *The Sun*, p. 9.

173 Emphasis original. 'Le Docteur Renon parlant d'une visite faite par lui à Leysin, disait: "J'ai été extrêmement impressionné de voir des malades *noirs* comme des nègres, avec des plaies bacillaires considérables et multiples cicatrisées, des tumeurs blanches guéries; sans les photographies des lésions avant le traitement, jamais on n'aurait pu croire que de pareils désordres aient pu exister auparavant."' Lamaison, *De l'Héliothérapie dans la tuberculose*, p. 62. Pertinently, the word *impressionné* here can mean both 'impressed' and 'upset'.

174 See John W. Brannan, 'Heliotherapy in Tuberculosis of the Bones and Joints', *Transactions of the American Clinical and Climatological Association*, 30 (1914), 149–64, at p. 160.

175 Dane, *Sunlight Cure*, pp. 10–11.

176 Maren Möhring, 'Working Out the Body's Boundaries: Physiological, Aesthetic, and Psychic Dimensions of the Skin in German Nudism, 1890–1930', in Christopher E. Forth and Ivan Crozier (eds), *Body Parts: Critical Explorations in Corporeality* (Lanham, Md.: Lexington, 2005), pp. 229–46, at pp. 234–5. There are significant correspondences and intersections with the German movements of *Lebensreform* (life reform), *Nachtkultur*, and *Freikörperkultur* (free body culture); see Karl Toepfer, *Empire of Ecstasy: Nudity and Movement in German Body Culture, 1910–1935* (Berkeley, Calif.: University of California Press, 1997).

177 Bernhard, *Light Treatment*, p. 62.

178 Bernhard, *Light Treatment*, p. 57.

179 'Algeria: The Land of Romance', *Times* supplement, p. xxvi.

180 Charles Brody, 'Technique de Brody', in Charles Brody (ed.), *Traité d'hélio- et d'actinologie: physique – biologie – thérapeutique*, 2 vols. (Paris: Maloine, 1938), vol. I, pp. 798–812, at p. 800.

181 'Il peut même arriver que l'apparition d'une pigmentation subite et intense soit l'élément d'un pronostic sévère et, quelquefois même, le prodrome d'un dénouement fatal et à brève échéance. C'est le cas des cachectiques. Chez eux, nous avons constaté qu'après une courte exposition, à dose insignifiante même, il se produisait une pigmentation subite et intense de couleur chocolat. Loin d'être de bon augure, chez eux, cette pigmentation rapide et foncée signifie une désintégration tissulaire de l'organisme en voie de destruction et est comparable, pour nous, comme signe avertisseur.' Brody, 'Technique de Brody', p. 799.

182 Brody, 'Technique de Brody', pp. 802, 804.

183 Brody, 'Technique de Brody', p. 812.

184 Thedering, *Sunlight as Healer*, p. 24.

185 Beaumont, *Fundamental Principles*, p. 95.

186 Surén, already well known for his nudist publications during the Weimar Republic, joined the Nazi Party in 1933 as a specialist in physical education in the Reich Labour Service. See Michael Hau, *The Cult of Health and Beauty in Germany: A Social History, 1890–1930* (Chicago, Ill.: University of Chicago Press, 2003), p. 189; Overy, *Light, Air and Openness*, p. 164; and Worpole, *Here Comes the Sun*, p. 44.

187 Alfred Noyes, *The Return of the Scare-Crow* (London: Cassell & Co., 1929), pp. 11, 88, 91, 131. On sunbathing and the 'noble savage', pastoralism, and primitivism, see Carter, *Rise and Shine*, p. 36; Sadar, '"Vita" Glass', p. 108; and Weart, *Nuclear Fear*, p. 41.

188 Analysing nineteenth-century American photographic portraits of black subjects, Sheehan similarly concluded, 'While light could rescue etiolated bodies from their pathological state, moreover, it also had the potential to close the perceived gap between the races, thus threatening to break down the crucial boundaries that defined social difference. As a result, phototherapeutic and photographic light had the power to darken and lighten, compose and decompose, as well as physically and chemically alter the complexion of a nation' (*Doctored*, p. 104).

189 It was already clear that X rays could (and were actively used to) sterilise the sexual organs, see Weart, *Nuclear Fear*, pp. 47, 52. The Nazis planned to secretly sterilise unsuspecting Jewish men and women at an estimated rate of 4,000 per day; see Kevles, *Naked to the Bone*, p. 123. Later, with the advent of atomic energy, some British writers playfully speculated on the possibility of 'atomic birth control' and 'atomic hereditary control' by means of 'controlled mutations', presenting an interesting reversal. See Christoph Laucht, '"Dawn – or Dusk?" Britain's *Picture Post* Confronts Nuclear Energy', in Dick van Lente (ed.), *The Nuclear Age in Popular Media: A Transnational History, 1945–1965* (New York: Palgrave MacMillan, 2012), pp. 117–48, at p. 135. Technologies designed to produce, inhibit, or control reproduction have caused and continue to cause controversy, see Michelle Stanworth (ed.), *Reproductive Technologies: Gender, Motherhood and Medicine* (Cambridge: Polity, 1987), pp. 10–11.

6

Dead points

In dealing with the effect of the Sun's rays on our bodies we have to bear in mind that every good thing in this world, whatever its nature – everything we come to regard as a blessing – contains within itself the power of its own destruction, if **misused**, that is wrongly used, or **abused**, that is, used in excess. A drug may cure – and the same drug may kill. [...] So it is with the Sun's rays.[1]

(Edward J. Deck, 1926)

The sun has got his hat on, hip-hip-hip-hooray.
The sun has got his hat on and he's coming out today.
Now we'll all be happy, hip-hip-hip-hooray.
The sun has got his hat on and he's coming out today.
He's been tanning niggers, out in Timbuktu.
Now he's coming back, to do the same to you.
So jump into your sunbath, hip-hip-hip-hooray.
The sun has got his hat on and he's coming out today.[2]

(Ralph Butler and Noel Gay, 'The Sun Has Got His Hat On', 1932)

FROM the din of a bare, expansive room, scattered white shapes and bright vermillion blotches emerge and demand our attention (Plate 8). It is an otherwise calm, even dull scene, the stillness conveyed by the rigid, upright poses of several composed nurses and their limp horizontal patients. Beatrice Langdon's oil painting, *The Finsen Light Treatment at the London Hospital* of c. 1938, is an unusual and mysterious work, now contained in the closed stores of the Wellcome Library. Little is known about Langdon, and there is no evidence as to why she made this painting.[3] Produced almost four decades after the institutionalisation of light therapy in Britain (1900), Langdon's painting depicts the original, and by now obsolete, versions of Finsen's carbon arc lamp at a moment when the London Hospital was to refit new, smaller, and more efficient lamps in its light department.[4] Acting as a kind of commemorative portrait of the Finsen lamp and its impact in the battle against lupus vulgaris, the painting included a choice, off-handed phrase by Queen Alexandra that was etched into the wall of the newly completed department in 1903: 'Nothing like perseverance.'[5] The remark was no doubt intended to encourage both patient and nurse. A year earlier, it was noted in the *BMJ* that,

> Each sitting lasts an hour and a quarter on, it may be, two or three hundred different days or even more. Thus the course of treatment for the [lupus vulgaris] patient means a substantial slice out of his life and the individual sitting for the nurse means an hour of constant strain of attention and a large amount of muscular fatigue.[6]

Prized for their meticulous attention to detail and high degree of skill, nurses were the primary operators of the Finsen lamp. Though Langdon's painting gives prominence to the large central lamps, detailing their metal supports, telescopic brass arms, red skirting, and scattered white light, the true figures of the work are the nurses. The patients, by comparison, appear ghostly and unfinished, barely noticeable next to their attendants' crisp white uniforms and goggled faces.

Langdon's choice of medium may be a rarity – it is the only British painting of light therapy I have seen – but her choice of subject is certainly not. The nurse is a ubiquitous figure in the visual culture of light therapy, ever present in archival photographs as an observant technophile or intimate carer (Figs. 1.3, 1.10, 2.6, 2.8–2.9, 3.1, 3.11–3.13, 3.16–3.17, 4.3, 4.15). Yet her role was only marginally discussed in the medical literature; highly visible in images, seemingly invisible in texts. The role of nurses in light therapy's development has only recently begun to be addressed, and they are among many 'invisibles' in its history that deserve further attention: Langdon, Edith Tudor-Hart, Dr Dora Colebrook, the all-female staff of the SLHWC, and even Queen Alexandra, these are important female agents who actively contributed to the therapy's development and dissemination in late nineteenth- and early twentieth-century Britain.[7]

Equally silent are the voices of patients, especially children, and of various members of the public who consumed home-use lamps and their emanating ultraviolet light.[8] Furthermore, who were the anonymous photographers providing images for key practitioners, institutions, and the press? Where are the archives of now-defunct manufacturers? And what of the therapy's 'other' subjects – those bodies of 'colour' in Chapter 5 – who proved so valuable to practitioners' perceptions of suntan? Was light therapy really only ever a 'white' therapy, the privilege of those whose skin readily consumed ultraviolet radiation and pigmented?

Dr Murray Levick, describing light-therapy experiments he carried out at St Thomas' Hospital on child patients exhibiting 'debility, with anorexia, listlessness, general malnutrition and fretfulness', stated in 1924: 'It was interesting to note that a little negro boy made very tardy progress alongside a white boy who made a rapid recovery.'[9] Since solar erythema (Chapter 1) and pigmentation (Chapter 4) on white skin became the visible standards with which to measure therapeutic progress, dark skin remained – and remains to this day – either a foil or a 'problem'.[10] With their resistant bodies and troubling skin, dark subjects refuse to assimilate to normative (white) treatments of light exposure, presenting a dead end to the practitioner.

In Chapter 5 I briefly mentioned another, related dead end for practitioners: excessive pigmentation in the white patient. For Dr Franz Thedering, too deep a suntan could inhibit further curative effect. The deep tan, acting as a protective 'coat of armour', impeded the body's absorption of ultraviolet radiation, signalling a dead end or plateau during treatment.[11] Dr William Beaumont called this the 'dead point'.[12] From this point treatment would stop, and the skin would be allowed time to rest and recover. Once the skin lost its tan, the treatment would start again, creating cycles of 'dead points' and recoveries.

Looking back on this today with hindsight, the phrase 'dead point' is particularly apt, especially in relation to messages from Cancer Research UK about sunburn and suntan as explicit, and potentially life-threatening, forms of bodily damage. As an initial inhibitor to progressing forward, the 'dead point' finds resonance with light therapy's numerous historical dead ends. In this book I have put medical practitioners in the driver's seat. This is not to say, however, that it was a smooth or easy journey for them, or an unaccompanied one. Artists, patients, members of the public, and manufacturers came along for the ride.[13] The difficulty of finding their voices revolves around access: limited or non-existent sources, restricted archives, and lost memories.[14] Silences, absences, loose threads, and dead ends are prevalent in this largely understudied topic.

So too could we view the key images discussed in each chapter as 'failures'. After being introduced to light therapy through images collapsing the distinction between medical and popular exposures in Chapter 1, we looked at poorly 'fixed' photographs of solar erythema in Chapter 2 and damaged photographs in Chapter 3. In Chapter 4, montages of lamps and their invisible emanating energies confounded us further, and in Chapter 5 we were dazzled by colour pamphlets of models less bronzed than fluorescent. All of these images might be said to have failed to disseminate the therapy's efficacies and methods clearly and legibly. Yet, as the book has argued throughout, the intersection of art and medicine need not be fluid or seamless. The images and objects are fascinating and significant precisely because they are problematic: confounding, ambiguous, and perplexing. Resistant and wily, they instead communicate vital information about practitioners' anxious investment to substantiate light therapy's many *values*: its medical 'worth', which practitioners struggled to establish through dosage standardisation amidst damning reports and contradictory exposure methods; its social 'aims', not least its claim to regenerate a 'sun-starved' nation of

'C3' citizens through the use of potentially lethal home-use lamps; and to do this aesthetically through gradations of 'luminosity', using black-and-white photographs to represent the variable red hues of sunburn, overexposed photographs and fantastical montages that obscure the therapeutic process, and saturated colour pamphlets in which white models become radioactive 'primitives'. Such values are embedded within these images, material objects shot, snipped, and printed to become complex and complicated things. As Alan Mayne put it:

> a great deal of material culture evidence – because it is fragmentary and incomplete, or because of its scale and volume, or its imperfect fit with other historical sources – is profoundly opaque and unfamiliar to interpreters in the present day. [...] That is their value. It is because material culture is not simple and transparent in its meanings that the effort required to comprehend its full complexity and to compare it usefully with other sources translates into open-ended research questions which [sic] can extend our understanding of past societies and habitats.[15]

What of the present? Can looking at the past, especially through images and objects, prove useful to thinking about our ambivalent relationship with natural and artificial sunlight today? Conversely, can contemporary images help us to rethink the past?

As of April 2011, UK legislation has prohibited sunbed usage to people under eighteen, in an effort to protect British youth from ultraviolet radiation exposure. It emerged amidst fears of a new beauty 'addiction' for the euphoric highs of tanning, termed 'tanorexia'.[16] Two years later, Cancer Research UK asked image-conscious British girls, 'R UV Ugly?' Its SunSmart campaign employed the terms 'ugly' and 'ageing' synonymously to educate the public about the damaging effects of ultraviolet light. It was a bold attempt to wrest apart the long-standing association between tanned skin, beauty, and youthfulness that continues to fuel a flourishing tourism industry to sunny locales abroad and the tanning industry in the UK. Meanwhile, rising concern about vitamin-D deficiency among children has forecast the 'return' of rickets, prompting mixed views from the medical community and the media.[17] Light therapy for mental health, in the treatment of SAD and depression, and its ongoing use for dermatological conditions indicates it remains within mainstream medicine. In 2016, *Prima* magazine informed its middle-class, middle-aged female readers that, among its '16 Simple Steps to Help You Feel Fitter, Healthier and Happier Every Day', number 7 was 'Wear sunscreen every day' and number 8 was 'Don't be D-ficient'.[18] It is but one of many examples of popular literature, sourcing the latest medical advice, recommending both protection from and exposure to sunlight. With such conflicting messages rife within the medical community and disseminated to the public, can we definitively answer the question: is sunlight good or bad for our health and that of our children?

Crucially, as I have argued in this book, the contemporaneous and contradictory array of attitudes – of fear versus desire – towards the therapeutic value of natural and artificial light is not a new phenomenon. 'Indeed the history of bodies and sunlight is one of controversy and disagreement', to quote Simon Carter.[19] Such controversy and disagreement can in part be attributed to competing conceptions of what light, and especially its ultraviolet radiation, is and how it acts upon our bodies: as a 'stimulant' analogous to a drug, according to Dr Edward Deck (epigraph); as a 'bandage' (*pansement*) for Dr Auguste Rollier; as a vital 'food' to be consumed; and as a destroyer, whether as a bactericide, disinfectant, or carcinogen. Little wonder light therapy's history is marked by ambiguities, tensions, and contradictions, it is a treatment premised upon harnessing an ephemeral, invisible, if not outright uncontrollable, natural source.

To conclude, I want to discuss two very different contemporary images about light exposure, both of which inform and are informed by light therapy's history (Figs. 6.1–6.2). The first is from Danish photographer Nicolai Howalt's series, 'Light Break' (Fig. 6.1).[20] Howalt gained intimate access to the Finsen archive in the Medical Museion (Copenhagen), borrowing pieces of original phototherapy

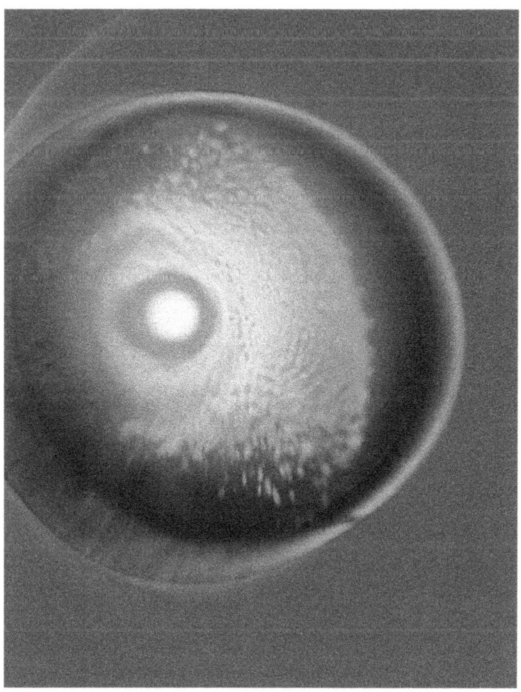

Figure 6.1 Nicolai Howalt, *Light Break #1*, 2013. Inkjet print. © Nicolai Howalt.

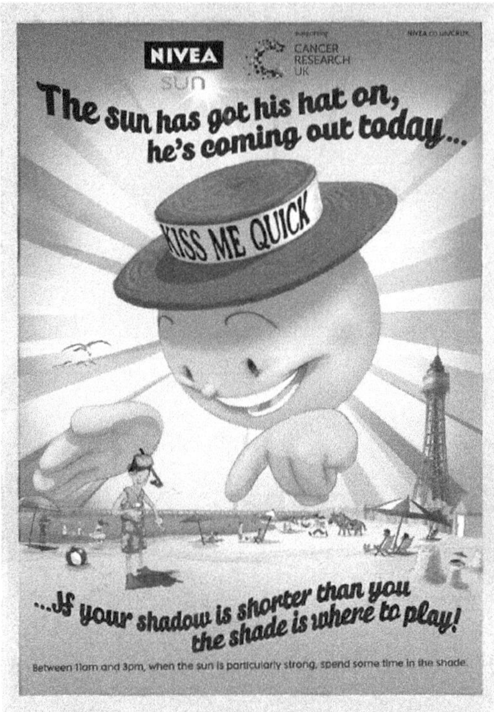
NIVEA
sun
CANCER
RESEARCH
UK
The sun has got his hat on,
he's coming out today...
KISS ME QUICK
...If your shadow is shorter than you
the shade is where to play!
Between 11am and 3pm, when the sun is particularly strong, spend some time in the shade.

Figure 6.2 Nivea and Cancer Research UK campaign poster, 2013
CRUK and Nivea SUN.

equipment such as lenses and telescopic arms from Finsen lamps, and produced photographs of them. Indeed, he did not simply make photographs of them, but *with* them, strapping the focusing lenses to his camera and aiming it at the sun. Beautiful aesthetic 'accidents' resulted, producing abstract swirls and scatterings typical of lens flare (Chapter 2).

Howalt's photographs and photograms visualise the 'injurious' rays and present them as the main photographic subject. These are as much portraits as Finsen's before and after photographs of his patients (Figs. 2.4, 2.7), but here Howalt made portraits of actinic light, of its fickle, powerful, and destructive character. The broken, shattered, refracted light made visible with Finsen's equipment signals Howalt's open engagement with chance and uncertainty. It is playful and uncontrolled in contrast to Finsen's rigorous experimentation with actinic light. Yet in doing so Howalt actively 'brings to light' the forgotten, obscure, and largely hidden archival equipment and documentation in the Finsen archive to a new audience. The hypnotising, swirling vortex of *Light Break #1* doubles as a transfixed pupil (Fig. 6.1). It is an unplanned but fitting likeness, since Howalt's project aestheticises therapeutic light's blinding action. Figure 6.1 is, put simply, a work of beautiful damage. It enables us to reconceptualise Finsen's healed lupus vulgaris patients as the same, their beautifully cicatrised skin produced by destructive light. Howalt's project is thus an instance of contemporary art allowing us to revisit medicine's past with fresh insight.

The second image is from a series of health campaign posters from 2013 created by the agency Draft FCB for a partnership between the skin-care company Nivea and Cancer Research UK (Fig. 6.2). Anthropomorphised with a button nose, gigantic smiling mouth, black eyes, and rosy cheeks, an enormous sun fills a third of the poster's composition.[21] It – or rather 'he' – is absurdly out of proportion with the scale of the rest of the landscape. With disembodied hands the sun benevolently instructs a white child, dressed for snorkelling in the sea, to observe the length of his shadow: the shorter the shadow, the stronger the sun's emanating rays. They burst forth in strong graphic blocks of white and yellow, reminiscent of the Art Deco rays in the 1936 'Vi-tan' pamphlet cover (Plate 1).

Not an advertisement per se, the poster promotes no actual product, unless we consider the shade a desirable commodity. There are subtle references to the Nivea brand, specifically the blue and white beach balls, and to Blackpool tourism, such as the inclusion of Blackpool Tower and a 'Kiss me quick' souvenir hat. The phrase 'Kiss me quick' is here cleverly employed both as a nostalgic signifier (of a bygone era of kitsch beach culture so strongly tied to Blackpool's history) and as another instruction, to literally make contact with the sun briefly (becoming 'sun-kissed'), an exciting and even naughty quick encounter of bodily contact with sunlight. Significantly, Draft FCB's creatives were inspired by the saucy seaside postcards of Donald McGill (1875–1962), an artist who faced charges for breaking the Obscene Publications Act (1857) in the 1950s.

The poster's caption reads, 'The sun has got his hat on, he's coming out today … If your shadow is shorter than you, the shade is where to play!' It is an excerpt of altered lyrics from Ralph Butler and Noel Gay's 1932 song, 'The Sun Has Got His Hat On'. The second epigraph above provides the original lyrics in full. Encouraging listeners to soak up the sun's rays by submerging themselves in a sunbath – and enjoy it – the song typifies interwar perceptions of bodily exposure to light as a liberating, pleasurable, and healthful act. Yet seeping through the negrophiliac joy (now offensive racism) in the third couplet is a forewarning characteristic of the ambivalence towards excessive exposures and deep tans as acts of racial transgression, even degeneration.[22] Like Baumer's *Punch* cartoon (Fig. 5.2), the sun's transformative power is at once desirable and worrying, unfixing the supposedly unalterable racial distinction between white and black.

The campaign's reference to the overly sexualised art of McGill (in a campaign directed towards children) and its use of Butler and Gay's negrophiliac song to communicate sun safety are puzzling, as is the 'voice' of instruction, that of the sun himself.[23] Deck likewise advocated practising moderation eighty-seven years earlier (see epigraph). Now the likes of Nivea facilitate, nay encourage, prolonged access to the sun through the consumption of sunscreen.[24] At once helpful and potentially lethal, the sun in this poster is represented as a jovial, carcinogenic force; he may appear benevolent, but can he truly ever be 'benign'?

This dual characterisation of the sun – as a source simultaneously of pleasure, happiness, and health but also of cancer, pain, and bodily damage – epitomises Britain's messy past and present relationship with sunlight. Like Rima Apple in *Vitamania*, I predict no simple resolution, only more contradictory data, and along with its many unanswered questions and mysteries (Langdon's painting included, Plate 8), surely why the subject will continue to fascinate practitioners and public alike. As Lavine put it, 'things that are controversial, or at least unsettled, are less likely to cede the spotlight'.[25] With a visual culture full of unstable representations, light therapy is nothing if not 'unsettled', and I encourage scholars to further explore, with new methods, fresh energy, and perseverance, the British body's fickle love of the light.

Notes

1 Bold original. Edward J. Deck, *The Sun and How to Use It* (London: Sunlight League, 1926), p. 3.

2 Originally performed by Ambrose and His Orchestra, with vocals by Sam Browne.

3 Born in Manchester (1898) and educated at the prestigious St Paul's Girls' School in Hammersmith (London), Langdon went on to study fine art at the Byam Shaw and Vicat Cole School of Art in Kensington. Her paintings were exhibited at the Royal Academy, Royal Institute of Oil Painters, Royal Society of British Artists, New English Art Club, and the Paris Salon, with one solo show at the Arlington Gallery in 1930. Regarding Plate 8, in 1952 she offered the painting to the Wellcome Trust, accepting £40 for it (approximately £1,100 in 2016, www.thisismoney.co.uk/money/bills/article-1633409/Historic-inflation-calculator-value-money-changed-1900.html [accessed 9 September 2016]). In its archival file there are letters describing her as a well-known artist during this period. She died in 1986, unmarried and childless. See David Buckman, *Artists in Britain since 1945* (Bristol: Art Dictionaries, 2006), vol. I, p. 17; *The Times*, 11 March 1930, p. 14; *The Times*, 10 January 1986, p. 24; Wellcome Library Archives, WA/HMM/Co/Chr/J.126, 'L, 1932–52', 'Langdon, Miss B'.

4 Anne Kinloch Jamieson, 'An Intolerable Affliction: A History of Lupus Vulgaris in Late Nineteenth- and Early Twentieth-Century Britain' (Ph.D. dissertation, University of Leeds, 2010), pp. 108–9.

5 P. H. Oakley Williams, 'A Day's Work at "The London"', *Pall Mall Magazine* (May 1903), pp. 68–2, at p. 73.

6 'The Present Position of the Light Treatment of Lupus', *BMJ*, 4 January 1902, pp. 44–7, at p. 44. See also Finsen, *Phototherapy*, p. 74; and Jamieson, 'An Intolerable Affliction', p. 74.

7 See Jamieson, 'An Intolerable Affliction'; Tanya Woloshyn, 'Nursing with Flare: The Operators of Light Therapy, *c*. 1890–1940', *Dermatological Nursing*, 15:1 (2016), 49–54; and Tanya Woloshyn, *The Kiss of Light: Nursing and Light Therapy in 20th-Century Britain* (London: Florence Nightingale Museum, 2015).

8 See also Susan E. Lederer, *Subjected to Science: Human Experimentation in America before the Second World War* (Baltimore, Md.: Johns Hopkins University Press, 1995), p. xvi.

9 Cited in Hill, 'The Physiological Effects of Light', *Proceedings of the Royal Society of Medicine*, 17 (1924), 15–21, at p. 20. See also Richard Dyer, *White* (London and New York: Routledge, 1997), pp. 1–2; and a photograph of Alma Smith modelling in lingerie under an unlit mercury vapour lamp, titled *Her Daily Sunbath*. The caption reads, 'Miss Alma Smith the 23-year-old actress who is considered to be the cleverest Soubrette of the coloured race and who recently arrived from America to join the cast of the "Blackbirds" at the London Pavilion snapped at her daily sunbath of ultra violet rays. For the past few months Miss Smith has been the sensation of New York where she has become known as "The Little Bunch of Personality." Her recent song hits "Banana Anna" and "Hot Poppa be Yourself" together with her Blackbottom dancing are the chief cause.' Greater Manchester County Archives, GB124.DPA/1129/15, [General Photographic Agency, Fleet Street], photograph, *c.* 1926.

10 A group of phototherapy nurses explained to me that dark skin remains a 'problem' when judging erythema and pigmentation production, since white skin is the 'norm'. The South-East of England Phototherapy Network's 21st Update Meeting, St Thomas' Hospital, 15 October 2015. See also Roberta Bivins, 'The "English Disease" or "Asian Rickets"? Medical Responses to Postcolonial Immigration', *Bulletin of the History of Medicine*, 81:3 (2007), 533–68.

11 Franz Thedering, *Sunlight as Healer: A Popular Treatise* (Slough: Sollux, 1926), p. 24.

12 William Beaumont, *Fundamental Principles of Ray Therapy* (London: H. K. Lewis & Co., 1931), p. 95. Similarly, Katherine Gamgee described the patient's tanned, unresponsive skin as 'stale' and recommended a similar cyclical pattern of alternating irradiation and rest. Katherine Gamgee, *The Artificial Light Treatment of Children* (London: H. K. Lewis & Co., 1927), p. 111.

13 On public appropriations of medical concepts, see Matthew Lavine, *The First Atomic Age: Scientists, Radiations, and the American Public, 1895–1945* (New York: Palgrave Macmillan, 2013), pp. 7, 9; and Nancy Tomes, *The Gospel of Germs: Men, Women, and the Microbe in American Life* (Cambridge, Mass.: Harvard University Press, 1998), p. 13.

14 On the difficulty of accessing silent voices, see also Margarete Sandelowski, *Devices and Desires: Gender, Technology, and American Nursing* (Chapel Hill, NC: University of North Carolina Press, 2000), p. 15; and Joel D. Howell, *Technology in the Hospital: Transforming Patient Care in the Early Twentieth Century* (Baltimore, Md.: Johns Hopkins University Press, 1996), p. 12.

15 Alan Mayne 'Material Culture', in Simon Gunn and Lucy Faire (eds), *Research Methods for History* (Edinburgh: Edinburgh University Press, 2012), pp. 48–65, at p. 56.

16 See, for example, Daniel Martin, 'The Tanorexia Timebomb: Sunbeds Blamed as Skin Cancer Soars in Young Women', *Daily Mail*, 8 April 2009, www.dailymail.co.uk/news/article-1168407/The-tanorexia-timebomb-Sunbeds-blamed-skin-cancer-soars-young-women.html (accessed 27 March 2016). See also Dorothy Porter, 'The Healthy Body', in Roger Cooter and John Pickstone (eds), *Medicine in the Twentieth Century* (Amsterdam: Harwood Academic Publishers, 2000), pp. 201–16.

17 Bivins, 'The "English Disease" or "Asian Rickets"?'

18 '16 Simple Steps to Help You Feel Fitter, Healthier and Happier Every Day', *Prima* (January 2016), p. 83. See also 'No Safe Way to Suntan, New NICE Guidance Warns', *BBC News*, 9 February 2016, www.bbc.co.uk/news/uk-35529596 (accessed 24 March 2016).

19 Simon Carter, *Rise and Shine: Sunlight, Technology and Health* (New York and Oxford: Berg, 2007), p. 27.

20 Nicolai Howalt, *Light Break: Photography / Light Therapy* (Copenhagen: Fabrik Books, 2015).

21 The sun has been anthropomorphised as a physician and photographer since the 1800s. See Melissa Miles, *The Burning Mirror: Photography in an Ambivalent Light* (North Melbourne: Australian Scholarly Publishing, 2008), pp. 82–4; Zane R. Kime, *Sunlight* (Penryn: World Health Publications, 1980), p. 36; and J. M. Andress and W. A. Evans, *Success and Health* (Toronto: Ginn & Co., 1925), p. 117.

22 In 2014, DJ David Lowe was fired for playing this song because of its racist language. 'BBC Radio Devon DJ David Lowe Loses Job over Racist Word', *BBC News*, 11 May 2014, www.bbc.co.uk/news/uk-england-devon-27360884 (accessed 24 March 2016).

23 By analysing this image I do not want to suggest that Nivea, CRUK, or this agency did anything necessarily 'wrong' or 'bad' in their choices for this campaign poster; rather, I want to make it clear that making historical references – to historical objects, places, songs, and artwork – when it comes to ultraviolet exposure and sun safety can only be ambiguous and unsettling because they are the products of a problematic past.

24 Dunne Romano posits sunscreen as the 'compromise between sun avoidance and sun worship', in Sally Dunne Romano, 'The Dark Side of the Sun: Skin Cancer, Sunscreen and Risk in Twentieth-Century America' (Ph.D. dissertation, Yale University, 2006), p. 257.

25 Lavine, *First Atomic Age*, p. 200.

Select bibliography

Major archives

British Library, London
Finsen Archive, Medical Museion, Copenhagen
London Metropolitan Archives, London
Manchester and Salford Hospital for Skin Diseases Archive, John Rylands Library Special Collections, Manchester
Royal London Hospital Archives, London
Thackray Medical Museum, Leeds
Treloar Archives, Hampshire Records Office, Winchester
Wellcome Library, London

Periodicals

British Journal of Actinotherapy
British Medical Journal
Lancet
Practitioner
Sunlight
Sun Bathing Review
The Times

Primary and secondary sources

Actinotherapy Technique (Slough: Sollux, 1933).
Actinotherapy Technique (Slough: Sollux, 1943).
Ades, Dawn, *Photomontage* (London: Thames & Hudson, 2000).
Alton 1908–1929–1937: The Unconventional Tribute of an Outsider (London: Treloar Hospital, 1937).
Anderson, Elizabeth, *The Essentials of Light Treatment for the Use of Masseuses* (London: Baillière, Tindall & Cox, 1935).
Apple, Rima, *Vitamania: Vitamins in American Culture* (New Brunswick: Rutgers University Press, 1996).

Barthes, Roland, *Camera Lucida: Reflections on Photography* (London: Vintage Books, 2000).

Batchelor, David, *Chromophobia* (London: Reaktion Books, 2005).

Batchen, Geoffrey, *Burning with Desire: The Conception of Photography* (Cambridge, Mass.: MIT Press, 1999).

Bazerman, Charles, *The Languages of Edison's Light* (Cambridge, Mass.: MIT Press, 1999).

Beaumont, William, *Fundamental Principles of Ray Therapy* (London: H. K. Lewis & Co., 1931).

Bernhard, Oskar, *Sonnenlichtbehandlung in der Chirurgie* (Stuttgart: Ferdinand Enke, 1917).

—— *Light Treatment in Surgery* (London: Edward Arnold, 1926).

Brody, Charles (ed.), *Traité d'hélio- et d'actinologie: physique – biologie – thérapeutique*, 2 vols. (Paris: Maloine, 1938).

Carter, Simon, *Rise and Shine: Sunlight, Technology and Health* (New York and Oxford: Berg, 2007).

—— 'The Medicalization of Sunlight in the Early Twentieth Century', *Journal of Historical Sociology*, 25:1 (2012), 83–105.

Cartwright, Lisa, *Screening the Body: Tracing Medicine's Visual Culture* (Minneapolis, Minn.: University of Minnesota Press, 1995).

Cleaves, Margaret, *Light Energy: Its Physics, Physiological Action and Therapeutic Applications* (London and New York: Rebman, 1904).

Cooter, Roger (ed.), *In the Name of the Child: Health and Welfare, 1880–1940* (London and New York: Routledge, 1992).

Cooter, Roger and John Pickstone (eds), *Medicine in the Twentieth Century* (Amsterdam: Harwood Academic Publishers, 2000).

Crary, Jonathan, *Techniques of the Observer: On Vision and Modernity in the Nineteenth Century* (Cambridge, Mass.: MIT Press, 1999).

Dane, Victor, *The Sunlight Cure: How to Use the Ultra-violet Rays* (London: Athletic Publications Ltd, 1929).

Daston, Lorraine and Peter Galison, *Objectivity* (New York: Zone Books, 2010).

Deck, Edward J., *The Sun and How to Use It* (London: The Sunlight League, 1926).

Dunne Romano, Sally, 'The Dark Side of the Sun: Skin Cancer, Sunscreen and Risk in Twentieth-Century America' (Ph.D. dissertation, Yale University, 2006).

Dyer, Richard, *White* (London and New York: Routledge, 1997).

Edwards, Martin, *Control and the Therapeutic Trial: Rhetoric and Experimentation in Britain, 1918–48* (Amsterdam and New York: Rodopi, 2007).

Ellenbogen, Josh, *Reasoned and Unreasoned Images: The Photography of Bertillon, Galton, and Marey* (University Park, Pa.: Pennsylvania State University Press, 2012).

Finsen, Niels R., *Phototherapy*, trans. J. H. Sequeira (London: Edward Arnold, 1901).

Flaskamp, Wilhelm, 'Light and Heat Therapy in Gynaecology', *Light and Heat in Therapy: The Proceedings of the 2nd International Conference on Light and Heat in Medicine and Surgery, University of London, October–November 1928* (London: The Actinic Press, Ltd, 1929), pp. 20–37.

Forbes, Duncan, 'Politics, Photography and Exile in the Life of Edith Tudor-Hart (1908–1973)', in Shulamith Behr and Marian Malet (eds), *Arts in Exile in Britain, 1933–1945: Politics and Cultural Identity* (Amsterdam and New York: Rodopi, 2005), pp. 45–87.

—— (ed.), *Edith Tudor-Hart: In the Shadow of Tyranny* (Osfildern: Hatje Cantz Verlag, 2013).

Forty, Adrian, *Objects of Desire: Design and Society since 1750* (London: Thames & Hudson, 1995).

Freund, Daniel, *American Sunshine: Diseases of Darkness and the Quest for Natural Light* (Chicago, Ill.: The University of Chicago Press, 2012).

Gamgee, Katherine, *The Artificial Light Treatment of Children* (London: H. K. Lewis & Co., 1927).

Gooday, Graeme, *Domesticating Electricity: Technology, Uncertainty and Gender, 1880–1914* (London: Pickering & Chatto, 2008).

Hanovia, *The New Light Treatment Department (Solarium) in the Public Health Centre, Bermondsey* (Slough: Hanovia Ltd, 1936).

—— *A Short Book of Instructions for Users of the 'Homesun' Sunlamp*, user manual, 1940 (Thackray Medical Museum, CAT HAN 1940 1089a, S.2249/340).

—— *Get Back in the Sun with a 'Homesun'*, pamphlet, 1940 (Thackray Medical Museum, CAT HAN 1940 1088, S.2434/240).

Harvie, David I., *Deadly Sunshine: The History and Fatal Legacy of Radium* (Stroud: Tempus, 2005).

Hennepe, Mieneke te, 'Private Portraits or Suffering on Stage: Curating Clinical Photographic Collections in the Museum Context', *Science Museum Group Journal*, Spring (2016), http://dx.doi.org/10.15180/160503.

Hentschel, Klaus, *Mapping the Spectrum: Techniques of Visual Representation in Research and Teaching* (Oxford: Oxford University Press, 2002).

Herzig, Rebecca, 'Removing Roots: "North American Hiroshima Maidens" and the X-Ray', *Technology and Culture*, 40:4 (1999), 723–45.

Hight, Eleanor M., *Picturing Modernism: Moholy-Nagy and Photography in Weimar Germany* (Cambridge, Mass.: MIT Press, 1995).

Hill, Leonard, *Sunshine and Open Air: Their Influence on Health, with Special Reference to the Alpine Climate* (London: Edward Arnold, 1925).

Hobday, Richard, *The Healing Sun: Sunlight and Health in the 21st Century* (Forres: Findhorn Press, 1999).

—— *The Light Revolution: Health, Architecture and the Sun* (Forres: Findhorn Press, 2006).

Hockberger, Philip E., 'A History of Ultraviolet Photobiology for Humans, Animals and Microorganisms', *Photochemistry and Photobiology*, 76:6 (2002), 561–79.

Howell, Joel D., *Technology in the Hospital: Transforming Patient Care in the Early Twentieth Century* (Baltimore, Md.: Johns Hopkins University Press, 1996).

Jamieson, Anne Kinloch, 'An Intolerable Affliction: A History of Lupus Vulgaris in Late Nineteenth- and Early Twentieth-Century Britain' (Ph.D. dissertation, University of Leeds, 2010).

—— 'More than Meets the Eye: Revealing the Therapeutic Potential of Light, 1896–1910', *Social History of Medicine*, 26:4 (2013), 715–37.

Jhally, Sut, 'Advertising as Religion: The Dialectic of Technology and Magic', in Ian Angus and Sut Jhally (eds), *Cultural Politics in Contemporary America* (London and New York: Routledge, 1989), pp. 217–29.

Jones, Caroline A. and Peter Galison (eds), *Picturing Science, Producing Art* (London and New York: Routledge, 1998).

Jones, Esyllt, 'Nothing Too Good for the People: Local Labour and London's Interwar Health Centre Movement', *Social History of Medicine*, 25:1 (2012), 84–102.

Jordanova, Ludmilla, *History in Practice* (London: Arnold, 2000).

Keller, Corey (ed.), *Brought to Light: Photography and the Invisible, 1840–1900* (New Haven, Conn.: Yale University Press with SFMOMA, 2008).

Kellogg, John Harvey, *Light Therapeutics* (Battle Creek, Mich.: The Modern Medicine, 1927).

Kelves, Bettyann Holtzmann, *Naked to the Bone: Medical Imagine in the Twentieth Century* (Reading: Helix Books, 1998).

Lavine, Matthew, *The First Atomic Age: Scientists, Radiations, and the American Public, 1895–1945* (New York: Palgrave Macmillan, 2013).

Lawrence, Christopher and George Weisz (eds), *Greater than the Parts: Holism in Biomedicine, 1920–1950* (Oxford: Oxford University Press, 1998).

Lederer, Susan E., *Subjected to Science: Human Experimentation in America before the Second World War* (Baltimore, Md.: Johns Hopkins University Press, 1995).

Littlewood, Ian, *Sultry Climates: Travel and Sex since the Grand Tour* (London: John Murray, 2001).

Luckiesh, Matthew and August John Pacini, *Light and Health: A Discussion of Light and Other Radiations in Relation to Life and to Health* (Baltimore, Md.: The Williams & Wilkins Company, 1926).

Lupton, Ellen, *Mechanical Brides: Women and Machines from Home to Office* (New York: Cooper-Hewitt National Museum of Design, Smithsonian Institute, and Princeton Architectural Press, 1993).

Miles, Melissa, *The Burning Mirror: Photography in an Ambivalent Light* (North Melbourne: Australian Scholarly Publishing, 2008).

Mitchell, W. J. T., *What Do Pictures Want? The Lives and Loves of Images* (Chicago, Ill.: University of Chicago Press, 2005).

Möhring, Maren, 'Working Out the Body's Boundaries: Physiological, Aesthetic, and Psychic Dimensions of the Skin in German Nudism, 1890–1930', in Christopher E. Forth and Ivan Crozier (eds), *Body Parts: Critical Explorations in Corporeality* (Lanham, Md: Lexington Books, 2005), pp. 229–46.

Morris, Hugh, *Physiotherapy in Medical Practice* (London: Edward Arnold, 1939).

Mould, Richard F., *A Century of X-rays and Radioactivity in Medicine* (Bristol and Philadelphia, Pa.: Institute of Physics Publishing, 1993).

Moynihan, G. S. E., *The Lord Mayor Treloar Hospital and College* (Southampton: Paul Cave, 1988).

Müller, Jørgen Peter, *My Sun-Bathing and Fresh-Air System* (London: Athletic Publications, 1927).

Otter, Chris, *The Victorian Eye: A Political History of Light and Vision in Britain, 1800–1910* (Chicago, Ill.: University of Chicago Press, 2008).

Overy, Paul, *Light, Air and Openness: Modern Architecture between the Wars* (London: Thames & Hudson, 2007).

Park, Bertram and Yvonne Gregory, *Sun Bathers* (London: George Routledge & Sons, Ltd, 1935).

Peebles Hotel Hydropathic: For Health & Pleasure, promotional booklet, undated (*c.* 1920s–1930s).

Rollier, Auguste, *La Cure de soleil* (Lausanne and Paris: Constant Tarin and Baillière & Fils, 1914).

—— *Le Pansement solaire: héliothérapie de certaines affections chirurgicales et des blessures de guerre* (Lausanne and Paris: Librairie Payot & Cie, 1916).

—— *Heliotherapy* (London: Henry Frowde and Hodder & Stoughton, 1923).

—— *Quarante ans d'héliothérapie* (Lausanne: F. Rouge & Cie, 1944).

Russell, Eleanor H. and William K. Russell, *Ultra-violet Radiation and Actinotherapy* (Edinburgh: E. & S. Livingstone, 1925).

Sadar, John Stanislav, 'Unpacking the Latent Bodies of Interwar Ultraviolet Health Glass' (Ph.D. dissertation, University of Pennsylvania, 2010).

—— '"Vita" Glass and the Discourse of Modern Culture', in Grace Lees-Maffei (ed.), *Writing Design: Words and Objects* (London and New York: Berg, 2012), pp. 103–17.

Saleeby, Caleb W., *Sunlight and Health* (London: Nisbet & Co., Ltd, 1923).

Sandelowski, Margarete, *Devices and Desires: Gender, Technology, and American Nursing* (Chapel Hill, NC: University of North Carolina Press, 2000).

Schivelbusch, Wolfgang, *Disenchanted Night: The Industrialization of Light in the Nineteenth Century*, trans. A. Davies (Berkeley, Calif.: University of California Press, 1995).

Sheehan, Tanya, *Doctored: The Medicine of Photography in Nineteenth-Century America* (University Park, Pa.: Pennsylvania State University Press, 2011).

The South London Hospital for Women and Children (Birmingham: Kynoch Press, 1935).

Stone, Dan, *Breeding Superman: Nietzsche, Race and Eugenics in Edwardian and Interwar Britain* (Liverpool: Liverpool University Press, 2002).

Suschitzky, Wolfgang, *Edith Tudor-Hart: The Eye of Conscience* (London: Dirk Nishen Publishing, 1987).

Teitelbaum, Matthew (ed.), *Montage and Modern Life, 1919–1942* (Cambridge, Mass.: MIT Press with the Boston Institute of Contemporary Art, 1992).

Thedering, Franz, *Sunlight as Healer: A Popular Treatise* (Slough: Sollux, 1926).

Thomas de la Peña, Carolyn, *The Body Electric: How Strange Machines Built the Modern American* (New York: New York University Press, 2003).

The Times, 'Sunlight and Health', special supplement, 22 May 1928.

Troup, W. Annandale, *Therapeutic Uses of Infra-Red Rays* (London: The Actinic Press, 1936).

Van Dijck, José, *The Transparent Body: A Cultural Analysis of Medical Imaging* (Seattle, Wash.: University of Washington Press, 2005).

Vaughan-Cowell, Myrtle, *Artificial Sunlight: Its Use and Application* (London: H. Edgar Smithers, 1928).

Vogel, Hermann, *The Chemistry of Light and Photography* (New York: D. Appleton & Co., 1875).

Wilder, Kelley, 'Photography Absorbed', *Bildwelten des Wissens: Kunsthistorisches Jahrbuch für Bildkritik*, 4:2 (2006), 43–53.

—— *Photography and Science* (London: Reaktion, 2009).

—— 'Visualizing Radiation: The Photographs of Henri Becquerel', in Lorraine Daston and Elizabeth Lunbeck (eds), *Histories of Scientific Observation* (Chicago, Ill.: University of Chicago Press, 2011), pp. 349–68.

Wilk, Christopher, *Modernism: Designing a New World, 1914–1939* (London: Victoria and Albert, 2006).

Williams, Raymond, 'Advertising: The Magic System', in *Problems of Materialism and Culture: Selected Essays* (London and New York: Verso, 1997), pp. 170–95.

Woloshyn, Tania, 'Patients Rebuilt: Dr Auguste Rollier's Heliotherapeutic Portraits, c. 1903 1944', *Medical Humanities*, 39:1 (2013), 38–46.

—— 'Regenerative Tanning: Pigmentation, Neo-Lamarckian Eugenics and the Visual Culture of the *Cure De Soleil*', in Fae Brauer and Serena Keshavjee (eds), *Picturing Evolution and Extinction: Regeneration and Degeneration in Modern Visual Culture* (Newcastle upon Tyne: Cambridge Scholars Publishing, 2015), pp. 193–216.

Woodruff, Charles E., *The Effects of Tropical Light on White Men* (London and New York: Rebman, 1905).

Worpole, Ken, *Here Comes the Sun: Architecture and Public Space in Twentieth-Century European Culture* (London: Reaktion, 2000).

Zweifel, Sophia, 'Pellicular Penetrations: The Skins of the Early X-Ray Image' (MA dissertation, University College London, 2012).

Zweiniger-Bargielowska, Ina, *Managing the Body: Beauty, Health, and Fitness in Britain, 1880–1939* (Oxford: Oxford University Press, 2010).

Index

EU authorised representative for GPSR:
Easy Access System Europe, Mustamäe tee 50,
10621 Tallinn, Estonia
gpsr.requests@easproject.com

www.ingramcontent.com/pod-product-compliance
Ingram Content Group UK Ltd.
Pitfield, Milton Keynes, MK11 3LW, UK
UKHW061933100926
8556IPUK00007B/903
* 9 7 8 1 7 8 4 9 9 5 1 2 6 *